Lessons from Medicolegal Cases in Obstetrics and Gynaecology

T0201407

Lessons from Medicolegal Cases in Obstetrics and Gynaecology

Improving Clinical Practice

Edited by
Swati Jha
Royal Hallamshire Hospital, Sheffield

Eloise Power
Sergeants' Inn, London

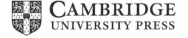

CAMBRIDGE
UNIVERSITY PRESS

University Printing House, Cambridge CB2 8BS, United Kingdom

One Liberty Plaza, 20th Floor, New York, NY 10006, USA

477 Williamstown Road, Port Melbourne, VIC 3207, Australia

314–321, 3rd Floor, Plot 3, Splendor Forum, Jasola District Centre, New Delhi – 110025, India

103 Penang Road, #05-06/07, Visioncrest Commercial, Singapore 238467

Cambridge University Press is part of the University of Cambridge.

It furthers the University's mission by disseminating knowledge in the pursuit of education, learning, and research at the highest international levels of excellence.

www.cambridge.org
Information on this title: www.cambridge.org/9781108995115
DOI: 10.1017/9781108993388

© Cambridge University Press 2022

First published 2022

Printed in Great Britain by Ashford Colour Press Ltd.

A catalogue record for this publication is available from the British Library.

Library of Congress Cataloging-in-Publication Data
Names: Jha, Swati, editor. | Power, Eloise, editor.
Title: Lessons from medicolegal cases in obstetrics and gynaecology : improving clinical practice / edited by Swati Jha, Eloise Power.
Description: Cambridge, United Kingdom ; New York, NY : Cambridge University Press, 2022. | Includes bibliographical references and index.
Identifiers: LCCN 2021048086 (print) | LCCN 2021048087 (ebook) | ISBN 9781108995115 (paperback) | ISBN 9781108993388 (epub)
Subjects: MESH: Obstetrics–legislation & jurisprudence | Malpractice–legislation & jurisprudence | Gynecology–legislation & jurisprudence | Obstetric Surgical Procedures–legislation & jurisprudence | Gynecologic Surgical Procedures–legislation & jurisprudence | England
Classification: LCC RG101 (print) | LCC RG101 (ebook) | NLM WQ 33 FE5 | DDC 618–dc23
LC record available at https://lccn.loc.gov/2021048086
LC ebook record available at https://lccn.loc.gov/2021048087

ISBN 978-1-108-99511-5 Paperback

....

This book is dedicated to my children, Shashwat and Sakshi, who give meaning to my life and have taught me the principle of carpe diem.

Swati Jha
Sheffield

Contents

List of Contributors

James Badenoch, 1 Crown Office Row, Temple, London EC4Y 7HH

Helen Bolton, DLM PhD MRCOG, Consultant in Gynaecology and Gynaecological Oncology, Department of Gynaecological Oncology, Cambridge University Hospitals NHS Trust

Joanna F Crofts, North Bristol NHS Trust

Ian Currie, FRCOG, Consultant in Obstetrics and Gynaecology, Buckinghamshire Healthcare NHS Trust, Stoke Mandeville Hospital, Aylesbury, Buckinghamshire

Alfred Cutner, Elizabeth Garrett Anderson Institute for Women's Health, University College London, United Kingdom

Kara Dent, Consultant Obstetrician, UHDB Foundation Trust

Professor Tim Draycott, Department of Obstetrics & Gynaecology, Southmead Hospital, North Bristol NHS Trust, Bristol, UK and Academic Women's Health Unit, School of Clinical Sciences, University of Bristol, UK

Andrew Farkas, Consultant Obstetrician and Gynaecologist, Sheffield Teaching Hospitals NHS Foundation Trust

Emma Ferriman, Consultant Obstetrician, Sheffield Teaching Hospitals NHS Foundation Trust

Anastasia Georgiou, BA (Oxon), Graduate Medical Student, University of Cambridge

Adam S Gornall, Shrewsbury and Telford Hospital NHS Trust

Janesh K Gupta, MSc, MD, FRCOG, Professor of Obstetrics and Gynaecology, University of Birmingham, Birmingham and Children's NHS Foundation Trust

Martin Hirsch, The John Radcliffe Hospital, Oxford University Hospitals NHS Trust

Emily J Hotton, North Bristol NHS Trust

David Howe, Princess Anne Hospital, Southampton

Swati Jha, MD, FRCOG, Consultant Obstetrician and Gynaecologist, Subspecialist in Urogynaecology, Sheffield Teaching Hospitals NHS Foundation Trust

Mark D Kilby, Dame Hilda Lloyd Professor of Fetal Medicine, University of Birmingham and Honorary Consultant in Obstetrics and Fetal Medicine Centre, Birmingham Women's and Children's Foundation Trust

Raj Mathur, Consultant Gynaecologist and Clinical Lead for Reproductive Medicine and Surgery, Manchester University NHS Foundation Trust, and Honorary Senior Lecturer, University of Manchester

John Mead, BA FCII, NHS Resolution, London, UK

John Murdoch, University Hospitals Bristol NHS Trust

Charles P O'Donovan, MB ChB MSc, Specialist Trainee Doctor, Bradford Royal Infirmary

Peter J O'Donovan, MB BCh BAO (NUI) FRCS England FRCOG, Consultant Gynaecologist and Professor of Medical Innovation, The Yorkshire Clinic, University of Bradford

Stephen Porter, Consultant Obstetrician and Gynaecologist, Airedale NHS Foundation Trust

Abdul H Sultan, MD (Res) FRCOG, Consultant Obstetrician and Urogynaecologist, Urogynaecology and Pelvic Floor Reconstruction Unit, Croydon University Hospital, and Honorary Reader, St George's University of London

Myles JO Taylor, BA (Oxon) PhD FRCOG, Obstetrician & Gynaecologist, Subspecialist in Fetal & Maternal Medicine, Royal Devon & Exeter NHS Foundation Trust

Preface

We learn best from our mistakes, but given the cost of litigation is going up year on year, maybe we are not paying heed to the lessons our errors teach us. The first step to learning from mistakes is acknowledging one was made. The subsequent steps include asking what we can learn from this and how we prevent it from happening in the future. It is also imperative to understand the legal principles that govern decisions made in cases reaching court or influencing out of court settlements. Insight into the law allows us to understand the legal rulings made in individual cases. Knowledge is power (*scientia est potentia*), and, through a better understanding of cases where errors occurred and the legal principles that govern our justice system, we can be better and safer doctors. Patient safety and well-being have got to be the basis of acquiring this knowledge, not defensive medicine.

The changing face of clinical negligence has meant that in 2019/2020 we paid out in litigation in excess of one billion pounds for NHS negligence in England alone, a sum that could have been used to improve patient care. At a time of significant financial difficulty, with cuts in all services, is it sustainable to divert such large sums away from essential services? And where will it all end?

Very few cases actually go to court, but when causation is disputed, it is because the experts for defendant and claimant are both confident they were in the "right". Whereas this can be a cause of significant consternation, clinicians should at least be aware that this is evidence that there was dispute about overt negligence. Disputes relating to quantum is another reason for cases going to court and leads to differences of opinion which can sometimes only be resolved by a judge. In the event of obstetric cases, litigation can ensue years, sometimes decades after the index event and judgements are based on reconstructions of events rather than recollection, hence the need for robust documentation and note keeping.

Reviewing past cases raises the question of whether tort litigation is the best means of dealing with claims. It is possible that a no-blame compensation scheme, as in some other countries such as New Zealand, may be a more equitable option for claimants without jeopardising existing healthcare services due to its spiralling costs. It should also be noted that to date there has been no robust evidence on the effectiveness of interventions aimed at reducing litigation.

No clinician sets out to deliberately harm a patient, but unfortunately there will occasionally be adverse outcomes. The aim of this book is to discuss the top causes of litigation, and through case studies of successful and unsuccessful claims related to these conditions, understand the key causes of litigation. I will present the case commentaries in each chapter. This will be followed by a legal commentary on these cases which is presented by my coeditor, Eloise Power. The clinical commentary is provided by the clinical experts in the relevant area of litigation and will focus on how best to avoid litigation from occurring.

Swati Jha
Sheffield

Foreword

A harsh reality of medicine is that those who choose to join the profession do so knowing they will face multiple avenues of complaint related to their practice when things go wrong or are alleged to have gone wrong.

This is not a new challenge. As far back as 1892, a group of doctors in the UK came together to establish what is now known as the Medical Protection Society, precisely for the purpose of providing support and assistance to members in the event that they needed to defend themselves.

The cost of clinical negligence claims is however a rapidly growing challenge, with much being written in recent years about the rising cost to the NHS. Of particular relevance to readers of this book is NHS Resolution's most recent annual report, which shows that the total value of maternity cerebral palsy and brain damage claims in England, over time, rose from £365 million in 2004/2005 to £1,822 million in 2019/2020.[1]

The impact of these claims of course goes much further than the financial cost.

Sadly, the huge cost of maternity claims reflects the fact that the patients concerned often need care and support for the rest of their lives. Birth injuries not only have wide ranging and devastating effects on the families, but also on the healthcare professionals involved, who may suffer significant stress and guilt.

The volume of complaints – and the nature of the claims process – requires a great number of patients and healthcare professionals to go through a painful and protracted legal process.

We also have to acknowledge that the cost of clinical negligence has a significant impact on the delivery of healthcare. For the NHS, the vast cost of clinical negligence claims is incurred by the state; money which could otherwise be made available for the provision of patient care. In the private sector, the cost of claims is largely incurred by healthcare professionals through the provision of their indemnity or insurance. If the cost of these claims continues to rise, there will come a point when it will have a detrimental impact on the viability of providing certain healthcare services.

So, what needs to be done to address this problem, and how could this book play an important contribution?

Prevention is, of course, better than cure. At Medical Protection we support safe practice by helping members to avoid problems happening in the first place via our risk prevention training programme. We work with members to identify areas where we can support them in reducing their medicolegal risk, increasing patient safety and enhancing the patient experience.

We also strongly advocate for the need to create an open learning culture in healthcare, where mistakes can be discussed and learnt from. Behind every case and claim are learnings that could help prevent other adverse incidents from occurring in the future. This is why we have published our own series of reports, each of which looks to

---

[1] NHS Resolution. Annual report and accounts 2019/2020. Available at: https://resolution.nhs.uk/wp-content/uploads/2020/07/NHS-Resolution-2019_20-Annual-report-and-accounts-WEB.pdf

understand the common themes that come through in the cases and claims where we have supported members. Our publication, *Learning from Cases: Specialty Focus – Gynaecology*,[2] will be of particular interest to readers of this text.

We hope this book can play a significant role in equipping those involved in delivering healthcare to women with knowledge that will drive improvements in patient safety and prevent adverse incidents from happening. Any intervention proven to help mitigate risk should be seriously considered. As such, we commend the efforts of the authors of this book in looking into the lessons that can be learned from a wide range of obstetrics and gynaecology cases.

Of course, despite the very best systems and training, things will still go wrong, and the cost of clinical negligence will remain very high. This is why Medical Protection will continue to call on the Government to introduce legal reforms that could help to control legal costs and make the compensation system more predictable, fair and transparent. It is also why it is important that healthcare professionals ensure that they are with an indemnity provider who has the experience and expertise to provide the best possible advice and support should they need it.

Simon Kayll
Chief Executive, Medical Protection Society

---

[2] Medical Protection Society. Learning from Cases: Specialty Focus – Gynaecology. Available at: www.medicalprotection.org/uk/articles/learning-from-cases-specialty-focus-gynaecology

Recent Trends in Clinical Negligence Claims in England

John Mead

Introduction

This chapter covers the period from 1990 to the present, with a focus on the most recent 10 years for statistical purposes. Necessarily, it focusses upon claims in obstetrics and gynaecology, the former specialty having produced undoubtedly the most significant judicial ruling on clinical negligence in the UK during the last decade in *Montgomery v Lanarkshire Health Board [2015] 2 All ER 1031.*

All statistics are from NHS Resolution, a special health authority which manages various risk pools on behalf of the Secretary of State for Health and Social Care in England. The data therefore cover England only and relate to secondary and tertiary care providers. Private healthcare cases, other than those where the defendant is an NHS trust in England, are excluded. Comparable data are not published by medical defence organisations (MDOs) or insurers who indemnify clinicians performing purely private work. References to claim numbers and breakdowns therefore need to be understood in that context.

NHS Resolution

This is the operating name of the NHS Litigation Authority (NHS LA), a public body formed in 1995 with the initial task of being scheme manager for the Clinical Negligence Scheme for Trusts (CNST), a role which it continues to fulfil in 2021.

The year 1990 saw the introduction of the concept of NHS indemnity. This meant that NHS organisations agreed to accept responsibility for clinical negligence committed by all employees arising out of and in the course of their employment. Previously, many NHS doctors purchased their own indemnity cover from MDOs and could be sued personally for negligence occurring during their NHS work. Health bodies were sued for system failures or equipment issues such as a faulty operating table which caused injury to a patient. This meant that litigation became unnecessarily complex and costly if negligence by both clinicians and hospital managers was alleged.

Between 1991 and 1995, NHS trusts were created in England. These replaced Health Authorities as the bodies responsible for managing NHS hospitals. New trusts did not inherit clinical negligence liabilities from their predecessors but started to incur their own from commencement. The government realised that trusts might suffer serious financial consequences if they developed substantial clinical negligence liabilities, because NHS bodies have never been allowed to insure against such risks. It was also apparent that a national approach to administering NHS clinical negligence claims was required, and so NHS LA was created with a remit to deal efficiently and fairly with claims, and to provide a measure of financial stability for the new trusts.

Shortly after its creation, NHS Resolution was also asked to take over historic clinical negligence cases where the alleged negligence was prior to 1 April 1995, the commencement date of CNST. In 1999 it took on most non-clinical liabilities for trusts, such as staff injuries and claims from members of the public other than patients. Initial claim excesses under CNST were abolished in April 2002, which means that NHS Resolution now has comprehensive data on NHS liability claims in England dating back almost 20 years, including, from April 2019, primary care cases. This is a rich resource, from which much important information can be gleaned and learning disseminated to the service.

Over the intervening years, NHS Resolution has been asked to take on a significant number of additional activities, most being outside the scope of this publication, including adjudicating on appeals against certain decisions of NHS England, and helping employers and clinicians resolve concerns about performance. A very important team in the context of obstetrics and gynaecology is Safety and Learning, which collates information and data from reported claims and publishes a series of thematic reviews, supported by seminars and online material, aimed at encouraging the NHS to learn from previous mistakes. This team also manages the Maternity Incentive Scheme, under which those trusts able to testify achievement of certain prescribed standards in their maternity function are entitled to receive a rebate of part of their CNST contribution.

Selected Legal Developments

This section does not attempt to present a comprehensive history of clinical negligence litigation, which would require a complete book of its own, but rather highlights a number of events which have been key milestones in the overall chronology.

Pre-action Protocol

Perhaps the best starting point is 1994, when Lord Woolf was asked by the Lord Chancellor to undertake a review of the civil justice system. This was a huge task, resulting in a final report in July 1996 [1]. In relation to clinical negligence, he concluded that there was often mistrust between the parties, entrenched positions were taken, delays were greater than in other areas of litigation and legal costs were often disproportionate to damages.

One of the many reforms advocated by Lord Woolf was a system of pre-action protocols for different types of claims, to encourage a "cards on the table" approach and co-operation between the parties. When the majority of Lord Woolf's reforms were introduced in April 1999, amounting collectively to the most significant change to civil litigation practice and procedure for over a century, the clinical disputes protocol had already been implemented. This has been amended several times over the intervening period, but its essence is unaltered. The current version came into effect on 6 April 2015 [2].

Full disclosure of relevant medical records, including scans and X-rays, is the first step. The claimant's lawyers are then required to explain in detail their case on breach of duty, causation and quantum. The proposed defendant has four months to provide a similarly detailed reply on all points. If there remains disagreement after these steps, the parties are encouraged to pursue appropriate methods of resolution.

This protocol has been successful in improving co-operation between parties to clinical negligence disputes. Each learns the case it has to meet, rather than being presented with generalities as often happened in pre-protocol times. Discussion is strongly encouraged, and litigation is very much a last resort. As a consequence, many of the problems identified by Lord Woolf in the 1990s have either disappeared or reduced. However, disproportionality of claimant legal costs to damages remains in many low-value cases.

Personal Injury Discount Rate

This is the mechanism by which damages for future losses are decreased, or in recent years increased, having regard to investment returns and the way in which claimants are deemed to invest their money. In 2001, the Lord Chancellor for the first time exercised his powers under the Damages Act 1996 and determined that this should be +2.5%. This meant that a claimant placing money in a secure investment such as Index-Linked Government Stock was expected to obtain an annual return, once inflation had been taken into account, of 2.5% per annum. That rate prevailed until March 2017 when it was altered to minus 0.75%, reflecting a marked reduction in investment returns owing to changes in the economic climate. There was a further revision, to minus 0.25%, in August 2019 and claimants are now deemed to invest in "low risk" rather than "no risk" portfolios. A negative discount rate means that claimants are supposed to make a loss on investments once inflation is factored into the calculation: a controversial assumption. To avoid a repeat of the 16-year absence of change in the early years of this century, the Civil Liability Act 2018 stipulates that subsequent reviews must take place at least every five years.

Whilst this might seem a relatively esoteric issue, it has profound implications for the level of damages in all medium- and high-value personal injury cases. Just one example serves to illustrate this point – a woman aged 25, earning £20,000 per annum nett, who is unable to work again in any capacity as a result of clinical negligence. The assumed age of retirement in normal circumstances is 65.

- With a +2.5% discount rate, the calculation for the 40-year period is £20,000 × 25.12 = £502,400
- At minus 0.75%, the calculation is £20,000 × 45.9 = £918,000
- At minus 0.25%, it is £20,000 × 41.4 = £828,000

The rise in damages for this head of loss, for precisely the same claim, is therefore 82.7% at minus 0.75% and 64.8% at minus 0.25%. By any measure, these are startling increases. The same rule applies in cerebral palsy cases, where typical annual claims for care costs are substantially higher than the earnings loss figure quoted. However, these are usually paid on an annual basis (periodical payments) until the claimant dies, and therefore the effect of the discount rate change is removed for defendants in the context of care costs; but any other future losses, such as therapies and items of equipment, are subject to the same level of increase. Overall, these changes have meant much higher payments since March 2017 on any clinical negligence claim where there are future losses paid by way of a lump sum.

Litigation Funding

When NHS Resolution was founded in 1995, many clinical negligence claims were brought with public assistance by way of Legal Aid. This form of funding has been progressively withdrawn over intervening years and is now available only in very limited situations, chiefly birth injuries to children in defined circumstances and claims under the Mental Health Act 1983 [3]. Conditional Fee Agreements (otherwise known as "no win-no fee" contracts or CFAs) have been available in clinical negligence cases since July 1995. Under such arrangements, lawyers can charge a mark-up on their usual fee for profit costs in successful claims, to offset the fact that they will not be paid at all on unsuccessful cases.

A key change was implemented by the Access to Justice Act 1999, whereby such uplifts in fees, together with "After the Event" (ATE) insurance premiums – covering claimants for potential liability to pay the defendant's costs if the defendant wins at trial – became recoverable from the unsuccessful party. This meant that claimants' lawyers could add up to 100% on top of their normal fee and seek to recover that from the defendant. Some ATE premiums were exceptionally high, in a few instances over £100,000, and the method of calculating them totally opaque to defendants. The effect of these changes was (a) to encourage increasing numbers of claimants to pursue claims via conditional fee agreements and (b) substantially higher payments by defendants for claimants' costs.

Such a situation became increasingly anomalous for defendants, and in a comprehensive report on the funding of civil litigation, Sir Rupert Jackson, a senior judge in the Court of Appeal, recommended major changes [4]. He concluded that the recoverability of success fees and ATE premiums was a major factor causing increases in litigation costs. As part of numerous reforms introduced by the Legal Aid, Sentencing and Punishment of Offenders Act 2012 (LASPO), the position on recoverability was altered with effect from 1 April 2013 to the extent that uplifts on fees and ATE premiums, on contracts entered into from that date, were no longer recoverable from the defendant. There was an exception, for clinical negligence claims only, allowing recovery of ATE premiums in respect of the cost of certain expert fees. Claimants' solicitors can still charge a success fee if they wish to, but this is now recoverable from their own client rather than the defendant and is restricted to a maximum of 25% of the amount the claimant received for pain, suffering and loss of amenity plus past pecuniary losses.

These 2013 changes had the effect of distorting NHS Resolution's claims data because many claimant solicitors endeavoured, prior to 1 April, to sign up numerous clients under "old-style" CFAs. Consequently, numbers of reported new clinical negligence claims peaked in the financial year 2013/2014 and only gradually reduced after that date, because some cases taken on by solicitors in the early months of 2013 were not lodged as formal claims for a lengthy period.

Case Law

Other chapters in this book cover important decisions in obstetric and gynaecology cases on breach of duty and causation, so those are not repeated here. In particular, no detailed account of *Montgomery v Lanarkshire Health Board* [2015] *2 All ER 1031* is given. Instead, this section focusses upon a small number of decisions which have had important implications for quantifying clinical negligence claims. In all these cases, rulings favouring the claimant's arguments have been made, thereby increasing the cost of claims for the NHS and other defendants.

Peters v East Midlands Strategic Health Authority and Others – Court of Appeal, 3 March 2009 – [2009] EWCA Civ 145; [2009] 3 WLR 737

The claimant was born with congenital rubella syndrome, causing severe disabilities, owing to failure by clinicians to offer her mother a rubella vaccination before she became pregnant. Liability was apportioned between the mother's general practitioner and the Health Authority. When the case reached the Court of Appeal, she was aged 20 and lived in a private care home, funded jointly by the local authority and Primary Care Trust. The trial judge, having visited the home in person, accepted that it met her reasonable needs. The question for determination was whether the negligent parties should be required to meet its cost (over £2,500 per week) when the fees were already being paid in full by a combination of public bodies. The court decided that there was no reason in policy why a claimant who wished to opt for self-funding in preference to relying upon public funding should not be allowed to do so. It was not open to the defendants to object to such a course of action. There was a risk of double recovery, but that could be dealt with by the claimant's deputy agreeing no longer to seek public funding and for the Court of Protection to be notified accordingly.

This is a problematical ruling for defendants because it means they potentially have to pay the full costs of care and accommodation even though the claimant is already receiving these in full from other sources. In essence, the court decided that as a matter of principle, the negligent parties should be responsible for such costs because they were the cause of the facilities being required. Significantly, the court did not *require* the deputy to cease claiming public funding, because it recognised that it could not remove from the claimant an entitlement which Parliament had granted her.

XXX v A Strategic Health Authority – High Court, 14 November 2008 – Jack J – [2008] EWHC 2727 (QB)

Breach of duty and causation were admitted in this cerebral palsy case. In dispute was the extent of the care claim. The claimant was almost 17 at the date of trial and considerably physically disabled, with no movement in his legs. His intellectual ability was reduced but he had been able to attend mainstream schools. Two carers were required to move him, but he did not need two at all times, for example, when reading or watching television. The judge awarded the cost of double-up care for 16 hours per day, on the basis that whilst this was not needed for many periods, the requirement for being lifted was relatively unpredictable so it was reasonable to have a second person on hand to cater for such a contingency.

James Robshaw v United Lincolnshire Hospitals NHS Trust – High Court, 1 April 2015 – Foskett J – [2015] EWHC 923 (QB)

This was also a cerebral palsy case where the only matter at issue was quantum. Numerous heads of loss were in dispute and the judgement runs to almost 500 paragraphs. It was uncontentious that the claimant had suffered serious brain damage as a consequence of the trust's negligence during the course of his birth and that he had numerous disabilities including jerky (athetoid) movements, limited ability to self-feed and the presence of a gastrostomy, plus significant communication problems. He does, however, possess a high level of retained intellect and insight.

The parties agreed that James's accommodation, a three-bedroom bungalow (including one for carers), was unsuitable. The defendant argued for adaptation of the existing property as a reasonable approach. Foskett J determined that it would be appropriate to award the costs of total demolition, estimated by the defendant to be an additional £50,000, such that a purpose-built bungalow suitable to James's needs could be constructed. He also decided that the new property should be built so as to permit access for James to all areas – including his mother's and carers' bedrooms – in his wheelchair, on the basis that the ability to go anywhere in his home was a facility he would have experienced if uninjured. This is a reference to the principle that compensatory damages are intended to place the claimant in the same position he or she would have enjoyed but for the negligence, so far as money can allow.

The cost of a home swimming pool was also awarded. Whilst swimming was not intended to be medically therapeutic, James enjoyed this activity and it helped him psychologically. The nearest public pool was situated in Horncastle, some 40 minutes' drive away from the family property, which the judge regarded as not unreasonable. However, it was maintained at too low a temperature for the claimant's needs. Consequently, the judge concluded that the case for a home pool was made out "on the basis of the real and tangible psychological and physical benefits" that swimming would afford the claimant. Foskett J stressed that it would not normally be reasonable to make such an award if the pool was for pleasure only – some real and tangible benefit needed to be demonstrated.

On the subject of transport, the cost of a mobile home totalling some £96,000 was awarded for use during holidays and trips. A small deduction was made, in the shape of one foreign holiday in three years, from the additional costs of leisure claim.

Overall, this case constituted the largest award in a clinical negligence at the time, although it has been superseded by other claims subsequently, owing to the effect of changes in the personal injury discount rate. Some of the decisions might be regarded as generous. However, Foskett J was at pains to point out in several places throughout his ruling that each case needs to be determined on its own individual facts, and that what might be regarded as an appropriate recovery for one claimant might not for another. This goes to the heart of what is "reasonable" – a debate at the centre of so many aspects of the law of negligence.

Manna v Central Manchester University Hospitals NHS Foundation Trust – Court of Appeal, 18 January 2017 – [2017] EWCA Civ 12; [2017] Med LR 132

This is another cerebral palsy case in which breach of duty and causation were accepted by the trust. The point at issue was the accommodation claim. The child's parents had divorced several years prior to trial but continued to look after him jointly until 2013. Shortly before the High Court hearing in 2015, they expressed a wish for shared care arrangements to resume. The Court of Appeal upheld the judge's ruling that the defendant meet the cost of adapting both the mother's and father's properties, so that their son could visit each. The trial judge expressed the view that it was very much in the child's best interests that he should resume his relationship with his father. Notably, the Court of Appeal characterised the judge's ruling on accommodation as generous, but intensely fact-dependent. It did not fall outside the ambit of reasonable decision-making but should not be regarded as setting a precedent.

Sadly, the birth of a child with serious disabilities not infrequently leads to the parents splitting up, and NHS Resolution is now seeing more claims of this nature. Adapting a home to accommodate wheelchairs can be very expensive, so significant extra costs will be incurred if a claim of this type is valid on the individual facts.

Swift v Carpenter – Court of Appeal, 9 October 2020 – [2020] EWCA Civ 1295

Not a clinical negligence case but one resulting from a motor vehicle accident, this decision is included because it has important ramifications for all personal injury claims where alternative accommodation is required as a result of negligence. For 30 years, this type of claim was quantified on the basis of loss of use of money required to purchase the replacement property over time and became linked to the personal injury discount rate. However, when that became negative in March 2017 this calculation turned negative too and resulted in courts awarding zero damages. That was clearly unfair to claimants, so the Court of Appeal decided upon this as a test case by which to create an alternative means of quantification.

It concluded that such claims should be determined by reference to the value of the reversionary interest in the property. This rather esoteric concept is the amount someone would pay, today, to purchase the property when the claimant dies. That sum depends upon the claimant's life-expectancy and the difference in value between their pre-existing property and the required replacement (namely the nett value). If the claimant has a life-expectancy of 10 years, a buyer would pay more for the reversionary interest than were the claimant expected to live for 30 years, assuming the property is the same. This amount is deducted from the nett value. Since there is a very small market in such interests, the court ruled that a 5% discount per annum would be applied in most cases, which was 1.6% below the average rate identified by the only expert giving evidence who had personal experience of the market. The consequence of this ruling is that the majority of alternative accommodation claims will increase in value over the old personal injury discount rate calculation. It should be added that this ruling only applies to the additional cost of the property itself: reasonable adaptations, occasioned by the claimant's disabilities, are paid in full.

Conclusions

Historic trends have suggested that damages inflation in personal injury claims runs at between 8% and 10% per annum. These decisions give some indication of why that should be – although changes to the personal injury discount rate can have a far greater one-off effect. Decisions based on the circumstances of individuals are unlikely, by themselves, to set precedents, but rulings of the Court of Appeal certainly do. Nevertheless, lawyers representing claimants understandably argue that what was appropriate for Z should be awarded to their client too. The concept of "reasonableness" in the context of damages therefore tends to be somewhat elastic, resulting in progressively higher payments by defendants' indemnifiers.

Claims Statistics

Introduction

It bears repetition that the following figures are taken exclusively from NHS Resolution's records (see Table 1.1). They relate to secondary and tertiary care in England, with inclusion of primary care from April 2019 only.

Table 1.1. Numbers of new clinical negligence claims, by specialty, reported to NHS Resolution per financial year (1 April to 31 March)

Speciality	Notification Year									
	2010/11	2011/12	2012/13	2013/14	2014/15	2015/16	2016/17	2017/18	2018/19	2019/20
Obsterics CP/BD	227	197	223	221	204	190	234	207	184	184
Obsterics Non CP/BD	865	868	952	1,081	975	914	886	881	887	834
Paediatrics	161	173	215	281	242	260	250	231	242	245
Emergency Medicine	1,136	1,154	1,333	1,494	1,430	1,341	1,318	1,389	1,410	1,401
Orthopaedic Surgery	1,242	1,453	1,581	1,763	1,638	1,501	1,381	1,284	1,264	1,361
General surgery	867	934	1,109	1,360	1,189	930	846	932	927	943
Neurosurgery	88	117	146	159	171	167	165	153	195	189
General medicine	724	672	509	666	534	585	534	516	496	468
Gynaecology	396	482	513	702	684	622	580	551	567	761
Radiology	127	154	234	325	349	379	354	387	390	426
Neurology	91	104	97	118	106	120	113	91	129	116
Psychiatry/Mental Health	188	179	257	273	235	246	283	306	313	386
Ophthalmology	177	159	204	238	229	253	271	255	242	272
Cardiology	158	142	159	185	214	204	186	218	215	231
Ambulanc	114	113	126	149	146	145	137	140	160	186
Gastroenterology	162	146	171	241	255	272	254	273	259	301
Urology	167	175	226	276	285	318	342	341	319	345
Other	1,766	1,921	2,074	2,413	2,611	2,518	2,552	2,513	2,473	3,033
Total	8,656	9,143	10,129	11,945	11,497	10,965	10,686	10,668	10,672	11,682

CP = cerebral palsy; BD = brain damage

New Clinical Negligence Claims

Numbers of new claims increased sharply in the years to 2013/2014, because of the availability of "old-style" conditional fee agreements under which claimants' lawyers could seek to recover up to 100% on top of their usual charge for profit costs. Numbers started to drop, albeit relatively slowly, following the reforms of April 2013, and overall totals were remarkably consistent for several years from 2015/2016. The increase in 2019/2020 was partly a consequence of NHS Resolution taking on the Clinical Negligence Scheme for General Practice, a state indemnity that covered primary care for the first time, which resulted in 401 new claims.

During these 10 years, numbers of new obstetric claims decreased slightly from a total of 1,092 in 2010/2011 to 1,071 in 2019/2020, the peak being 1,302 in 2013/2014. On the other hand, gynaecology started at 396 in 2010/2011 and totalled 761 in 2019/2020, a rise of no less than 92%. A great part of this increase is attributable to large numbers of claims in respect of vaginal mesh, together with groups of cases against certain clinicians such as the disgraced Ian Paterson, who was jailed for his crimes against patients.

Emergency medicine and orthopaedic surgery have competed for the largest number of new claims consistently over this period. Obstetrics has usually, but not invariably, been in third place. However, if obstetrics and gynaecology are deemed to constitute a single speciality, this produces the highest number of claims per annum for every year covered, quite a startling outcome.

As of 30 June 2020, the following numbers of claims per speciality were open:

Obstetrics: 3,669

Emergency Medicine: 2,775

Orthopaedic Surgery: 2,712

Gynaecology: 1,167

The chief reason why these figures do not follow the same pattern as numbers of new claims received is that many obstetric cases involve brain-damaged babies, which take far longer to resolve than claims from other specialties, due to the need to allow children to reach at least the age of five, and often much older, before medical experts can assess prognosis with a fair degree of certainty.

Interestingly, numbers of new cerebral palsy claims reported per annum have been remarkably consistent over the last 10 years, at around 200. Indeed, during the period since 2006/2007, the number has only varied between 179 and 234. Quite why this might be is a matter for speculation. However, such claims can be difficult to prove because they often turn upon activity, or the lack of it, during a relatively short period at the end of labour plus the necessity to demonstrate that the child's disabilities were caused as a consequence of that delay rather than being due to events earlier in the pregnancy or unrelated factors.

This picture is, however, beginning to change, as a result of the Early Notification Scheme, which commenced on 1 April 2017, where maternity cases falling within the RCOG Each Baby Counts criteria are reported to NHS Resolution as soon after birth as possible. Latterly, this reporting has been undertaken by the Healthcare Safety Investigation Branch (HSIB). NHS Resolution triages those cases and investigates where (a) there is identified hypoxic brain damage and (b) breach of duty and causation may exist, with a view to concluding enquiries swiftly. If breach and causation are demonstrated on the balance of probabilities, admissions are made and financial help given to the parents, even if they have not made a formal claim. That will usually happen much quicker than via standard arrangements, where solicitors acting for disabled children can take years or even decades to bring a claim. Under Early Notification, parents are strongly urged to obtain legal assistance where they have received admissions – not least because the court must approve any substantial payments in the interests of the child. Early Notification cases are excluded from the above figures, save where solicitors have lodged a formal claim.

Payments

Obstetrics is consistently, by a very large measure, the specialty with the highest payments per annum (see Table 1.2). For example, in 2019/2020, the sum in round terms was £905 million against overall outlay of £2,267 million, some 40% of the total amount. This is explained by the very high level of damages in cerebral palsy cases, with £15 million plus being common, rising to £30 million or even more in the most severe cases where there is also a long life-expectancy. Virtually all cerebral palsy cases settled by NHS Resolution are concluded on the basis of periodical payments. These entail a lump sum in respect of past losses, pain and suffering, plus certain future losses such as speech therapy and equipment, together with an annual payment, index-linked for life, in relation to care and case management. The courts recognise that such arrangements are very much in the best interests of affected children, because their ongoing care needs are catered for irrespective of how long they live. Parents are reassured that their disabled child will have sufficient funds to be looked after even following their own death.

Gynaecology, by contrast, usually accounts for around 2% to 3% of total outlay. This is because individual claims, although these can be very serious for those involved, tend not to entail the need for extensive ongoing care or expensive therapies and equipment, albeit some cases are settled well into six figures.

Unsuccessful Claims

Inevitably, there are claims which do not succeed, either because the defendant is able to demonstrate that no breach of duty occurred, or that any alleged breach did not cause the patient additional harm, or both. The following Table 1.3 depicts such cases.

It can be misleading to compare numbers of new claims per annum with numbers closed that year without damages, because these figures will often not represent the same cases – in other words, a claim reported in 2017/2018 may not be closed, following detailed investigation, for a year or two – say until 2019/2020. Nevertheless, bearing that caveat in mind, unsuccessful obstetric claims numbered 394 per annum on average over this 10-year period. The equivalent figure for gynaecology was 164. Average numbers of new claims were 1,121 and 586 respectively. This means that, on average, the failure rate for obstetric claims was 35.1%, and for gynaecology 28%.

Conclusions

Relative stability in the numbers of new obstetric, and especially cerebral palsy, claims over 10 years contrasts markedly with the steep increase in claims against gynaecologists. Whether the former will continue is uncertain, given the ongoing Ockenden review

Table 1.2. Total payments (damages plus legal costs) by NHS Resolution on clinical negligence claims, by specialty, per financial year (1 April to 31 March)

Speciality	2010/11	2011/12	2012/13	2013/14	2014/15	2015/16	2016/17	2017/18	2018/19	2019/20
Obsterics CP/BD	260,905,996	451,150,978	409,661,006	366,240,989	302,192,516	396,078,615	440,955,961	768,348,774	773,902,452	712,116,565
Obsterics Non CP/BD	68,868,574	104,247,036	96,643,512	93,191,925	90,824,924	112,622,614	142,828,593	147,828,179	178,723,058	192,773,682
Paediatrics	51,027,862	84,878,450	71,797,249	71,554,109	98,225,133	79,061,296	94,697,474	149,126,442	175,548,767	167,115,244
Emergency Medicine	70,425,411	101,959,764	107,798,422	97,698,479	110,858,058	113,719,849	156,800,710	176,579,550	198,887,112	181,229,250
Orthopaedic Surgery	95,572,293	119,057,095	121,930,686	116,364,557	126,540,134	179,784,687	192,828,073	178,630,067	168,071,528	166,004,815
General surgery	59,236,129	70,770,560	82,256,755	78,040,005	79,063,165	102,077,225	121,553,720	117,687,521	118,829,198	114,410,794
Neurosurgery	25,526,435	28,063,384	33,434,499	32,788,963	31,663,118	49,532,233	58,357,538	68,201,528	75,615,518	74,993,031
General medicine	31,584,137	50,876,466	47,012,909	45,535,668	37,526,133	43,020,751	45,109,991	62,441,252	54,809,186	48,405,458
Gynaecology	22,561,807	32,104,896	23,511,918	28,817,396	36,081,767	50,491,538	54,841,250	56,657,698	61,820,420	54,816,392
Radiology	16,116,008	15,433,113	12,688,720	19,599,138	19,442,820	27,626,964	35,856,734	54,011,356	68,755,049	53,140,400
Neurology	18,226,305	14,808,586	21,511,307	24,540,870	18,974,541	20,535,466	25,648,808	24,985,892	38,201,749	35,201,281
Psychiatry/Mental Health	14,099,074	18,768,004	21,933,545	19,335,782	16,040,923	21,099,947	25,813,830	31,545,620	40,260,158	42,521,914
Ophthalmology	11,903,939	13,219,227	15,970,338	15,250,308	17,242,205	16,715,905	26,483,820	27,033,525	31,380,142	37,998,912
Cardiology	8,106,042	16,337,963	19,281,951	10,365,386	13,084,124	25,991,183	22,051,309	19,403,174	28,511,323	25,692,669
Ambulance	6,004,123	6,713,495	8,152,650	6,972,025	9,548,381	15,698,659	14,325,663	15,257,021	24,786,429	18,858,655
Gastroenterology	10,288,727	13,071,326	13,776,222	16,872,984	12,898,695	14,968,891	25,482,688	22,318,461	30,504,549	29,103,112
Urology	8,512,939	10,824,168	11,368,915	11,655,699	13,151,432	15,588,778	19,228,890	26,749,416	26,796,662	27,011,839
Other	102,298,650	135,492,914	137,176,377	135,278,171	137,360,695	203,544,521	209,921,059	280,713,019	261,777,661	285,229,639
Total	881,264,452	1,287,777,427	1,255,906,981	1,190,096,455	1,170,718,762	1,488,159,121	1,712,786,113	2,227,518,495	2,357,180,961	2,266,623,652

CP = cerebral palsy; BD = brain damage

11

Table 1.3. Numbers of clinical negligence claims, for selected specialties only, closed by NHS Resolution per financial year (1 April to 31 March) on which no damages were paid

Year of closure	Specialty		
	Gynaecology	Obstetrics	Grand Total
2010/2011	68	290	358
2011/2012	75	320	395
2012/2013	100	306	406
2013/2014	157	357	514
2014/2015	211	444	655
2015/2016	211	416	627
2016/2017	198	435	633
2017/2018	213	378	591
2018/2019	181	412	593
2019/2020	227	581	808
Grand Total	1,641	3,939	5,580

regarding Shrewsbury and Telford Hospital NHS Trust together with other maternity service investigations in East Kent and elsewhere. What is abundantly clear though, is that many of these cases involve women and families whose lives have been profoundly affected by their experiences. That is why the learning which comes from studying the causes of claims is so vital in helping to reduce harm, and hence claim numbers, by not repeating past mistakes.

References

1. Woolf, Lord H. *Access to Justice Final Report and Draft Rules of Court*. London: HMSO; 1996.

2. Ministry of Justice. Pre-Action Protocol for the Resolution of Clinical Disputes – Annex to the Civil Procedure Rules for England and Wales. Available at: www.justice.gov.uk/courts/procedure-rules/civil/rules

3. Legal Aid, Sentencing and Punishment of Offenders Act 2012, Schedule 1, Part 1.

4. Jackson, Sir Rupert. *Review of Civil Litigation Costs: Final Report*. London: TSO; 2009.

2

From Complaint to Litigation

Eloise Power

Introduction

Obstetrics and gynaecology claims account for 20% of the number of all clinical negligence claims notified to the NHS Litigation Authority (predecessor to NHS Resolution) and 49% of the total value of clinical negligence claims.[1] Many clinicians in the field of obstetrics and gynaecology will be involved in the litigation process at some point in their career, whether as a defendant, as a witness or as an expert. The purpose of this chapter is to provide an overview of the pre-litigation and litigation process.

Not every clinical error is actionable. Clinical negligence claims have traditionally been divided into three elements: breach of duty, causation and loss. This tripartite analysis is something of a simplification. In *Khan v Meadows*,[2] the majority of the Supreme Court established a more comprehensive six issues which fall for consideration, incorporating the concept of scope of duty. *Khan v Meadows* is considered in more detail in the legal commentary to Chapter 5. However, the tripartite distinction between breach of duty, causation and loss remains a helpful starting point for analysing many clinical negligence claims.

The standard of proof applicable to clinical negligence claims is the normal civil standard, which is the balance of probabilities. This is often expressed as the need to prove that it was "more likely than not" that an event occurred.[3] The burden of proof is on the claimant.

Element 1: Breach of Duty

Breach of duty in clinical negligence cases (other than cases involving informed consent) is assessed by reference to principles which derive from the cases of *Bolam*[4] and *Bolitho*.[5] Put briefly, McNair J in *Bolam* held that a doctor:

> is not guilty of negligence if he has acted in accordance with a practice accepted as proper by a responsible body of medical men skilled in that particular art……Putting it the other way round, a man is not negligent, if he is acting in accordance with such a practice, merely because there is a body of opinion who would take a contrary view.

---

[1] "Ten Years of Maternity Claims, An Analysis of NHS Litigation Authority Data": section 2.
[2] [2021] UKSC 21 (on appeal from: [2019] EWCA Civ 152).
[3] Contrast the criminal standard of proof, where facts need to be proved "beyond reasonable doubt".
[4] *Bolam v Friern Hospital Management Committee* [1957] 1 WLR 582.
[5] *Bolitho v City and Hackney Health Authority* [1998] AC 232.

Lord Browne-Wilkinson in Bolitho clarified that the body of opinion relied upon must be based upon logic:

> The court is not bound to hold that a defendant doctor escapes liability for negligent treatment or diagnosis just because he leads evidence from a number of medical experts who are genuinely of opinion that the defendant's treatment or diagnosis accorded with sound medical practice......The use of these adjectives – responsible, reasonable and respectable – all show that the court has to be satisfied that the exponents of the body of opinion relied upon can demonstrate that such opinion has a logical basis.

A discussion about the application of the Bolam/Bolitho principles to cases involving pure diagnosis rather than treatment can be found in the legal commentary to Chapter 25.

Where the breach of duty involves a failure to obtain properly informed consent, the legal principles differ from *Bolam/Bolitho*. Chapter 4 contains a detailed discussion of the landmark case of *Montgomery v Lanarkshire Health Board* [2015] UKSC 11 and the law relating to consent.

Element 2: Causation

Causation in clinical negligence claims is often described as "but for" causation: in other words, the claimant needs to prove, on the balance of probabilities, that "but for" the breach of duty, s/he would not have suffered a particular injury. This can be something of an oversimplification, although it is a helpful starting point.

In certain circumstances, causation can be established by proving that the breach of duty made a material contribution to the claimant's injury. In the case of *Williams v Bermuda Hospitals Board*,[6] the Court held that *"where a defendant has been found to have caused or contributed to an indivisible injury, she will be held fully liable for it, even though there may well have been other contributing causes"* and that *"As a matter of principle, successive events are capable of each making a material contribution to the subsequent outcome." Williams* is discussed in more detail in the legal commentary to Chapter 12.[7]

In relation to consent, there have been various attempts by claimants to depart from "but for" causation: the key recent authorities are discussed in detail in the legal commentary to Chapter 18.

In some circumstances, claimants are unable to succeed even if they can demonstrate "but for" causation. A key example of this is the Supreme Court's judgement in *Khan v Meadows*,[8] which is discussed in more detail in the legal commentary to Chapter 5. In a situation where, due to negligence, a mother had not undergone a termination of a fetus with haemophilia, the mother was only allowed to recover for the costs associated with the child's haemophilia, and was not allowed to recover for the costs associated with the child's autism. The autism was unrelated to the negligence and was held to be outside the

---

[6] [2016] UKPC 4.

[7] See also the recent first-instance judgement in *Davies v Frimley Health NHS Foundation Trust* [2021] EWHC 169 (QB), which contains a comprehensive review of the authorities on divisible and indivisible injuries and on material contribution: a full review would be outside the scope of this chapter.

[8] [2021] UKSC 21 (on appeal from: [2019] EWCA Civ 152).

scope of the duty owed by the defendant to the claimant even though, on a simplistic "but for" level, the child would never have been born if it were not for the defendant's negligence.

Element 3: Loss or Damage

The claimant must have suffered some form of loss or damage, and the loss or damage must be measurable or quantifiable. In *Tahir v Haringey Health Authority and another*,[9] the Court held that it was not sufficient to show a *"general increment"* from a delay in providing treatment: the claimant *"must go further and prove some measurable damage"*. The loss of a chance (rather than a probability) of a more favourable outcome will not suffice: see Chapter 26 for a discussion of the House of Lords' judgement in *Gregg v Scott*.[10]

Complaints Procedure

Many clinical negligence matters originate from a complaint brought under the internal complaints procedure of the Trust or other health body. The NHS Constitution provides that patients have the right to make a complaint about any aspect of NHS services. The complaint should be acknowledged within three working days and should be properly investigated.[11] In the event that patients are dissatisfied with the response to their complaint, the matter can be referred to the independent Parliamentary and Health Service Ombudsman. The Ombudsman does not have the power to investigate complaints in circumstances where patients have the option to take legal action, and does not have the power to award compensation (although it can award some out-of-pocket expenses).[12]

Complaints are typically far wider in scope than clinical negligence claims: they may well include issues which are not legally actionable, such as failings of communication which do not result in injury, or poor standards of accommodation on hospital wards. Few letters of complaint will be drafted by legal professionals, although patients and families sometimes have assistance from organisations such as the NHS Complaints Advocacy Service. It is nevertheless important to take all complaints seriously and to instigate early and thorough investigations; in the minority of cases which reach trial, complaint responses are typically included in the court bundle and considered in evidence.

Duty of Candour

One of the main developments of the last decade has been the introduction of a statutory duty of candour in 2014. The relevant legislation[13] was passed following recommendations which were made in the Report of the Mid Staffordshire NHS Foundation Trust

---

[9] [1998] Lloyd's Rep Med 104; [1995] 1 WLUK 382.
[10] [2005] UKHL 2; [2005] 2 AC 176.
[11] www.gov.uk/government/publications/the-nhs-constitution-for-england/the-nhs-constitution-for-england
[12] www.ombudsman.org.uk/
[13] Regulation 20, Health and Social Care Act 2008 (Regulated Activities) Regulations 2014, SI 2936/2014.

Public Inquiry by Sir Robert Francis QC (the Francis report[14]). The statutory duty of candour applies to all health and social care organisations registered with the Care Quality Commission (CQC).

The key statutory provision is that health service bodies must notify patients (or persons lawfully acting on their behalf) both in person and in writing when a *"notifiable safety incident"* has occurred.[15] A *"notifiable incident"* is defined as follows:[16]

> ... any unintended or unexpected incident that occurred in respect of a service user during the provision of a regulated activity that, in the reasonable opinion of a health care professional, could result in, or appears to have resulted in –
>
> (a) the death of the service user, where the death relates directly to the incident rather than to the natural course of the service user's illness or underlying condition, or
>
> (b) severe harm, moderate harm or prolonged psychological harm to the service user.

The regulations also contain a definition of *"moderate harm"*, which means harm that requires a moderate increase in treatment and significant but not permanent harm.

Where an organisation has failed to comply with the duty of candour, the Care Quality Commission can impose fixed penalty fines or bring prosecutions. The first prosecution of an NHS Trust for breach of the duty of candour regulation was heard on 23 September 2020.[17]

The statutory instrument relating to the duty of candour does not make provision for a civil remedy in damages for patients in the event of a breach. In the unreported case of *Linehan v East Kent Hospitals University NHS Foundation Trust* (3 July 2018), a claimant attempted to argue that she should recover damages for psychiatric injury consequent upon a breach of the statutory duty of candour. The submission failed on the facts: please see the legal commentary at Chapter 7 for a more detailed discussion of the case. At the time of writing, there is no legal authority which supports the existence of a free-standing right to claim damages for breach of the statutory duty of candour. However, failures of candour may well be taken into account as part of the evidence relating to other causes of action, such as cases raising the failure to obtain informed consent.

Individual clinicians should be aware that their regulatory bodies are likely to impose professional duties upon them which go beyond the statutory duty of candour. By way of example, the General Medical Council (GMC) and Nursing and Midwifery Council (NMC) have produced joint guidance in this area: *"Openness and honesty when things go wrong: the professional duty of candour."*[18] The joint guidance provides that *"Every healthcare professional must be open and honest with patients when something that goes wrong with their treatment or care causes, or has the potential to cause, harm or distress."* This guidance goes somewhat further than the statutory duty of candour: the statutory duty of candour does not cover "near misses" or harm which falls below the "moderate harm" threshold, whereas the GMC/NMC guidance covers situations which merely have

---

[14] www.gov.uk/government/publications/report-of-the-mid-staffordshire-nhs-foundation-trust-public-inquiry, published 6 February 2013.

[15] There are strict statutory requirements as to the matters which should be included in the notification, which can be found at Regulation 20 (3) and 20 (4), SI 2936/2014, supra

[16] Regulation 20 (7), SI 2936/2014, supra

[17] www.cqc.org.uk/news/releases/care-quality-commission-prosecutes-university-hospitals-plymouth-nhs-trust-breaching

[18] www.nmc.org.uk/standards/guidance/the-professional-duty-of-candour/

the *potential* to cause harm or distress. In order to ensure compliance with regulatory obligations as well as statutory obligations, practitioners would be well advised to err on the side of caution and follow the GMC/NMC guidance where appropriate.

Pre-action Protocol and Qualified One-Way Costs Shifting

Before issuing formal Court proceedings, the parties are expected to follow the Pre-Action Protocol for the Resolution of Clinical Disputes.[19] In most cases, the Protocol is followed after claimants have instructed solicitors. The key provisions of the Protocol include:

(a) A 40-day period for a response to requests by the claimant for copied medical records;

(b) Suggested content of a Letter of Claim (this should include details of the claimant, dates and events, an outline of the allegations of negligence, an outline of causation, information as to injuries, condition and future prognosis, the likely value of the claim/an outline of the main heads of loss, and information about funding[20]);

(c) A four-month period for a substantive response to the Letter of Claim;

(d) Suggested content of a Letter of Response;[21]

(e) Advice upon what to do if a limitation period is approaching: the Protocol does not alter the statutory time limit, so Court proceedings should be issued if necessary and the parties should apply to the Court for a stay of proceedings in order to enable them to follow the Protocol.[22]

Since 1 April 2013, personal injury claims are subject to the Qualified One-Way Costs Shifting (QOCS) regime. This provides that an unsuccessful claimant will not have to pay the defendant's legal costs unless one of the QOCS exceptions applies.[23] Unsuccessful defendants will, however, have to pay the claimant's legal costs.

The QOCS exceptions include: cases where the claimant has disclosed no reasonable grounds for bringing a claim; proceedings which are an abuse of the Court's process; cases where the conduct of the claimant or their representative is likely to obstruct the just disposal of proceedings; or cases where the claimant has been found by a Court to have been fundamentally dishonest. QOCS is also disapplied in cases where a claimant fails to beat a defendant's Part 36 offer.[24]

At first blush, the QOCS regime seems unfair to defendants, and it can indeed cause unfairness to defendants in individual cases – particularly in circumstances where a claimant discontinues an unmeritorious claim shortly before trial, leaving the defendant with a high and irrecoverable costs bill of several hundred thousand pounds or more.

---

[19] www.justice.gov.uk/courts/procedure-rules/civil/protocol/prot_rcd. Note that there are separate Protocols for Scotland and for Northern Ireland.

[20] C2, Pre-Action Protocol, supra.

[21] C3, Pre-Action Protocol, supra.

[22] 1.6.1, Pre-Action Protocol, supra.

[23] Civil Procedure Rules 44.14–44.16.

[24] Part 36 refers to Part 36 of the Civil Procedure Rules, which provides a set of Court rules governing offers of settlement. Where a claimant fails to beat a defendant's Part 36 offer, they are at risk of having to pay the defendant's costs from 21 days after the offer is made. This is capped at the level of damages recovered by the claimant.

However, when viewed across the board, the QOCS regime was welcomed by many insurers and defendant bodies. This was because various additional liabilities which they would previously have paid under the old system were abolished: in particular, defendants no longer have to pay "success fees" on no-win, no-fee agreements, nor do they have to pay for claimants' after-the-event insurance premiums.

A point in favour of the QOCS system is that it encourages early resolution of cases, as defendants will receive costs protection if they make an early Part 36 offer of settlement, and they will not recoup their costs if they seek to defend an indefensible claim. A point against the QOCS system is the concern that it could encourage claimants to bring unmeritorious claims (as they are unlikely to face costs sanctions if they lose). Notwithstanding this concern, claim numbers have not increased since 2013–2014,[25] and most defendants remain willing to contest unmeritorious claims to trial where appropriate.

It is clear that the QOCS regime has increased the importance of the early stages of claims, and that all parties would be well advised to identify the issues which are worth fighting and the issues which should be conceded as soon as possible – preferably at the pre-action protocol stage.

Vicarious Liability and Non-delegable Duty

The identification of the appropriate defendant(s) at the earliest possible stage is crucial. In many cases, this will be a straightforward exercise: for example, in a case involving an NHS patient treated by a single NHS Trust, the defendant will be the relevant NHS Trust. Other cases can raise difficulties and will require consideration of issues of vicarious liability and non-delegable duty. Three examples from the present author's recent practice include:

(a) A claim against a private consultant gynaecologist and an NHS Trust arising out of the failure to manage a post-operative infection after a gynaecological procedure. The gynaecologist was a Trust employee at the same hospital where he had a private practice. Following her private surgery, the patient was attended by a number of Trust employees and by the gynaecologist. Was the gynaecologist acting as a member of Trust staff or as a private consultant after the surgery?

(b) A claim alleging the failure to obtain informed consent for elective gynaecological surgery. There were two consultations prior to surgery. The patient paid privately for the first consultation but underwent the second as an NHS patient. The gynaecologist was not adequately covered by insurance in respect of the first consultation. To what extent should the NHS Trust be responsible for the claim?

(c) Civil actions brought against a former General Practitioner who sexually assaulted female patients in the course of performing internal examinations. The General Practitioner had been found guilty in criminal proceedings, was in prison and had no resources. Should his surgery be responsible for the claim?

As is the case in many areas of clinical negligence work, many cases settle rather than reach trial, so there is no single right answer to the examples set out above.

---

[25] There were 11,945 claims reported in 2013–2014, which was the peak year for clinical negligence claims. By 2018–2019 there were 10,678 claims: www.statista.com/statistics/893770/number-of-claims-reported-to-nhs-england-by-type/.

The legal principles relating to vicarious liability have been considered in several Supreme Court judgements in recent years.[26] The most recent Supreme Court judgement (at the time of writing) is *Barclays Bank plc v Various Claimants* [2020] UKSC 13. Giving unanimous judgement, Lady Hale observed that there are two elements which have to be shown before one party can be made vicariously liable for a tort committed by another: (1) a relationship between the parties which makes it proper for the law to make one pay for the fault of another. This includes employment relationships as well as *"relationships akin or analogous to employment"*, but does not cover independent contractors;[27] (2) the connection between the relationship and the tort.

As Lady Hale observed,[28] *"the key... will usually lie in understanding the details of the relationship."* On the facts in the *Barclays Bank* case, the bank engaged a doctor to perform medical examinations upon prospective employees between 1968 and around 1984. In the course of the unchaperoned examinations, which took place at the doctor's home, the doctor was alleged to have committed sexual assaults upon 126 claimants. Lady Hale looked at the detail of the relationship between the doctor and the bank. She took into account that the doctor had a portfolio of clients and patients and was in business on his own account, probably with his own insurance. He was not paid a retainer and was free to refuse work. Her conclusion was that the bank should not be held vicariously liable for the doctor's wrongdoing.

The key lesson which emerges from the *Barclays Bank* case is the importance of looking at the detail of the relationship between the parties as well as the connection between the relationship and the tort. It is essential to obtain all relevant documentation. This will differ from case to case but is likely to include agreements (such as practising privileges agreements or contractual documentation), together with policies and protocols covering work arrangements. To prevent disputes from arising in the first place, it can be helpful for doctors and organisations to ensure that lines are clearly drawn to demarcate between private and NHS work.

A related but different concept to vicarious liability is the concept of a non-delegable duty of care. This concept often arises in cases involving outsourced services – particularly where the outsourced provider is uninsured or under-insured. The landmark Supreme Court case of *Woodland v Swimming Teachers Association* [2013] UKSC 66, a case involving a catastrophic accident in the course of a swimming lesson run by an independent contractor, contains a key summary of the principles. Vicarious liability did not apply, as it was clear that there was no relationship with the independent contractor which was "akin to employment". The Court held that the education authority could not delegate its duty of care to the independent contractor: *"the respondent education authority assumed a duty to ensure that the Appellant's swimming lessons were carefully*

---

[26] Detailed consideration is beyond the scope of this book, but the cases of *Various claimants v Catholic Child Welfare Society* [2012] UKSC 56 (generally known as "Christian Brothers"), *Cox v Ministry of Justice* [2016] UKSC 10, *Mohamud v WM Morrison Supermarkets* [2016] UKSC 11, *Armes v Nottinghamshire County Council* [2017] UKSC 60 are important.

[27] Para 24; see also the "five incidents" which will assist in doubtful cases in distinguishing between relationships akin to employment and independent contractor. The "five incidents" are set out at para 15 and discussed at para 27.

[28] At para 27.

conducted and supervised, by whomever they might get to perform these functions".[29] The following principles arose from the case law in relation to the circumstances where a non-delegable duty of care will arise:[30]

(1) The claimant is a patient or a child, or for some other reason is especially vulnerable or dependent on the protection of the defendant against the risk of injury. Other examples are likely to be prisoners and residents in care homes.

(2) There is an antecedent relationship between the claimant and the defendant, independent of the negligent act or omission itself, (i) which places the claimant in the actual custody, charge or care of the defendant, and (ii) from which it is possible to impute to the defendant the assumption of a positive duty to protect the claimant from harm, and not just a duty to refrain from conduct which will foreseeably damage the claimant. It is characteristic of such relationships that they involve an element of control over the claimant, which varies in intensity from one situation to another, but is clearly very substantial in the case of schoolchildren.

(3) The claimant has no control over how the defendant chooses to perform those obligations, i.e. whether personally or through employees or through third parties.

(4) The defendant has delegated to a third party some function which is an integral part of the positive duty which he has assumed towards the claimant; and the third party is exercising, for the purpose of the function thus delegated to him, the defendant's custody or care of the claimant and the element of control that goes with it.

(5) The third party has been negligent not in some collateral respect but in the performance of the very function assumed by the defendant and delegated by the defendant to him.

The principles in *Woodland* are clearly of relevance to clinical negligence cases involving the outsourcing of services to patients. Prior to *Woodland*, the Court of Appeal had rejected the imposition of a non-delegable duty of care in circumstances where the Ministry of Defence had sub-contracted procurement of secondary healthcare in Germany for service personnel and their families: *Re A (A child) v Ministry of Defence and another* [2004] EWCA Civ 641. Following *Woodland*, there have been a number of first-instance decisions involving healthcare:

(a) In *Gallardo v Imperial College Healthcare NHS Trust* [2017] EWHC 3147 (QB), a judge held that a surgeon had a responsibility to inform his patient of the outcome of a surgical procedure, and that this responsibility did not end when the patient moved to a private wing of the hospital. *Woodland* was considered, but the relevant duty arose when the patient was under the NHS Trust in any event and had not been discharged at the point of transfer.

(b) In *Ramdhean v Agedo and another* (28 January 2020, unreported), a County Court judge applied *Woodland* and found that a dental practice owed a patient a non-delegable duty of care in relation to advice and treatment provided by a self-employed dentist engaged by the practice.

(c) In *Hopkins (a child) v Akramy* [2020] EWHC 3445 (QB), a judge found that a primary care trust (PCT) did not owe a non-delegable duty of care to protect NHS patients from harm. The case involved alleged negligence at an outsourced "Out of Hours" service based in an NHS hospital but managed under a contract between a

---

[29] Para 26.
[30] Para 23.

PCT and a private company. The *Woodland* principles were not applied, as the Court found that Parliament had provided for a statutory delegable duty to secure provision of primary medical services.

(d) In *Breakingbury v Croad*, 19 April 2021,[31] a County Court judge applied *Woodland* and found that the owner of a dental practice owed a non-delegable duty of care to a patient. In the alternative, the owner was vicariously liable for the torts of the associate dentists. The judge held that *"The setting of targets seems to me to be important"*, finding that this amounted to the kind of control which was sufficient to form the basis of vicarious liability.

At the time of writing, a first-instance decision of the High Court in this area is awaited.[32] It is likely that the appellate courts will need to give further consideration to the concept of a non-delegable duty of care in the healthcare context in the future, particularly in the light of the growth of outsourcing and the inadequate insurance cover held by some outsourced providers. A powerful argument in favour of liability in these circumstances (whether by the imposition of a non-delegable duty of care or by way of the law relating to informed consent) is that patients are often unaware that they are receiving services from outsourced providers rather than the NHS and may not have given their properly informed consent to the receipt of such services. An alternative approach, which would require legislation rather than developments in the common law, would be to ensure that all outsourced providers are required to have comprehensive insurance cover sufficient to meet the highest value claims. The Government is currently in the process of establishing a Patient Safety Commissioner,[33] and it is to be hoped that the ambit of this role will include outsourcing issues.

Limitation

The concept of limitation[34] is deceptively simple. Assessing the correct limitation period can pose considerable difficulties. In the event of a dispute, the courts have the power to direct that limitation should be dealt with as a preliminary issue, which means that it is considered at a separate hearing rather than left for trial.

The normal limitation period in personal injury cases, including clinical negligence cases, is three years from either the date on which the cause of action accrued or (if later) the claimant's date of knowledge.[35] Both of these concepts require some further consideration.

The date on which the cause of action accrued refers to the date upon which all of the elements of the cause of action have occurred: breach, causation and damage. Damage must be real rather than minimal.[36] In some cases, breach, causation and damage will occur at around the same time, but this is not always the case: for example, in the event of

---

[31] Unreported at time of writing; due to be reported in *Medical Law Reports*.

[32] *Hughes v Rattan* (Heather Williams QC, sitting as a Deputy Judge of the High Court).

[33] www.gov.uk/government/publications/medicines-and-medical-devices-bill-overarching-documents/medicines-and-medical-devices-bill-patient-safety-commissioner

[34] In other words, a time period for starting claims after which a claim is not permitted to be brought.

[35] Section 11 (4), Limitation Act 1980.

[36] *Haward and others v Fawcetts (a firm) and others* [2006] UKHL 9.

a prescribing error leading to a catastrophic drug overdose some days later, the date on which the cause of action accrued would be the date of the drug overdose.

The date of knowledge is defined[37] as the date upon which the claimant had knowledge of the following matters: (a) that the injury was significant; (b) that the injury was attributable (in whole or in part) to the act or omission alleged to constitute negligence;[38] (c) the identity of the defendant; (d) if the act or omission was that of a person other than the defendant, the identity of that person and the additional facts supporting bringing an action against the defendant. By way of an example, if a radiologist negligently misses a tumour when reporting a scan and a patient suffers a worsened prognosis as a result, the date of knowledge is likely to be the date when the patient gains awareness that she has cancer *and* that the tumour was missed on the scan by the radiologist.

In the landmark *Atomic Veterans* case,[39] the claims brought by servicemen who alleged that they had suffered injury as a result of exposure to radiation during nuclear tests carried out in the 1950s were held to be time-barred. The servicemen argued that prior to 2007, they only had a belief (as distinct from knowledge) that their injuries were attributable to exposure to radiation; things changed in 2007 when they received a crucial expert report. The Supreme Court held that a claimant was likely to have acquired knowledge of the required facts when he first came reasonably to believe them. The claimant's belief had to have been held with sufficient confidence to justify embarking on the preliminaries to the issue of proceedings. On the facts, the servicemen's position was made more difficult because the majority of their claims had been issued in 2005, before the claimed date of knowledge: Lord Wilson observed that it was *"heretical"* for a claimant to argue that he did not have the requisite knowledge after he had started Court proceedings.

Where an injured person has died before the expiry of the three-year period, the limitation period for claims on behalf of the estate under the Law Reform (Miscellaneous Provisions) Act 1934 is three years from the date of death or three years from the date of the personal representative's knowledge, whichever is later.[40] Similarly, the limitation period for claims under the Fatal Accidents Act 1976 is three years from the date of death or three years from the date of knowledge of the person for whose benefit the action is brought, whichever is later.[41] The legal commentary to Chapter 26 contains further information about post-death and lost years claims.

Where an injured person is a child, the limitation period expires 3 years after the child turns 18. Where the injured person lacks capacity to conduct legal proceedings under the Mental Capacity Act 2005 at the date when the cause of action accrued, the limitation period expires three years after the date when the injured person regains capacity or dies.[42] In practice, where a claimant is unlikely to regain capacity (e.g. in cases of serious brain injury), this means that limitation is effectively disapplied within the claimant's lifetime. The result is that historic claims sometimes reach trial: an example of a case which reached trial in April 2016 but dealt with events in May 1986 can be found in the legal commentary to Chapter 16.

---

[37] Under section 14 of the Limitation Act 1980.
[38] Or nuisance, or other breach of duty.
[39] *AB & Others v Ministry of Defence* [2012] UKSC 9.
[40] Section 11 (5), Limitation Act 1980.
[41] Section 12 (2), Limitation Act 1980.
[42] Section 28, Limitation Act 1980.

Finally, the Court retains a discretion to disapply the limitation period even where a claim is time-barred if it is regarded as *"equitable"* to allow the claim to proceed.[43] In exercising its discretion, the Court has regard to all the circumstances of the case, including prejudice to both parties, the length of the delay, the reasons for the delay, the effect of the delay on the cogency of the evidence, the conduct of the defendant, the duration of any period when the claimant lacked capacity after the cause of action accrued, the extent to which the claimant acted promptly and reasonably after gaining knowledge that the defendant's acts/omissions "might be capable" of giving rise to a claim, the steps taken by the claimant to obtain expert advice and the nature of the advice received.

Needless to say, the existence of the Court's discretion to disapply the limitation period has generated a large amount of case law in various contexts. In the context of clinical negligence, the case of *Pennine Acute Hospitals NHS Trust v Simon de Meza* [2017] EWCA Civ 1711 is of interest: the Court of Appeal overturned a trial judge's decision to disapply the limitation period in a case against a Trust which had been delayed for 28 years. The Court held that it was relevant to take the weakness of the underlying claim into account. Further, the defendant Trust would suffer prejudice if the claim were allowed to proceed: in particular, key records had been destroyed due to the lapse of time. By way of a contrast, in *Azam v University Hospital Birmingham NHS Foundation Trust* [2020] EWHC 3384 (QB), a High Court judge (on appeal) upheld a trial judge's decision to allow a clinical negligence claim to proceed 18 years out of time in circumstances where the operating surgeon had died; on the facts, the Trust had failed to prove that prejudice flowed from the surgeon's death.[44]

In a nutshell, limitation can be complex and may require specialist advice.[45] It is unsafe (to say the least) to make the assumption that a potential claim will vanish after the initial three-year period.

Court Timetable[46]

Figure 2.1 outlines the different stages in formal Court proceedings. The first stage in formal Court proceedings involves issuing a Claim Form at Court and payment of a Court fee. The Claim Form must be served upon the defendant within four months of the date of issue at the latest. Particulars of Claim (a formal document setting out the facts and allegations upon which the claimant relies), a Schedule of Loss (a document setting out details of the damages sought by the claimant) and a medical report on condition and prognosis must be served upon the defendant within the four-month period.[47]

---

[43] Section 33, Limitation Act 1980.

[44] See also the similar decision in *Estate of Mohammed Mossa v Wise* [2017] EWHC 2608 (QB) involving a deceased gynaecologist.

[45] The information in this chapter is only intended as an overview of the issues which are most relevant in clinical negligence practice; other issues which can affect limitation include fraud, concealment and mistake, and there are different limitation periods for different causes of action.

[46] This section is inevitably something of a simplification for reasons of space. The authoritative guide to civil Court proceedings is the White Book, published by Thomson Reuters, current edition 2021.

[47] These documents can be served together with the Particulars of Claim or up to 14 weeks later, provided that this is within the four-month period: Civil Procedure Rules 7.4.

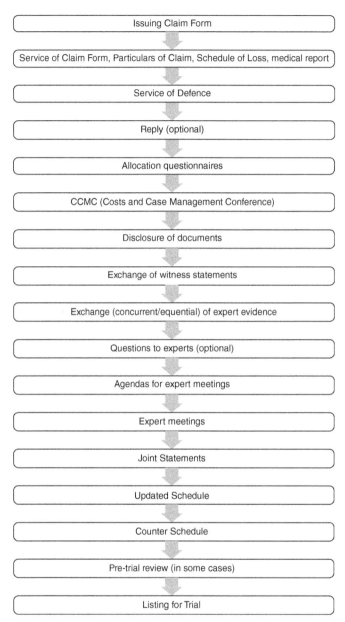

Figure 2.1

Unless the defendant wishes to admit the claim, a Defence must be served within 14 days after service of the Particulars of Claim, or alternatively 28 days if an Acknowledgment of Service has been filed. In the Defence, the defendant must state: (a) which allegations in the particulars of claim it denies, (b) which allegations it requires the claimant to prove, (c) which allegations it admits.[48] The claimant thereafter has the option of serving a Reply, although this is not compulsory.

After the parties have served their respective statements of case,[49] the Court issues the parties with an allocation questionnaire, after which the case is allocated to a track: small claims, fast track or multi-track. The majority of clinical negligence cases are allocated to the multi-track, which is designed for more complicated and/or higher value matters. The matter is then listed for a procedural hearing called a Costs and Case Management Conference (CCMC).

At the CCMC, directions are set on a case-by-case basis for the onward management of the matter. Typical directions will include:

(a) Provision for disclosure

(b) Exchange of factual witness evidence

(c) Permission for expert evidence in specific disciplines

(d) Timetable for exchange (simultaneous or sequential) of expert evidence

(e) Timetable for experts' discussions, including the provision of Agendas and a date by which the experts should provide Joint Statements: please see Chapter 3 for further consideration of experts' discussions and Joint Statements

(f) Permission for an updated Schedule of Loss and a Counter Schedule (i.e. the defendant's response to the Schedule)

(g) Listing for trial (and for a pre-trial review hearing in some cases).

Some cases raise further procedural issues: for example, there might be a dispute as to whether limitation should be dealt with as a preliminary issue, or there might be a dispute as to whether the case should proceed as a "split trial" (separating the liability stage from the quantum stage). The Court will also consider the parties' respective costs budgets[50] at the CCMC.

Once formal Court proceedings have begun, all of the stages of the case take on great importance both for claimants and for defendants. There can be significant sanctions for parties who do not comply with Court directions or miss deadlines, particularly if no application has been made for an extension of time.

Alternative Dispute Resolution

Alternative Dispute Resolution (ADR) simply refers to the resolution of disputes without going to court. There are various well-known methods of ADR, which include:

(a) Negotiation between legal representatives, which can include the making of offers of settlement under Part 36[51] or any other form of offer of settlement.

(b) A Joint Settlement Meeting or Round Table Meeting: these meetings are usually attended by legal representatives and clients, and can take whatever form the parties

---

[48] Civil Procedure Rules 16.5.

[49] "Statement of case" is a generic term for pleadings, including Claim Forms, Particulars of Claim, Defences, Replies, Part 20 claims (counterclaims and claims made by defendants against additional parties) and responses to requests for further information.

[50] Costs Budgets are essentially a detailed estimate of the legal costs which are likely to be incurred at the various stages between the CCMC and trial.

[51] I.e. the formal process set out by Part 36 of the Civil Procedure Rules.

wish. These meetings are very common in practice and often lead to settlements, particularly where all parties have effective representation and are motivated to achieve a sensible resolution of the matter.

(c) Mediation, which is discussed below.

(d) Arbitration: this involves the parties agreeing that an independent third party[52] should resolve the dispute. Arbitration is rarely used in clinical negligence cases but is used more frequently in other contexts such as product liability matters.

(e) Early Neutral Evaluation, which involves the parties agreeing to obtain an opinion from an independent third party. Unlike arbitration, the parties do not agree that the opinion will be binding.

Importantly, the parties can enter into ADR at any stage in the claim. It is not necessary to wait for formal Court proceedings to be issued – indeed, it may well be more commercially attractive for defendants to start ADR before the issue of proceedings. Having said that, it can be difficult or impossible to assess the value of claims at the early stages, particularly where matters are complex or high value. Where parties want to enter into ADR, it is sensible to engage in constructive discussions beforehand about the evidence which is needed to value the claim.

The Court system encourages ADR, and a failure to engage in ADR can be taken into account at the costs stage, particularly where no reasons have been given for the lack of engagement.

A key trend in recent years has been the increased use of mediation in clinical negligence cases. Mediation involves the appointment of a neutral third party (the mediator) whose role is to facilitate discussions between the two opposing parties.

NHS Resolution (under its previous name, the NHS Litigation Authority), established a mediation panel focusing on resolving clinical negligence and personal injury claims in December 2016. An evaluation report published in February 2020[53] concludes that *"the power of mediation as a resolution tool cannot be overestimated."*

In appropriate cases, mediation can be very effective, particularly in cases where emotions understandably run high, or where one or more parties have demonstrated intransigence towards settlement, or where an extra-legal remedy such as an apology is sought. On the other hand, criticisms of mediation have included the additional costs which it tends to involve (in comparison with settlement meetings), and the focus (or perceived focus) on achieving any settlement rather than the most appropriate settlement. The present author's view is that it is important to consider suitability for mediation on a case-by-case basis and that mediation should not be seen as a silver bullet.

Trial

Only a small minority of clinical negligence claims reach trial; the majority are either settled through ADR or discontinued by the claimant. In the event that a case reaches

---

[52] E.g. a barrister or retired judge.

[53] https://resolution.nhs.uk/wp-content/uploads/2020/02/NHS-Resolution-Mediation-in-healthcare-claims-an-evaluation.pdf

trial, the claimant and defendant prepare skeleton arguments in advance, which are written documents setting out the key points in favour of their respective cases. In many cases, the barristers acting for the claimant and the defendant will come to an agreement about the Court timetable, which should make provision for the following:

(a) Any applications which are outstanding by the date of trial

(b) Each party's opening (oral submissions in favour of their respective cases)

(c) Factual evidence

(d) Expert evidence

(e) Each party's closing submissions

(f) Judgement

At Court, each witness (whether they are a witness of fact or an expert witness) is invited to take the oath or to affirm that they will tell the truth. In most circumstances, their witness statement or report will stand as their evidence in chief, although permission is sometimes given for supplementary questions. The witness is then cross-examined by the opposing party's barrister: please see Chapter 3 for guidance to expert witnesses facing cross-examination. The witness is thereafter re-examined by their side's barrister. Re-examination should be confined to issues which emerge in cross-examination. The judge can intervene and ask the witness questions at any point during their evidence.

After closing submissions are heard, judgement is sometimes given *ex tempore* (at the time of trial). Alternatively, the judge can decide to reserve judgement and hand it down at a later date.

When reading the legal commentaries contained in this book, it is important to bear in mind that they mainly relate to cases which have come to trial. Such cases are not necessarily representative of the majority of clinical negligence work. As might be expected, the small group of cases which reach trial tend to pose particular difficulties either of legal principle or (more commonly) of evidence.

Professional Disciplinary Proceedings

This chapter has focused on clinical negligence proceedings in the civil courts. In certain circumstances, healthcare professionals may also face Fitness to Practise proceedings before their regulators.[54] Providing a detailed account of Fitness to Practise proceedings is beyond the scope of this book.[55] However, the following points should be borne in mind:

(a) Referrals to professional regulators can originate from a variety of sources, including but not limited to employers, official bodies, fellow-professionals and patients. In some circumstances, healthcare professionals have a duty to refer themselves to their

---

[54] Such as the General Medical Council, the Nursing and Midwifery Council or the Health and Care Professions Council.

[55] A readable account of the relevant law can be found in *Professional Discipline and Healthcare Regulators: A Legal Handbook* (published by Legal Action Group, 2018): by way of a disclaimer, I am the author of an individual chapter and have a (minimal) financial interest in the book.

regulator. Clinical negligence claims, in contrast, can only be brought by the injured person, those acting on behalf of the injured person, or by the estate or dependants of a deceased person.

(b) The concept of "misconduct" in healthcare regulatory law is different from the concept of negligence in civil proceedings. Misconduct has been defined as follows: *"It must be linked to the practice of medicine or conduct that otherwise brings the profession into disrepute, and it must be serious."*[56] There is support in the case law for seriousness to be given proper weight and to be characterised as *"conduct which would be regarded as deplorable by fellow practitioners."*[57] In broad terms, misconduct is likely to involve worse behaviour than mere negligence. As Jackson LJ observed in *R (on the application of Calhaem) v General Medical Council* [2007] EWHC 2606: *"Mere negligence does not constitute 'misconduct' within the meaning of section 35C(2)(a) of the Medical Act 1983. Nevertheless, and depending upon the circumstances, negligent acts or omissions which are particularly serious may amount to 'misconduct'."*[58]

(c) Most clinical negligence cases do not generate a referral to a professional regulator, particularly where the case relates to an isolated error. Single incidents are less likely to cross the threshold for misconduct than multiple incidents. However, it is possible for a single incident to amount to misconduct if it is particularly grave.[59]

(d) Misconduct may relate to matters which could not form the subject of a clinical negligence claim: for example, serious failings of record-keeping which have not led to patient harm, or criminal conduct which has nothing to do with a healthcare professional's clinical practice.

(e) Professional regulators are empowered to instigate Fitness to Practise proceedings on the basis of "deficient professional performance" as well as/in the alternative to misconduct: *"'Deficient professional performance'. . . is conceptually separate both from negligence and from misconduct. It connotes a standard of professional performance which is unacceptably low and which (save in exceptional circumstances) has been demonstrated by reference to a fair sample of the doctor's work.*[60]*"* Professional regulators are also empowered to instigate Fitness to Practise proceedings on the basis of health issues.

(f) Professional regulators do not award compensation to patients. They are empowered to impose sanctions on practitioners in circumstances where a healthcare professional's fitness to practise has been found to be impaired: these sanctions can include warnings/cautions, conditions of practice (e.g. working under supervision, training requirements, etc.), suspension and erasure from the Register.

---

[56] *Meadow v General Medical Council* [2007] 1 All ER 1, Auld LJ, para 200.

[57] *Nandi v General Medical Council* [2004] EWHC 2317 (Admin), Collins J, para 31.

[58] Para 39.

[59] *R (on the application of Calhaem) v General Medical Council* [2007] EWHC 2606, Jackson LJ, para 39.

[60] Para 39, *Calhaem*, supra.

(g) Professional regulatory hearings take place before specialist panels or committees rather than courts, although healthcare professionals have a statutory right of appeal to the High Court against certain decisions, including the decision to impose sanctions. Unduly lenient decisions can be appealed by the Professional Standards Authority.

Specialist legal advice should be sought in the event that a healthcare professional faces Fitness to Practise proceedings; these proceedings can raise complex legal and evidential issues, and their impact on professionals' lives can be grave.

Being a Medicolegal Expert and Report Writing

Swati Jha

Introduction

The Civil Procedure Rules (CPR) defines an expert in general terms as a "person who has been instructed to give or prepare expert evidence for the purpose of proceedings". A "single joint expert" is an expert instructed to prepare a report for the court on behalf of two or more of the parties (including the claimant) to the proceedings. When making decisions in negligence claims, the courts rely heavily on the advice and opinions of the experts, and in clinical negligence claims this is provided by clinicians. Experts should be used appropriately, and their duty is always to the court rather than as an advocate of either party. But as medicine is not an exact science, often there will be a difference of opinion even with the views of experts.

The GMC [1] has issued guidance on acting as an expert witness, and all clinicians considering this line of work should familiarise themselves with this guidance.

For a medical negligence claim to be successful there is a requirement to fulfil the following criteria:

1. Demonstrate that the defendant owed a duty of care. In clinical negligence claims it is a given, as the healthcare provider owes their patient a duty of care.
2. That duty of care was breached, which implies that the care fell below a reasonable standard and that expected of a reasonably competent body of medical practitioners. This is referred to as Liability.
3. The breach led to the avoidable harm that subsequently ensued. This is referred to as causation.

All clinicians have a duty of care to the patients they are treating but in cases of litigation where care was in an NHS hospital, the claim is brought against the hospital where treatment was provided rather than the clinician. The NHS hospital is vicariously liable for all its employees including doctors, nurses, embryologists, midwives, radiographers, cytologists etc. The exception to this being cases of criminal negligence and cases that go to the coroner.

The standard applied for duty of care in clinical cases is the Bolam principle. This applies to all cases related to technique in carrying out surgery, subsequent complications and their management. In cases of consent however, the standard of proof is now Montgomery, as discussed in Chapter 4.

Proving causation is usually the most intricate aspect of a negligence claim. In several cases described in this book, whereas liability was proven, causation was not. For causation to be proven, it needs to be established first that the clinical problem did not predate the commencement of treatment. The main issues of causation in clinical negligence claims include: the difference in outcomes if alternative treatment had been offered; the difference in outcomes if different treatment had been given and what difference the competent treatment would have made to the condition and prognosis of the patient.

Need for an Expert

The need for an expert arises in specific situations. For a court to accept evidence, the courts must be assured of the following:

- The evidence provided by the expert will assist the courts and is needed to reach a decision. In other words, the knowledge is out with the experience of the tribunal (judge/jury). This is to allow the evidence to be made intelligible to them.
- The expert needs to be able to demonstrate they have the knowledge to act as the expert in a particular case. They need to have an understanding of the relevant area of expertise.
- Experts must be able to demonstrate they are impartial and have no conflicts of interest, hence should be independent.

The role of the expert is not to give a verdict on the facts, this is the role of the judge. The expert is required to explain the basis of their evidence; hence weightage is in the reasoning not the conclusions reached.

It is important for experts to formulate their opinion following due consideration of the facts, as instructing solicitors may not take kindly to a change of opinion late in the day. However, if the experts for the alternative party give compelling reasons to change an opinion, it is reasonable to concede this early in the day rather than adhering to an opinion simply to please the instructing team. When the expert's view changes, this should be communicated to all parties without delay and where appropriate to the court. Providing a partisan report can result in severe criticism and in other parties refusing to instruct experts in future.

Principles of Report Writing

A medicolegal expert does not need to have any legal qualifications, but they should familiarise themselves with Part 35 of the Civil Procedure Rules [2], the practice directions to Part 35 of the Civil Procedure Rules and the Civil Justice Council's guidance for the instruction of experts in civil claims. The salient issues that an expert should be aware of are shown in Table 3.1.

All reports should include details of the expert's qualifications. The report should make clear which facts are out with the expert's area of practice. There should be a statement setting out the instructions and facts, and the report should always have a brief summary of the claim at the start and the opinions which will be addressed in the report.

Published literature which supports a viewpoint should be adequately referenced in the report and a reference list of literature or material relied on to reach an opinion. Where unpublished literature is relied on, this must be served at the same time as the report.

Where there is a range of opinions, these should be laid out and the reasons for reaching one opinion over the others clearly stated. Where an opinion cannot be given without qualification, this should be stated. The report should state that the expert is

Table 3.1. Legal framework for expert witnesses (Civil Procedure Rules Part 35)

- Expert's evidence is restricted to that which is reasonably required to resolve the proceedings.
- The duty of experts to assist the courts overrides any obligation they have to the person from whom they have received instructions. They are independent and are not advocates.
- Experts can only be asked to provide evidence when invited by the court.
- Parties inviting experts must provide an estimate of costs of instructing the expert.
- They should confine their opinion to matters which are relevant to the dispute.
- They should confine their opinions to matters within their expertise.
- Evidence is given in a written report and must comply with Practice Direction 35, 3.1–3.3. Compliance should be stated in the report.
- All facts should be taken into account but should be kept separate from opinions.
- Where a range of opinions are expressed, these should all be taken into account, summarised and the expert should present their own opinions while giving reasons for this.
- When facts are in dispute between experts, individual experts should express their own separate opinions based on the facts.
- A summary of the conclusions should be presented.

aware of the requirement of the Part 35, this practice direction and the guidance for the instruction of experts in civil claims. It should state they understand their duty to the court and have complied with their duty.

Subheadings within a report are shown in Appendix 1 and 2.

The expert report must include a CV with a statement of qualifications and the current post of the expert. The Court will require a full CV if the case goes to trial, and this should therefore be supplied as an appendix. The CV should be updated regularly to ensure it is current.

The report that is prepared should be in keeping with Practice Direction 5A, which concerns the preparation of all Court documents and requires that reports are:

- On A4 paper
- With a 3.5 cm margin
- With pages numbered consecutively (ideally centre bottom or top corner)
- With numbered paragraphs
- All numbers, including dates, are in figures.

Font size should be no smaller than 11. When cross-referencing the medical records, it is helpful to refer to the page number of the document. When it is necessary to quote from medical reports, embedded screen shots may be used. It is essential to make a distinction between what is being quoted from the medical record, a narrative or summary opined from the report and the expert comment provided.

Medicolegal Expert Indemnity Cover

In the past, experts were immune from prosecution or civil action for views expressed in their reports when undertaking preliminary work for courts or giving evidence in court and tribunals. The stance taken previously was articulated by the common law, and that no action will be taken against a witness in the course of giving evidence. Initially, this applied only to evidence given orally in court but was extended to reports, affidavits and other statements by experts. In the case of *GMC v Meadows [2006] EWCA Civ 1390*, a prominent paediatrician wrote reports which were used in proceedings against Sally Clark (a solicitor herself) to prove she killed two of her children. This conviction was later quashed on appeal and the reports prepared by Professor Meadow were found to be misleading and held responsible for the prior convictions. He had failed to familiarise himself with all relevant data and published work relating to the incident. This should have been sufficient to provide a competent, impartial, balanced and fair expert opinion of scientific validity. In addition, he gave expert evidence on matters beyond his competence. This was found to be sufficiently serious for his name to be struck off from the medical register, even though he was an internationally acclaimed specialist. In this case, which attracted a lot of media attention, the English Court of Appeal determined that the principle of "witness immunity" does not protect experts from accountability to their regulatory bodies for substandard forensic work in court or in preparation for court. This is consistent with the law in both the United States and Australia

Another case in which lack of immunity was emphasised was that of Jones v Kaney. This case highlighted that experts can be sued by their clients for negligence for non-contentious work. The case also considered the issue of whether preparation of a joint statement by experts was immune from suit. An expert's overriding duty is to the court. However, clients may find it hard to accept that the expert paid by their legal team has a duty which overrides that owed to him. This only applies to the client's own expert action; a client cannot sue the other side's expert for their evidence.

For these reasons, it is now imperative, when undertaking work as an expert in medical negligence claims, that clinicians have adequate medical indemnity. Medical indemnity policies provide cover for claims arising from delivery of medical services and medical incidents. To provide cover for work undertaken as an expert witness in clinical negligence claims, this needs to be specifically declared, endorsed and incorporated into the indemnity policy.

Types of Report Writing

Broadly speaking, clinical negligence reports are of three types:
1. Breach of Duty reports, also referred to as Liability reports
2. Causation reports
3. Condition and Prognosis reports

Breach of Duty (Liability) and Causation reports are usually written in conjunction, and the Condition and Prognosis report is required to determine quantum, i.e. value of the pay-out. The function of the two are therefore very distinct. As clinicians carrying out medicolegal work, it is imperative to understand the principles of breach of duty and causation. It is a common misconception that in order for litigation to succeed, it is enough if the defendant admits that there was a breach of duty of care, but there is much more to a medical negligence claim than this. If the breach did not result in the injury (causation), then a case may well be successfully defended, even when there was harm to the patient.

Breach of Duty Report (Liability Report)

For a negligence claim to succeed, it must be proven that a doctor's actions caused or contributed to the injury. This addresses the issue of whether or not the care provided fell below a reasonable standard of care. The test used to establish breach of duty is the Bolam Test, except in cases of consent where the standards are judged against Montgomery. This means that clinicians should be able to demonstrate that they provided care that a reasonable clinician would have provided.

When writing a Breach of Duty report, it is important to bear in mind the following:

- Irrespective of who the instructing party is, the report should be able to opine independently and prepare their report for the Court.
- Opinions should be restricted to the expert's area of practice. For example, it would not be appropriate for a gynaecologist to comment on a case of mismanaged labour if they do not practise obstetrics in their routine day to day work, or for a generalist who does not carry out incontinence work to comment on issues of liability related to incontinence surgery.
- When presenting a view within the report, the expert must scrutinise carefully what the basis of their opinion is. A good test of this is whether they would be comfortable being cross-examined on their opinion, and what supports their opinion.
- Where specific queries are not answerable, this should be flagged by the expert.
- If an expert view changes on account of further information coming to light, this should be discussed with the instructing solicitor as soon as possible.
- If further records are required to formulate an opinion, this should be proffered early so that these can be retrieved.
- Experts are expected to be aware of all relevant guidelines or protocols in place at the time of the said negligence, as this is evidential support.
- Experts need to be aware of the technical issues that need to be explored and those that are outside of their own expertise. Those aspects outside of the expert's specialism should be flagged early.
- Though not a requirement of the litigation process, one of the by-products of a liability report is an explanation and understanding of the situation in which the parties (particularly the claimant) find themselves.
- There should be good communication with instructing solicitors to ensure that the evidence provided is complete and clear.

Causation Report

The main point of interest in establishing causation is whether the injury suffered by the claimant was a direct result of the breach of duty. Having a clear understanding of causation is a key requirement of a good medicolegal expert.

The tests for causation are:

- Would the injury have happened anyway, in which case the claim will fail.
- The "but for" test, i.e. the injury would not have happened "but for" the negligence, in which case the claim will succeed.
- If it can be shown that the breach of duty contributed to the injury to some extent, the claim will succeed, although other conditions may have made the injury worse.

Leading on from this, it therefore follows that one of the main objectives of a medical report is to distinguish which symptoms, effects, consequences have been caused directly from the breach of duty and which have not. Occasionally, there is a requirement for multiple experts in different disciplines to address the different aspects of the injury being alleged. If a symptom/consequence would have happened anyway, this cannot be recovered in damages. One of the main attributes of a medicolegal expert therefore is being able to establish causation which needs to be presented accurately and precisely in language that is understandable immediately to the solicitors.

Confusion arises when a patient has a pre-existing condition and the symptoms arising after the event are superimposed on these underlying conditions. Further confusion can arise from conditions that are likely to affect the claimant in later life anyway e.g., menopause impacting on sexual function, or persisting degenerative conditions which tend to be progressive and would have continued to impact on an individual. These may have been asymptomatic at the time of the injury but present after the injury, making the principle of causation challenging to apply. These symptoms can wrongly be attributed to the breach of duty.

Another problem for medical experts is that we are trained to provide opinions on the current status of a medical problem, but providing an opinion on hypothetical situations based on what the situation would have been had the injury not occurred is far more complicated. It is the opinion dealing with the "but for" scenario that allows a claim to be valued. The report should clearly identify the current situation, and also the situation had the breach of duty not occurred, while explaining and describing the difference between the two situations.

When writing a Causation report it is important to bear in mind the following:

- The balance of probabilities argument is used to establish causation. The balance of probability test means that, based on the evidence available, the occurrence of the event was more likely than not. The inherent probability of an event occurring is a matter taken into account when weighing the probability of the event occurring. In judicial terms, if a judge reaches the conclusion that it was 50% or more likely that the injury was caused by the breach, then the judgement will be for the claimant.
- When there are multiple possible causes that may have brought about the injury, it has to be shown that the breach of duty was the cause of the injury. If there are multiple factors which are cumulative, then a claim can still succeed if it can be shown that by acting together, the injury occurred.
- If the chain of causation is broken, this is difficult to prove. This is where an unforeseeable event occurs after a breach of duty which worsens the effect of the injury.
- In causation claims, injuries are categorised as divisible and indivisible, based on whether the injury is the product of one or more than one cause and whether it is possible to quantify how much cause is attributed to each cause.
- In causation claims, the person who is injured must be taken as they are, so even though they have pre-existing conditions which may make them more vulnerable to the effects of injury, the defendant is liable for all the consequences of the injury. This is referred to as the "Egg-Shell Skull" principle of causation.

Condition and Prognosis Report

This is a report dealing with the claimant's current situation and the purpose is to shed light on how the claimant's injury will impact on their prognosis. This will usually require the expert to meet with the claimant and examine them. It is important to be clear that this is not a doctor–patient relationship and should not be treated as a medical consultation. This report is usually obtained pre-action and allows a solicitor to establish if there is any merit in the claim and give an indication of its value. These reports allow a value to be placed on a claim and is based on the claimant's present condition and the medical prognosis.

When preparing a Condition and Prognosis report, it is important to bear in mind the following:

- It is essential to maintain a distinction between injury, symptoms, effects and consequences of the said breach of duty or injury. "Symptoms" is used to refer to the physical/psychological impact of the injury. "Effects" refers to limitations experienced as a result of the injury/symptoms, and "consequences" refers to the restrictions on daily activities since the injury, both current and future, arising from the injury/symptoms/effects. This allows the formulation of the financial claim.
- A detailed examination and the findings from it should be included in the report.
- It helps to use quality of life questionnaires where appropriate.
- The claimant's needs, which are qualitatively or quantitatively different owing to the injury, should be specified.
- The severity and duration of symptoms as a result of the breach of duty should be clearly stated.
- Future treatment requirements, and any ongoing assistance that may be needed should, be included in this report.
- Details of the costs of future treatments should be included. Restrictions on future activities, with its likely impact, should also be covered.
- In the presence of comorbidities, the impact of this should be differentiated from the effect of the negligence.
- A deferment to an appropriate specialist should be made where areas outside one's expertise are raised.

Pitfalls in Report Writing

All relevant documentation should be read in advance of acceptance of instructions. This is to ensure that all conflicts are identified and declared upfront. It is important to be able to demonstrate complete objectivity, which may be lost if the case involves past colleagues, friends or trainees.

Where documentation is missing, this should be requested at the earliest or a reference made to missing records in the report.

As previously mentioned, instructions should only be accepted when a case falls within the remit of the expert's area of clinical practice.

Cases should not be discussed with colleagues and details of the case should be kept completely confidential.

Avoid the temptation to cut and paste from one medical report to another as it calls into question the validity of the report.

A report should never be amended under duress from the instructing solicitors. Opinions should be formed on the basis of the facts available and should be well founded and defensible with evidence and reasoning in court where necessary. Counter arguments should be considered from the start.

Going to Court

When an expert is asked to attend Court to give evidence, it is essential to be familiar with proceedings.

In all cases leading to trial, read the report prepared and any exhibits being used. All other relevant documents should be read in advance as well. Check the time attendance at Court is required and the address relevant to the type of Court. There may be a fair amount of waiting so it is useful to have reading material while waiting.

It is important to address all statements to the decision maker (judge/coroner/district magistrate), even when questioned by the legal representative of the opposing party. It is advisable therefore to stand in the witness box with feet pointing to the judge. It is usual practice to address the decision maker as "Your Honour", "My Lord/My Lady", "Sir/Madam" depending on the court in which the case is being tried.

Witnesses are asked whether they wish to affirm or swear and are given a card from which they read out their oath or affirmation. This will typically state:

Oath: I swear by Almighty God that the evidence I shall give shall be the truth, the whole truth and nothing but the truth.

Affirmation: I do solemnly, sincerely and truly declare and affirm that the evidence I shall give shall be the truth, the whole truth and nothing but the truth.

It is usual in civil proceedings for the expert to give their full name and address, qualifications and relevant expertise as stated in their report.

When in the witness box, it is important to be comfortable and natural when responding. If there are any questions an expert wishes to ask the solicitors, these can be directed to the decision maker, who can then pose the question to the solicitors, thereby reducing the contact and the possibility of disputes with them in Court. When responding to queries by the solicitors, answers should still be addressed to the decision maker.

From the time that the oath/affirmation is taken to the time that the expert leaves the court, they should not speak to the solicitors or anyone else about their evidence. The sequence of questioning is as follows:

i) **Examination in Chief:** The solicitors calling you as a witness will ask questions first. These are non-leading and open-ended questions usually. It is therefore important to be familiar with the evidence and contents of the report, statements, notes and exhibits that have been provided. Usually, the report that has already been served and is the evidence, therefore only a few questions will be asked at this stage.

ii) **Cross Examination:** Is the cross questioning by the other party. At this stage, caution is required, as the solicitors may attempt to undermine the expert's evidence, character or put forward their client's alternative explanation of what happened. At this point, several tactics can be employed to trip up the witness and make them doubt their evidence. If the question being asked is confusing, it is reasonable to ask the judge that Counsel simplify the question.

iii) **Re-examination:** When there are queries arising from the cross-examination, the solicitors who performed the examination in chief may have further points that need clarification. At this stage the Judge too may have questions.

Where there is doubt about the Court proceedings, it is advisable to ask the solicitors prior to the trial.

In all proceedings, experts are given a copy of their report. There are also bundles of relevant documents and all attendees work from identical copies of the hearing bundles which are also available to the expert when in the witness box.

The role of the expert in Court is to assist the Judge in reaching a decision by answering questions truthfully and completely. Explanations may be given where necessary.

Conclusion

Doctors wishing to undertake expert witness work should consider attending courses or some formal training such as those run by Bond Solon [3], which is affiliated to Cardiff University. This will provide training in writing different types of reports, give a better understanding of the legal system and familiarise them with the rules to follow when attending court for trials. Many expert witnesses will obtain advice and experience from colleagues undertaking this work, as well as the instructing solicitors. It is advisable to undertake both defendant and claimant work to avoid bias and to be able to demonstrate a neutral stance if ever required to present evidence in Court. Experts should only undertake work that is within the remit of their practice and expertise, as this provides a solid foundation should their experience ever be called into question in Court. All clinicians undertaking this work should be familiar with the GMC guidance on acting as an expert witness. Established experts will receive regular instructions from solicitors both for the claimant and defendant to provide an opinion as they become recognised as an expert in their respective fields.

Appendix 1: Subheadings for Breach of Duty (Liability) and Causation Report

1. Introduction and Instructions.
2. Factual Background: Review of medical records and chronology of events. This will involve a review of the paginated records to create a timeline.
3. Aspects related to Breach of Duty and Causation: The issues the solicitors wish the expert to discuss will usually be highlighted.
4. Opinion on Breach of Duty and Causation: Based on the review of the medical records and issues of breach of duty, causation is established and the expert opines on the facts available, providing arguments for the viewpoint as well as alternative viewpoints and the reasoning behind these.
5. Summary: Overall conclusions regarding breach of duty and causation.
6. Documents and records reviewed.
7. Statement of Truth/Compliance/Awareness and Conflicts.
8. Expert's CV.
9. Glossary of terms.
10. References.

Appendix: CV; any relevant papers, supporting tools.

Appendix 2: Subheadings for Condition and Prognosis Report

1. Introduction and Instructions.
2. Factual Background: Review of medical records and chronology of events. This will involve a review of the paginated records to create a timeline.
3. Condition: This is based on the examination of the patient and questionnaires being completed. This requires the current problems be established and the association, if any, to the alleged negligence be established.
4. Prognosis: The aims are to comment on the following aspects:

   i) To consider to what extent their current condition is related to the injury/breach of duty.
   ii) To comment on the likely future condition and prognosis including socio-recreational activities/activities of daily living/psychological and general well-being/longevity and ability to obtain gainful employment.
   iii) How will current and future medical problems arising from the injury impact on the patient's ability to care for themselves and carry out everyday tasks both currently and in the future?
   iv) What would the situation have been with alternative treatments?

5. Summary.
6. Documents and records reviewed.
7. Statement of Truth/Compliance/Awareness and Conflicts.
8. Expert's CV.
9. Glossary of terms.
10. References.

Appendix: CV; any relevant questionnaires used to assess the patient; any investigations performed as part of the patient review.

References

1. www.gmc-uk.org/ethical-guidance/ethical-guidance-for-doctors/acting-as-a-witness/acting-as-a-witness-in-legal-proceedings

2. www.justice.gov.uk/courts/procedure-rules/civil/rules/part35

3. www.bondsolon.com/expert-witness/courses/

Consent: Legal and Clinical Implications

James Badenoch

CASE COMMENTARY

Swati Jha

Successful Claim

Montgomery v Lanarkshire Health Board [20115] UKSC 11

The Claim

Mrs Montgomery was booked for consultant-led care antenatally as she was a type 1 diabetic. She brought a claim for damages for severe injuries suffered by her child as a result of his problematic delivery following shoulder dystocia. She alleged inter alia negligent failure to disclose the risks of dystocia, or to explain or offer the option of elective C-S to avoid it, that this failure vitiated her consent to induction of labour, and that if adequately informed, she would have chosen C-S and her child would have been born unharmed.

The Summary

This was Mrs Montgomery's first pregnancy. She worked for a pharmaceutical company as a hospital specialist. She was of small stature (just over five feet) and a type 1 diabetic. Her pregnancy was therefore classed as high risk, requiring increased monitoring in the antenatal period and during labour. Diabetes carries increased risk of particularly large [macrosomic] fetuses, with increased concentration of weight around the shoulders, and so of dystocia during vaginal birth, albeit usually mild and quite easily manageable. Frequent serial ultrasound measurements provided clear evidence of fetal macrosomia and the baby, when eventually delivered, weighed 4.25 kg (9 lbs 6 oz). The risk of shoulder dystocia of any grade is 9–10% in a diabetic woman, and if it occurs, extraction may prove difficult. Resultant delay in delivery can result in asphyxial brain damage and even death of the fetus. The risk of such an outcome is less than 0.1%, though which dystocia cases will end in serious injury cannot be predicted.

Mrs Montgomery became naturally very anxious about her ability to safely deliver vaginally, and questioned it with the obstetrician more than once, but was given no information at all about the known risks of dystocia in her case, or about avoiding it by elective C-S. It was in total ignorance therefore that she consented, or more accurately submitted, to the effective imposition upon her, without any choice, of induction with prostaglandin.

During her delivery there was significant shoulder dystocia, with the need to perform a range of manoeuvres and a 12-minute delay before delivery was completed. In the process the baby sustained an Erb's palsy and asphyxial brain damage which caused dyskinetic cerebral palsy affecting all four limbs.

Crucial to the issue of "consent" were admissions and assertions made by the obstetrician in charge. She said that she deliberately chose not to disclose the risk of shoulder dystocia in labour; not to discuss elective C-S as an option; to end serial ultrasound measurements before the due date (to conceal their likely trajectory *"so as not to alarm her more"*); and to *"reassure her"* that if there were problems in labour they could go to C-S (without explaining that if shoulder dystocia occurred that would be impossible). She justified her silence about risks and elective C-S on the grounds that the mother would have chosen it if offered, but C-S was in her opinion *"not in the maternal interest"*. Perhaps surprisingly, she also maintained that *"shoulder dystocia is often overcome without the mother being aware of it."*

The Judgement

The case was tried initially in the courts of Scotland. It was defended by reliance on evidence from obstetric expert witnesses that they approved the withholding of all relevant information from this mother in the given circumstances. That meant, so it was contended, that her purported consent to induction and the pursuit of vaginal delivery (on the admitted facts in total ignorance and with no other choice) was legally valid, because those witnesses represented a responsible body whose approval established a cast-iron *Bolam* defence against the charge of inadequate disclosure. [For discussion of *Bolam*, see below].

The Scottish trial judge ruled that the *Bolam* test applied to the adequacy of disclosure for consent, and that in light of professional approval in this case it was not negligent to withhold all relevant information from the mother. He held also (precisely contrary to the evidence of all the witnesses on both sides of the case) that if she had been offered elective C-S she would have refused it. The *Bolam* defence succeeded, the mother's entirely uninformed purported consent to induction of labour was held valid, and the claim was dismissed. On her appeal in Scotland the three Appeal Court judges endorsed and upheld the Trial judge's decision in every particular, asserting inter alia that: *"too much in the way of information ... may only serve to confuse or alarm the patient, and it is therefore very much a question for the experienced practitioner to decide, in accordance with normal and proper practice, where the line should be drawn in a given case"*. The case then came on its final appeal to the Supreme Court in London.

The seven Supreme Court Justices unanimously reversed and overruled the decisions of the Scottish courts in a judgement which radically corrected and restated the law of disclosure for consent as it had hitherto (wrongly) been said to be. In their ruling, which now governs the practice of all healthcare professionals, they removed the *Bolam* test altogether as the yardstick of adequate disclosure, because *"it is the right of the patient to decide whether or not to submit to treatment recommended by the doctor, and even to make an unbalanced and irrational judgment."* They recognised *"the imbalance between the knowledge and objectivity of the doctor and the ignorance and subjectivity of the patient,"* and said it was illogical that a patient should have to make the decision based on information *"known to the doctor but not to the patient."* They held that the doctor's duty in law is to explain the treatment proposed, and any alternatives (including refusing treatment altogether which is the patient's absolute right), and the potential benefits, risks, burdens and side effects of each choice. Doctors may recommend one option over another, but it is for the patient to weigh these up. The duty is thus to ensure that a patient is aware of "all material risks" inherent in a procedure, and the legal definition of "material" in this context was set out in the judgement [see Legal and Clinical Commentary below]. The overarching principles which informed the decision were (a) that it is the patient's right to decide what, if any, risks they are willing to take, and (b) that consent is not the doctor's but the patient's decision to make, as a matter of free and genuine choice.

By these correct legal principles, the obstetrician should have advised Mrs Montgomery of the substantial risk of shoulder dystocia if vaginal delivery was pursued and discussed with her the option of C-S to avoid the risk altogether. With adequate information she would, if given that option, have accepted it and her child would have been delivered unharmed. The claim was therefore upheld.

Unsuccessful Claim

A v East Kent Hospitals University NHS Foundation Trust [2015] EWHC 1038

The Claim

Mrs A delivered a baby suffering from an unbalanced chromosome 4 and 11 translocation, resulting in severe disabilities to the child. It was alleged that when she saw the consultant obstetricians at 32 and 35 weeks of gestation and was found to have asymmetric intrauterine growth restriction, the material risk of a chromosomal abnormality should have been considered and she should therefore have been offered further testing with an amniocentesis. This would have identified the chromosomal abnormality and Mrs A would have opted for a termination of the pregnancy at 32 or 35 weeks. Mrs A claimed that the failure to offer and perform further testing had therefore caused the birth of a severely disabled child, and sought damages for the extra cost burden which care for such a child imposed.

The Summary

Mrs A conceived following the second round of ICSI in 2009. Previous tests had shown that the morphology of some of the Mr A's sperm was poor, though the count was normal. Mrs A had suffered an earlier miscarriage and failed ICSI the first time, so Mr A had DNA fragmentation tests which ruled out the common aneuploidies.

At the start of the trial, Mrs A sought an anonymity order to protect the child's sensitivities if she became aware of her parents' attitude to her birth, and the judge directed that the names of claimant and child should not be revealed.

Mrs A had a normal dating and anomaly scan, and nuchal translucency and biochemistry both demonstrated only a "background" risk of chromosomal abnormality, less than 1 in 1,000. Mrs A wished not to have a disabled child, but the judge found that she had at that time considered that level of risk acceptable.

During pregnancy it was noted that there was evidence of a constitutionally small fetus, with growth on the fifth centile, tailing off at 32 weeks. RCOG Guideline No.31 in place in November 2002 stated: *"When a small fetus is diagnosed, assess for risk of chromosomal defects,"* and reported that *"up to 19% of fetuses with an AC and EFW less than the fifth centile may have chromosomal defects ... Therefore, all growth-restricted fetuses need an ultrasound anatomical survey as a minimum. It may also be appropriate to offer karyotyping".* There was no evidence of anatomical abnormality on the scans, which meant only that "background risk" of chromosomal defects which the judge held did not mandate chromosome analysis. The pregnancy was extensively monitored with CTH, Dopplers and scans, and in light of the diagnosis of placental insufficiency and IUGR, preparations were made for premature delivery, with steroids administered.

The Judgement

On several grounds, the material risk of a chromosomal abnormality presenting at 32 or 35 weeks was held to have been prospectively small. Mrs A carried the pregnancy to term, which is unusual in babies with chromosomal abnormalities; the nuchal translucency (NT) and biochemistry in early pregnancy were normal; and the USS showed no abnormality. The risks in question were *"negligible, theoretical, or background"* according to the judge, and so were not *"material"* within the *Montgomery* definition. It followed that they did not have to be disclosed, and that there had been no sufficient reason to offer amniocentesis. The judge further held that because the risks of chromosomal abnormality were at or below the level of risk Mrs A had previously been willing to accept, she would probably not have wanted amniocentesis if it had been offered, and also that it was questionable whether Mrs A would have accepted a termination at such a late stage of the pregnancy in any event.

The case was dismissed.

Legal and Clinical Commentary

James Badenoch

The case of *Montgomery v Lanarkshire Health Board* is of the very greatest importance for all healthcare professionals. This is because in it the Supreme Court laid down binding legal principles which now define and govern the type and the extent of the information which must be disclosed to patients from whom, in whatever area of practice, consent to treatment is sought. It is a major legal landmark ruling in which the Court did more than decide a specific issue of alleged obstetric negligence; it significantly redefined the doctor–patient relationship.

The principles expressed in the judgement reflect and give effect to the twin imperatives of respect for patients as autonomous human beings, and for their consequent absolute right to make a free and unfettered (and so real) choice whether to consent or not. This was long ago expressed by the American Justice Cardozo in the case of *Schloendorff v Society of New York Hospital*, in 1913, in these famous words:

> *Every human being of adult years and sound mind has the right to determine what shall be done with his own body. . . .*

The legal requirements for valid patient consent, as now redefined, are of such great importance, not least because by the law of the United Kingdom, any interference with the body of another, even where part of otherwise legitimate medical treatment, is unlawful if done without that other's true consent – indeed is in strict law an assault, though nowadays characterised as negligence unless done with criminal intent. It follows that a patient injured by a bad outcome of treatment which was in clinical terms properly given will win a claim for damages if they prove two things: first that their consent to it was nullified by negligent failure to make adequate disclosure of the legally required information, and second that if sufficiently informed, they would have refused to consent to it and so would have avoided its harmful effects.

For these reasons, it is vital for clinicians to know the nature and extent of the information they must provide about a proposed treatment to ensure that consent to it is legally valid. That is the question which the Supreme Court in *Montgomery* has authoritatively answered – in a decision which overruled existing legal precedent and radically restated the relevant law. Discussed below will be: (a) the special features of consent in maternity care; (b) the legal background to the *Montgomery* decision; (c) examination of the facts and litigation history of Mrs Montgomery's case; and (d) the decision in *A v East Kent*. At the end are presented guides to the *Montgomery* law of consent and to its application in practice which are based on the Montgomery decision itself, and also on the way the courts have interpreted and applied it since. Here is first set out the *Montgomery* definition of the information which must in every case be disclosed to patients about any proposed clinical procedure, without which the consent will be invalid.

The Montgomery Test of Information Disclosure Required for Valid Consent

Did the doctor take reasonable care to ensure that the patient was made aware, before consenting, of any material risks, and of any reasonable alternative or variant treatments?

The legal test of the materiality of risks is:

Whether in the circumstances of the particular case, *a reasonable person in the patient's position* would be likely to attach significance to the risk? (an objective test); OR

the doctor is or should reasonably be aware that *the particular patient* would be likely to attach significance to it (a subjective test).

To this duty there are a few closely confined exceptions, namely:

(i)   The so-called *"therapeutic privilege"*, by which the doctor may withhold or limit information if he believes on reasonable grounds that disclosure will harm the patient's health (physical or mental).

(ii) Cases of necessity, e.g. when treatment is essential but the patient is unconscious or otherwise incapable of understanding.

(iii) Presumably also [though not covered by *Montgomery*] where an adult patient of sound mind has expressed a considered and determined wish not to be told about risks or about uncertainty of outcome.

Consent in Maternity Care: Special Features and Clinical Considerations

Consent in maternity care can present problems unusual in other fields, and also opportunities which are elsewhere generally lacking. These special features stem from the fact that pregnancy is not an illness and is relatively seldom complicated by serious abnormality. The role of professionals is most commonly therefore not to treat, but rather to monitor and supervise a normal process, by helping and guiding the mother in a task which is essentially hers and not theirs to accomplish, the delivery of her baby.

Other clinicians, by contrast, deal constantly with the diagnosis and treatment of disease, in patients who are largely passive recipients of their ministrations and have no active role to play. These are differences which can significantly affect the consenting process.

Maternity care, with or without complications, does of course necessarily involve a variety of physical interventions to which the mothers' attendants will or may have to subject them, some uncomfortable or painful, and some requiring quite major interference with their bodily integrity. Among them are abdominal palpation, vaginal examination, methods of monitoring, changes of position, cervical sweep, rupture of membranes, manual manipulation, drugs to initiate or to augment labour and for pain relief, episiotomy, delivery by ventouse, forceps or Caesarean Section [C-S]. All require consent, which depending on the circumstances may be easier, can become more complicated, and is often more nuanced, than it is in other fields of clinical practice.

On the one hand, the long lead-in time, sequential ante-natal visits, and presentation in early labour afford more opportunities than in other fields to inform mothers about interventions which will or may become necessary, and to do so in advance when they are calm, unhurried and unaffected by the exertions, pains and psychological stresses which accompany normal labour and most emergencies. Ideally, this allows time to weigh up risks and benefits, to think things through, and to make reasoned, informed and so true choices about what they are willing to agree to in the given event. On the other hand, if those opportunities are not available or taken, or when an unforeseen emergency occurs, a mother may be asked urgently to consider vital, sometimes complex, information, and to make a rational decision about consenting, while in the throes of labour or panicked by a sudden frightening situation. In such a case, her capacity for considered and reasoned decision-making may be substantially reduced by the over-whelming physiological imperatives of childbirth, or by the distractions of pain, alarm and fear.

As for the nuances, there is here a delicate balance to be struck in respect of the (ideal) provision of information to mothers in advance of events, and the desire not to burden them with concern and apprehension about abnormalities and emergencies which are unlikely in the given case and will probably not have to be faced. Professionals must be mindful of this tension, which is not easy to resolve, and must decide with each mother whether there is a particular need now to address unhappy possibilities, and to assess her ability to cope psychologically with their anticipation. These points were all of particular relevance in Mrs Montgomery's case, in which there were pressing reasons to address potential risks with her in advance, and ample opportunities to do so, which were not taken. The facts in her case are instructive, and will be examined below, but a look first at what had previously been thought to be the law will serve to illustrate and explain the changes made by the decision of the Supreme Court, and their significance for healthcare professionals.

The Law of Consent before *Montgomery*: *Bolam*

Before *Montgomery*, much trouble had resulted from a tendency in some quarters to see consent as an inconvenient formality to be got out of the way ("just sign here"), but more especially from the effects of the long-standing and hitherto binding precedent of the case of *Sidaway v Board of Governors of Bethlem Royal Hospital* [1985] 871 AC, which had established the supposed principle which *Montgomery* finally removed and replaced. The Law Lords (now called Supreme Court Justices) had ruled in *Sidaway* that there must be applied to every aspect of clinical practice, including adequacy of information disclosure, the so-called *"Bolam test"* of the clinician's standard of care, named for the case in which it was first propounded, namely *Bolam v Friern Hospital Management Committee* [1957]. By this test, no matter how little or how much information about risk, benefit or likely outcome a clinician might have chosen to provide, and regardless of what the patient themselves might have wanted to know, their consent would be held incontrovertibly valid in law – provided only that a responsible body of professional opinion could be found to approve and support the disclosure in fact made. The profession was thereby effectively made judge in its own cause.

In *Sidaway*, the expression and approval even of the most extreme end of the spectrum of views among clinicians was found in the assertion made by Lord Diplock in his judgement that:

> The only effect the mention of risk can have on the patient's mind, if it has any at all, can be in the direction of deterring the patient from undergoing the treatment which in the expert opinion of the doctor it is in the patient's interest to undergo.

That was a proposition from a judge of the old school, which most clinicians would nowadays find insupportable. It reflected a condescending and patronising approach which assumes in the patient a lack of capacity for rational and independent thought, and expects unquestioning subservience to the doctor's superior status and abject surrender of personal autonomy – although astonishingly not if the patient happened to be Lord Diplock himself or one of his kind, as he made clear in a separate passage in that judgement in which he said:

> But when it comes to warning about risks, the kind of training and experience the Judge will have undergone at the Bar makes it natural for him to say (correctly) it is my right to decide whether any particular thing is done to my body, and I want to be fully informed of any risks there may be involved of which I am not already aware from my general knowledge as a highly educated man of experience, so that I may form my own judgment as to whether to refuse the advised treatment or not.

The exception to the rule which the judge thus unashamedly made for his own kind exposed the nowadays unacceptable disdain for popular intelligence which underpinned the judicial application of *Bolam* to disclosure for consent. It was a disdain which derived from the belief that patients can be divided into two distinct and very different categories, one being an elite group for whom it is obviously the wrong test because they are capable of independent thought and reasoned decision-making, and the other comprising the rest of the population for whom it is the right test, because they all supposedly lack the capacity to make up their own minds about their priorities and the degree of risk they are willing to accept. The existence of one law for the judge and his kind and another for everyone else went surprisingly unchallenged and unremarked over the many years before *Montgomery* came to the Supreme Court, throughout which time the *Bolam* principle in this context prevailed.

The Need and Rationale for Change

The problem of *Sidaway* for aggrieved patients was that a purportedly responsible body of practitioners could in the past quite easily be found professing to sanction even the most limited disclosure of information about risks, benefits and prospects of treatments. Given the wide variety of idiosyncratic views which certainly used to exist among clinicians about what was right or necessary to tell patients, such approval was offered for almost any withholding or rationing of information, however important it might have been to patients themselves to know more when deciding whether to consent. Crucially, the approval of such a body was as a matter of law conclusive of the issue, no matter how small a minority it represented, and however strongly the majority would disagree with them.

The profession was thus by the imposition of *Bolam* made judge in its own cause in respect of information disclosure for consent, and the judges were effectively disqualified from performing their normal judicial function of deciding in disputed cases which of the opposing contentions have the greater merit and which should be rejected. And yet, while it may be one thing in logic to make professional approval decisive where negligent diagnosis or treatment is alleged (which are the practitioners' decisions based on their specialised learning), it is quite another to apply it to allegedly inadequate disclosure of information on which the patient is asked to consent (which is the patient's own decision to make based on their personal priorities and attitude to the risks and benefits). That important distinction proved decisive in *Montgomery* when *Sidaway's* application of the *Bolam* test to consent was challenged and finally overthrown. But until then, the dominance of *Bolam* as the governing law of patient consent persisted, despite the fact that minority professional approval sometimes, when viewed objectively, seriously distorted justice, and notwithstanding that its acceptance as decisive sometimes required extreme intellectual gymnastics from judges faced with objectively illogical defence "expert" positions.

The Supreme Court Decision: Its Justification and Effects

The decision of the Supreme Court in *Montgomery*, following the lead of judges in other countries, now belatedly reflects the major changes which have occurred in modern times in societal norms and in public attitudes to the doctor–patient relationship. The *Bolam test* is removed altogether from the question of the validity of consent and is replaced by what is often called the *"patient-centred test"* set out at the beginning of this chapter. This logically defines the legal obligation of disclosure for consent entirely from the point of view of the patient – whose sole decision it is to consent or not, and so on whose entirely personal preferences, priorities and attitudes that choice must be based. That this change was just and necessary is well illustrated by the facts of Mrs Montgomery's case, summarised at the head of this chapter. She had induction imposed upon her in total ignorance of its implications, and so without any real choice in the matter. Her case was that, if adequately informed, she would not have consented to it, and would have opted instead for elective C-S.

The Supreme Court ruled that the risks of dystocia and the means of avoiding them by elective C-S should have been disclosed to her as a matter of legal principle, because that information would have been "material" to her independent personal choice whether to consent to induction and pursuit of labour. "Material" in this context means, put simply, *the facts which a reasonable patient in her situation would be expected to consider significant and relevant to her decision*, without which her purported consent to proposed treatment is nullified. To put it another way, the question on the answer to which the validity of consent will now depend is essentially: *What is it that my patient would reasonably want and need to know about the proposed treatment before deciding to accept or to refuse it?* Choice without that information is no true choice at all, and by *Montgomery*, a clinician's failure to provide it will be held negligent, the purported consent invalid, and the treatment administered in reliance on it unlawful.

The decision of the Supreme Court Justices went further. They reversed the trial judge's "finding of fact" that if offered C-S the mother would have refused it, because it was a finding contrary to all the evidence in the case – quite apart from offending common sense and logic. Appellate courts do not often reverse findings of fact made by trial judges because they alone see and hear the witnesses in person, and so are best placed to assess their evidence. The reversal here meant that legal causation was established. If adequately informed, as the law required, this intelligent and rightly anxious mother would have opted for C-S, and her healthy full-term baby would have been spared his serious and thereby avoidable injuries. It followed that the negligent withholding of material information had been the cause of those injuries, for which he was entitled to damages (which have subsequently been paid in a sum agreed between the parties).

United Kingdom Consent Law Is Now Aligned with that of Other Jurisdictions

The principle which has thus been established belatedly reflects in United Kingdom law the modern ideas of the rights and the autonomy of the adult, which had long since been accepted and endorsed in the courts of the United States, Canada and Australia. Indeed, in *Montgomery*, the following passages from judgements in those countries were influential, and clearly illustrate the reasoning of the Supreme Court Justices in *Montgomery*, who cited them with approval in their decision:

From the American case of *Canterbury v Spence* in 1964:

> *Respect for the patient's right of self-determination on particular therapy demands a standard set by law for physicians, rather than one which physicians may or may not impose upon themselves.*

From the Canadian judgement in *Reibl v Hughes* in 1980:

> *Expert medical evidence is, of course, relevant to findings as to the risks that reside in or are a result of recommended surgery or other treatment. It will also have a bearing on their materiality, but this is not a question that is to be concluded on the basis of the expert medical evidence alone. The issue under consideration is a different issue from that involved where the question is whether the doctor carried out his professional activities by applicable professional standards. What is under consideration here is the patient's right to know what risks are involved in undergoing or foregoing certain surgery or other treatment.*

And from the Australian case of *Rogers v Whittaker* in 1993:

> *The choice [to consent] is in reality meaningless unless it is made on the basis of relevant information and advice. Because the choice to be made calls for a decision by the patient on information known to the medical practitioner but not to the patient, it will be illogical to hold*

that the amount of information to be provided by the medical practitioner can be determined from the prospective of the practitioner alone or, for that matter, of the medical profession.

So, while professional approval is still, for the time being at least, the test by which the courts will judge the standard of clinicians' diagnosis and treatment decisions, *Montgomery* has radically restated the law of patient consent in the United Kingdom by removing the *Bolam* as the test of the adequacy of disclosure for consent, and since it was a decision of the Supreme Court, it is binding on all judges in every case. How the courts can be expected to interpret and apply the new *"patient-centred test"* has emerged gradually from the cases on disputed consent issues which have followed *Montgomery*, and the key findings in those cases are the basis for the practical guidance for clinicians offered at the end of this chapter, in particular those which have the precedent-establishing authority of the Court of Appeal.

It is important to note, however, that individual findings made by judges at lower levels must be approached with a degree of caution. In the case of *A v East Kent Hospitals Trust*, for example, which is summarised at the head of this chapter, the judge held that a less than 1:1000 risk of chromosomal abnormality, viewed prospectively, was no more than *"theoretical"*, *"negligible"* or *"background."* Such a risk, said the judge, was not *"material"* per Montgomery, and its non-disclosure to the expectant mother was accordingly not (on the particular facts of her case) negligent, though the judge observed that for a risk of 1–3% his ruling would have been different. Caution is required here because, by the authority of *Montgomery*, percentages of risk are not in and of themselves decisive of materiality, though they may quite often be so. Each case is fact-sensitive, which means in different circumstances, with a different individual patient, a similarly small risk will not necessarily be held to have been negligible and non-material.

The Importance of Legal Causation and Its Comfort for Practitioners

It is important to always bear in mind, when these issues arise, that a patient who proves (a) negligent failure of adequate disclosure about a proposed intervention to which they consented, and (b) that its outcome caused themharm, will not succeed in a damages claim unless theycan also prove (c) that if they had been correctly informed they would have refused to consent to it and so avoided the harm. That is the hurdle of "legal causation". It is a hurdle which can be very difficult for aggrieved patients to surmount, as decided cases show, because the issue is judged prospectively, by reference to the patient's likely views at the time the treatment was proposed (when by definition they needed and wanted professional help), and not from the standpoint of sad hindsight after things have turned out badly.

For in normal circumstances, clinical interventions are reasonably expected, at the time they are proposed, to be both safe and effective and are offered for that reason, (leaving aside wrongly chosen or badly administered treatments for which there is a separate remedy in law). There is accordingly a *prima facie* presumption that they would prospectively, before their bad outcome was known, have been consented to. Proof of legal causation of the harm suffered in such cases often therefore requires extraneous corroborative evidence of attitudes held or previous experiences which were likely to have influenced the patient when their consent was sought and caused them to refuse it.

There are, for example, decided cases of mothers of babies damaged in labour, who prove negligent information disclosure and denial of the option of C-S, and succeed also in proving (where disputed) that they would have chosen C-S if offered it by demonstrating a history of unhappy experiences or bad outcomes in their own or in some instances close relatives' previous confinements.

Conclusion

This chapter concludes with a tabulation of the central principles of the *Montgomery* law of consent, followed by a practical guide for clinicians to the way they should be applied. The responsibility for these is the author's, and they do not of themselves have the force of law, but they are expected to be reliable. The first presents an account of the law as restated by the Supreme Court Justices, mainly taken directly from the wording of their judgements. The second offers practical guidelines for professionals on the consenting process and how to get it right, based on the *Montgomery* principles and the way the courts have applied them in subsequent cases (and so can be expected broadly to apply them in future). At first sight, these may appear difficult and demanding of time and thought, but it is hoped that such perceived difficulties will diminish with familiarity. Experience suggests that applying them correctly in practice does quite quickly become second nature for professionals, if it is not already, with the recognition that their requirements are founded on common sense and a sensitive appreciation of the expectations and rights of their patients.

A Guide to the Law of Consent Following *Montgomery*

1. **The doctor's duty of disclosure** by which to ensure valid patient consent is **to take reasonable care to ensure that the patient is aware of any material risk of proposed treatment** (whether in respect of outcome or of potentially intervening complication), **and of any reasonable alternative or variant treatments**. This is a *legal test*, which means that conformity or otherwise with this duty will in disputed cases be judged by the courts and not by the professions, though expert evidence from professionals will always be relevant, often persuasive and sometimes conclusive.

2. **A material risk is now defined in law as**: (a) a risk that *a reasonable person* in the patient's position would be likely to attach significance to; OR (b) a risk that the doctor is or should reasonably be aware that *the particular patient* would be likely to attach significance to.

3. **The assessment of materiality** of risk is fact sensitive. Statistics/percentages of risk are relevant, but not necessarily decisive.

4. **A small risk of serious harm** may be expected to be of significance to most patients, and particularly significant to a patient undergoing minor, and/or non-urgent, avoidable, or purely cosmetic treatment.

5. By contrast, **a relatively large risk of very minor harm** would not be expected to weigh heavily or at all in the minds of patients, especially when the proposed treatment was vital or strongly indicated.

6. **A risk, however remote**, may be of particular significance to a patient whose life or livelihood would be especially adversely affected if the risk materialised, e.g. threat to fertility for a childless young woman, or risk of damage to the voice of a singer or the finger of a concert pianist.

7. **The purely "mechanical" approach**, (getting the patient to read and sign a pro-forma consent form, without explanation) of itself proves only that the patient can write his/her own name. That will not suffice save possibly for the most simple and minor routine procedures.

8. There must be **genuine dialogue** between doctor and patient in every case save those where:

   (a) the patient is a young [non-Gillick competent] child or mentally incapacitated (e.g. because of unconsciousness or intoxication) and therefore judged reasonably to be incapable of understanding; or

   (b) the patient is so endangered by his condition that urgent need for immediate treatment allows no safe opportunity (**the "emergency proviso"**).

9. In the case of **a patient** who is **a young [non-Gillick competent] child or who is unconscious or otherwise judged incapacitated** by reason of some impairment or disturbance in the mind or brain, the dialogue must take place where possible and time allows with a parent (for a child) or lasting power of attorney/deputy for personal welfare (for adults). Alternatively, those close to the adult patient (family/friends) must be consulted for the doctor to make a best interests decision (s4 Mental Capacity Act 2005). In any such case, and in particular the emergency, the facts and the doctor's reasoning should be carefully recorded. If a patient is incapacitated, any advance decision to refuse treatment (ss24–26 Mental Capacity Act 2005) must be respected if valid and applicable to the circumstances.

10. Genuine **dialogue** about risk requires the doctor:

    (a) to use understandable language and check it is understood;

    (b) to avoid excessively detailed information – keep it simple;

    (c) so far as possible to avoid technical jargon;

    (d) to tailor the discussion to the individual patient.

11. The **"therapeutic exception"** will in rare cases allow a doctor to avoid disclosure if he decides on reasoned and carefully noted grounds that the patient is so psychologically fragile or otherwise vulnerable that disclosure would present a real threat to the patient's mental health or stability.

12. **Sensitive and frank disclosure in advance** of risks and benefits, including acknowledgement of any real uncertainty of a successful outcome, may be expected to engender less anger and recrimination in the patient if things do not turn out well.

13. **Information which displaces ignorance** will (as the GMC have asserted and the Supreme Court agreed) make it less likely that the patient will have recourse to lawyers in the belief that a bad outcome must be the result of bad performance, and this should ultimately reduce litigation.

A Practical Guide to the Consenting Process

1. The steps the practitioner must take, following Montgomery, can be summarised as follows:

   (i) First **identify the risks of the proposed treatment** about which a reasonable patient in this patient's position would need and want to know [**the objective test**], and disclose accordingly, explaining the balance of those risks with the expected benefits of what is proposed and the likely prospects if untreated.

(ii) Next **consider the particular patient's individual characteristics and situation in life**, e.g. age, intellectual ability, nature and demands of employment, family and other responsibilities, social and other problems etc., and having done that:

(iii) **Personalise the issues** so as to identify what this patient, with his/her personal characteristics and situation, would reasonably need and want to know [**the subjective test**] and adapt the disclosure accordingly. Patients are not "standard issue".

(iv) Next **identify any reasonably available and potentially effective alternative treatments/procedures**, describe them and their relative risks and benefits (explaining if wished why they are not the doctor's first choice).

(v) **Explain** the patient's **absolute right to choose** between alternatives, and to refuse treatment altogether, detailing the risks of that choice.

2. **The required extent of disclosure is *reasonable* not exhaustive**. Accordingly, the recitation of a catalogue of risks of very minor and/or transient side-effects (such as is found in the small print of drug data sheets) will not be required and should generally be avoided altogether. Reasonableness is the key, and the courts can be expected to apply the test of reasonableness in all cases. Common sense should prevail.

3. **Personnel:** The person who advises/prescribes/carries out the treatment should whenever practicable provide the information and obtain the consent. It may sometimes be reasonable to delegate this, but only to one sufficiently informed and trained for the task.

4. **Communicating with patients:** A doctor who is not good at communication, whether because inexpert or unwilling, must recognise the fact and take steps to acquire the necessary skills.

5. **Lack of time** for adequate dialogue with the patient may seem an ever-present or insuperable obstacle. It must be overcome, because what is at issue is the patient's most basic and fundamental right to make a true and free choice, which requires adequate information, whether to submit or not to proposed treatment, or which of alternatives to choose.

6. **The "recusant" patient**: If a patient of adult years and with mental capacity adamantly insists on not being told about the benefits and risks, and the prospects or uncertainties of outcome, the doctor:

(i) Should first decide whether there is nevertheless a compelling need to disclose a risk (e.g. a recognised complication which would result in very serious harm), the withholding of which could vitiate consent.

(ii) May, absent such a compelling need, accept the patient's wish not to be told, and limit disclosure accordingly, but should in either case make a careful note of the matter.

7. **The doctor's own position**: If asked directly by the patient what choice he would make for himself or e.g. for his child, the doctor may answer truthfully, but with words carefully chosen to avoid exerting or appearing to exert undue pressure, such as: *"It is entirely a matter for you. You and I are quite different people, but I would choose, and I would want my loved ones to choose, to undergo this treatment"*.

8. **Findings from screening tests and other investigations** may be distressing, and may have grave implications, e.g. mandating abandonment or alteration of planned

treatment, to which consent is required afresh. Disclosure will require tact and sensitivity, and withholding under the "therapeutic exception" may need to be considered (see the Guide to the law).

9. **When test results require patient choices**, e.g. to cease or to pursue or to alter treatment, or to terminate or to continue a pregnancy, even-handed information about the implications and effects of each available choice should be provided, so allowing to the patient the freedom to make a genuine choice between the options without partiality, pressure or persuasion from the practitioner.

10. **Pre-prepared leaflets, and/or illustrative diagrams or CDs** are useful, especially where the material information is substantial or complex (e.g. for open heart surgery), with patients asked to acknowledge by signature that they have read or watched them. It is also helpful to patients and staff to prepare and offer explanatory material about common procedures and treatments, even those which are minor or mundane.

11. **A note should always be made of the consenting process**, when possible, at the time or shortly thereafter. In difficult or unusual cases, the disclosure made and the reasoning for it, as well as the patient's response, should be recorded in particular detail.

Chapter 5

Prenatal Diagnosis, Screening and Wrongful Birth

David Howe

CASE COMMENTARY

Swati Jha

Successful Claim

Mordel v Royal Berkshire NHS Foundation Trust [2019] EWHC 2591 (QB)

The Claim

The claimant had a baby with Down's syndrome in her first pregnancy. It was stated by the claimant that two opportunities to carry out screening for Down's syndrome were missed, and that had this been offered and detected the underlying abnormality, it would have led to a termination of the pregnancy.

The Summary

Down's syndrome is one of the commonest chromosomal abnormalities and it is routine to offer all women screening for this abnormality. In the first trimester this is by an ultrasound scan of the fetal neck area in conjunction with a blood serum test of the mother (combined test). Combining the results gives a statistical risk which if more than 1:150 is considered high risk and is an indication for more invasive diagnostic testing. In the second trimester, screening is usually only offered if this has not already been done in the first trimester and involves a blood test (quadruple test). Invasive tests carry a risk of miscarriage. In this particular case, at the time of booking the visit at the GP surgery, the claimant accepted all the screening tests. When she attended for her dating scan however, the sonographer ticked the box indicating 'Down's screening declined'. When the patient subsequently attended for her second trimester anomaly scan, given she had not had the combined test, the patient should have been offered the quadruple test.

The Judgement

It was ruled that when offering the combined test, it was the sonographer's duty to satisfy themself that the patient was consenting to the procedure. This required (i) checking that there had been a discussion between the patient and midwife, (ii) checking that the patient had been supplied with the NHS booklet and (iii) ascertaining by brief questioning that the patient understood the essential elements and purposes of screening for Down's syndrome. Merely ticking a box limited to recording the patient's decision of acceptance or declination of the Down's screening was inadequate.

Additionally, in women who had not received the combined test, it was substandard to fail to offer the quadruple test when the claimant attended in the second trimester. As a consequence, two opportunities for prenatal diagnosis were missed.

It was also accepted that on balance, had the claimant been given a high risk of Down's syndrome, she would have undergone invasive screening and proceeded to a termination.

The judgement was for the claimant.

Unsuccessful Claim

Lindsey Shaw v South Tees [2019] EWHC 2280 (QB)

The Claim

The claimant had a baby diagnosed with a rare genetic disorder called Aicardi syndrome which is characterised by agenesis of the corpus collosum (ACC) which connects the two halves of the brain. The presence of the cavum septum pellucidum (CSP) rules out an ACC. As a result of this syndrome the child born to the claimant suffered microcephaly, severe learning difficulties, visual abnormalities and seizures. It was claimed that if this had been detected at the time of the anomaly scan, the claimant would have terminated the pregnancy and failure to do so was substandard. As a consequence, the costs of bringing up a child with such severe disabilities would be significantly more than those required for a healthy child.

The Summary

This was the claimant's third pregnancy and she was 27 years old at the time. She had a termination in her first due to fetal anomaly followed by a birth of a healthy baby. Her BMI was raised at 36. In the index pregnancy, the claimant underwent dating scans at 7 and 13 weeks. Due to her history of past fetal abnormality, she was scheduled for an additional scan at 16 weeks which was undertaken at 17+6 weeks due to her obesity to allow for greater clarity of the images. At this scan it was stated that the head, brain, spine, neck, skin and other structures had been visualised and appeared normal. No attempt was made to visualise the CSP as it is not sufficiently formed at this stage. This was followed by an anomaly scan at 21+6 weeks gestation. The standards considered reasonable for an anomaly scan had been identified in guidance issued in 2010 (Fetal Anomaly Screening Programme) to ensure an agreed level of quality. The relevant standard in this guideline was standard 6, which identifies which anatomical structures should be assessed during the anomaly scan. The standard stipulates that where the image quality is impeded by raised BMI (or other factors) a further single scan should be offered at 23 weeks. However, women also need to appreciate that the scan is a screening test and has limitations. At the anomaly scan, the biparietal diameter, the occipitofrontal diameter, the head circumference, the posterior ventricle, the transcerebellar diameter, the cisterna magna, the nuchal fold, the abdominal circumference and the femur length were recorded. It was not recorded that the CSP had been seen, but noted that all the brain measurements and signs were normal. The report went on to state, "The following were visualised and appear normal: head, brain, spine, neck and skin, chest, abdominal wall, gastro-intestinal tract, kidneys and bladder, extremities, skeleton".

It was admitted that had the CSP been detected on the anomaly scan at 21 weeks, the claimant would have been referred for further investigations in the form of an MRI allowing the diagnosis to be made antenatally. Hence the test of negligence came down to whether reasonable care and skill had been used when carrying out the scan.

The consultant obstetrician performing the scan stated that they had seen the CSP, and given multiple images were taken during the procedure, these were scrutinised at some length during the court hearings.

The Judgement

The evidence presented demonstrated that signs of ACC are difficult to detect at the time of the anatomy scan. The signs that would suggest this abnormality present in later gestation, and in addition there are artefacts that may mimic the CSP and give a false impression that it was present and normal. It was also admitted that a range of factors influence visualisation. It was accepted that if a scan was carried out to a competent standard and all the relevant structures were seen, it was reasonable to sign it off as being complete rather than requiring a further scan. Even experts in specialist centres could miss an ACC. This is not an easy task and it is a matter of judgement and subjectivity.

This case of wrongful birth following a missed diagnosis of ACC on ultrasound scan was therefore dismissed.

Legal Commentary

Eloise Power

Statutory Framework for Proceedings Brought by Children: Congenital Disabilities (Civil Liability) Act 1976

The 1976 Act sets out provisions relating to civil liability in the case of children born disabled in consequence of another person's fault. At section 1, the 1976 Act provides that a child can sue for damages in respect of disabilities arising from occurrences which:

> 1 (2)(a) affected either parent of the child in his or her ability to have a normal, healthy child; or
>
> (b) affected the mother during her pregnancy, or affected her or the child in the course of its birth, so that the child is born with disabilities which would not otherwise have been present.

The liability of a defendant under the 1976 Act is derivative: in other words, the child's right to sue the defendant derives from the duty owed by the defendant to the parent(s) of the child. The parent does not need to have suffered an injury herself/himself for liability to arise under the Act. Liability does not arise where a parent knew, at the time of conception, of the existence of the risk that a child conceived as a result of the intercourse would be disabled (unless the father is the defendant and he knew of the risk but the mother did not know).

The standard of care as set out at section 1 (5) of the 1976 Act is equivalent to the *Bolam/Bolitho* standard:

> The defendant is not answerable to the child, for anything he did or omitted to do when responsible in a professional capacity for treating or advising the parent, if he took reasonable care having due regard to then received professional opinion applicable to the particular class of case; but this does not mean that he is answerable only because he departed from received opinion.

In cases involving fertility treatment, liability arises under section 1A of the Act where a child is born disabled and where:

> the disability results from an act or omission in the course of the selection, or the keeping or use outside the body, of the embryo carried by her or of the gametes used to bring about the creation of the embryo.

The standard of care relating to fertility treatment cases is the same as the standard set out at section 1(5) of the Act (quoted above).

Wrongful Life and Wrongful Conception: Cases Brought by Children

In *McKay v Essex Area Health Authority* [1982] 2 All ER 771, the Court of Appeal considered a claim brought by a child who had suffered disability as a result of her mother contracting rubella during her pregnancy. The child argued that, but for the negligent management of her mother's pregnancy, her mother would have been informed of the risk of disability to the fetus due to rubella and would have terminated her pregnancy. The Court of Appeal struck the claim out. It was held to be a claim for wrongful life. Such a claim was regarded as untenable on policy grounds as it was regarded as being inconsistent with the sanctity of human life, as well as being impossible to quantify. In the words of Ackner LJ (and Shakespeare):

> But how can a court begin to evaluate non-existence, 'the undiscovered country from whose bourn no traveller returns?' No comparison is possible and therefore no damage can be established which a court could recognise. This goes to the root of the whole cause of action.

Although the claimant in *McKay* was born before the 1976 Act came into force, the Court made clear observations to the effect that the matter would have been decided in the same way under the 1976 Act: Griffiths LJ observed that *"claims for 'wrongful life' in all cases subsequent to the Congenital Disabilities (Civil Liability) Act 1976 are excluded by the wording of section 1 (2) (b) of that Act"*.

For almost four decades after *McKay*, the law relating to wrongful life claims was generally regarded as settled. In a recent judgement of Lambert J handed down on 21 December 2020 in *Toombes v Mitchell* [2020] EWHC 3506, further consideration was given to the issue of wrongful life/wrongful conception. The claimant alleged that she had suffered a congenital development defect causing spinal cord tethering as a result of the defendant's negligent failure to advise her mother to take folic acid before her conception. Although the underlying facts were disputed, the Court considered the preliminary issue of whether the claim disclosed a lawful cause of action if the facts were proved. The defendant relied upon *McKay* and argued that this was a wrongful life claim and, as such, was expressly excluded both under the 1976 Act and at common law. The claimant argued that this was not a wrongful life claim but was rather a wrongful conception claim: the submission was that the claim fell squarely within subsection 1 (2) (a) of the 1976 Act, i.e. an occurrence which *"affected either parent of the child in his or her ability to have a normal, healthy child"*.

The Court held that the claim did indeed disclose a lawful cause of action. Upon detailed consideration of the Law Commission's Report which gave rise to the 1976 Act, the Court held that wrongful life cases falling within subsection 1 (2) (b) (i.e. occurrences which *"affected the mother during her pregnancy, or affected her or the child in the course of its birth, so that the child is born with disabilities which would not otherwise have been present*") were indeed excluded. On the other hand, wrongful life/wrongful conception cases falling within subsection 1 (2) (a) of the 1976 Act – such as Ms Toombes' case – were not excluded.

At the time of writing, it is possible that an appeal to the Court of Appeal, or alternatively a leapfrog appeal direct to the Supreme Court, might be brought by the unsuccessful defendant. The law in this area should consequently be regarded as in flux.

Wrongful Birth: Cases Brought by Parents

Many cases are brought by parents rather than by children arising out of births which, for a variety of reasons, would not have occurred but for a particular act of negligence. These cases can broadly be divided into three categories: (1) where a non-disabled child is born to a non-disabled parent (e.g. after a failure of sterilisation), (2) where a disabled child is born to a non-disabled parent (e.g. after a failure of sterilisation or a failure of prenatal screening, such as arose in the two case examples considered above), (3) where a non-disabled child is born to a disabled parent. The basic legal principles are now well-established, although there have been some interesting developments in recent years.

In *McFarlane v Tayside Health Board* [2000] 2 A.C. 59, the House of Lords considered a failed vasectomy case in which negligent advice had been given to a husband and wife to the effect that the vasectomy had rendered the husband infertile. They stopped using contraception, and the wife conceived and delivered a healthy child. A majority of the House of Lords held that no duty of care was owed to the parents in relation to the pure economic loss of raising a child. The mother was, however, permitted to recover for the *"pain and discomfort and inconvenience of the unwanted pregnancy and birth"*, together with certain pecuniary losses: *"extra medical expenses, clothes for herself and equipment on the birth of the baby. She does not claim but in my view in principle she would have been entitled to prove compensation for loss of earnings due to the pregnancy and birth"* (Lord Slynn).

In the case of *Parkinson v Seacroft and St James University Hospital NHS Trust* [2001] EWCA Civ 530, the Court of Appeal considered the applicability of *McFarlane* in a situation where a child was born with a disability following a failed sterilisation. The Court held that the additional expenses attributable to the disability were recoverable, whereas damages for the expenses which would inevitably be incurred in bringing up any child were disallowed. In relation to the timing and type of disability which could form the basis for recovery, Hale LJ (as she was) observed as follows: *"I conclude that any disability arising from genetic causes or foreseeable events during pregnancy (such as rubella, spina bifida, or oxygen deprivation during pregnancy or childbirth) up until the child is born alive, and which are not novus actus interveniens, will suffice to found a claim."*

In the case of *Rees v Darlington Memorial Hospital NHS Trust* [2003] UKHL 52, the House of Lords considered the applicability of *McFarlane* to the situation where a healthy child is born to a disabled parent. The Claimant in *Rees* suffered from a severe visual disability and underwent a sterilisation procedure because she was concerned that she could not fulfil the duties of a parent. The sterilisation failed due to negligence and she gave birth to a healthy son. A majority of the House of Lords held that the claimant could not recover for the costs of bringing up her child. However, an award of £15,000 was made to reflect the loss of the claimant's opportunity to live the life which she had planned to live.

In *ARB v IVF Hammersmith and another* [2018] EWCA Civ 2803, *McFarlane* and *Rees* were considered in an entirely different context. A heterosexual couple underwent fertility treatment and froze five embryos. They subsequently separated. The female ex-partner attended the clinic alone for fertility treatment, claiming that the couple had agreed to have another child. She was allowed to take away the consent form to obtain a signature from her partner. She forged the male ex-partner's signature on the consent documents, underwent embryo implantation and gave birth to a healthy child. The male ex-partner brought an action in contract against the clinic and the female ex-partner. The Court of Appeal found that – regardless of the significant failings on the part of the clinic – the legal policy barring damages for the pure economic loss of raising a child should apply in breach of contract as much as in tort. Accordingly, the father was not entitled to damages.

In *Khan v Meadows*,[1] the Supreme Court considered a case which raised the key issue of whether the concept of scope of duty was applicable to clinical negligence cases. A doctor negligently failed to determine that a female patient (the claimant) was a carrier of haemophilia. The claimant became pregnant and gave birth to a child who suffered from haemophilia and also from autism. It was common ground that, but for the negligence, the claimant would have undergone a termination. It was also common ground that the claimant was entitled to recover for the additional costs associated with the condition of haemophilia. The question for the Court was whether the defendant was liable for the additional costs associated with the child's autism, which was agreed to be a risk which existed with every pregnancy and was not increased by the failure to manage the risk of haemophilia. On a simplistic level, "but for" causation was made out on the facts: but for the defendant's negligence, the child would not have been born. On the other hand, the child's autism was an entirely coincidental injury.

The Supreme Court held that the concept of "scope of duty" was applicable to clinical negligence claims. The majority[2] set out a six-part analysis as follows[3]:

(1) *Is the harm (loss, injury and damage) which is the subject matter of the claim actionable in negligence? (the actionability question)*

(2) *What are the risks of harm to the claimant against which the law imposes on the defendant a duty to take care? (the scope of duty question)*

(3) *Did the defendant breach his or her duty by his or her act or omission (the breach question)*

(4) *Is the loss for which the claimant seeks damages the consequence of the defendant's act or omission? (the factual causation question)*

(5) *Is there a sufficient nexus between a particular element of the harm for which the claimant seeks damages and the subject matter of the defendant's duty of care as analysed at stage 2 above? (the duty nexus question)*

(6) *Is a particular element of the harm for which the claimant seeks damages irrecoverable because it is too remote, or because there is a different effective cause (including novus actus interveniens) in relation to it or because the claimant has mitigated his or her loss or has failed to avoid loss which he or she could reasonably have been expected to avoid? (the legal responsibility question).*

---

[1] [2021] UKSC 21 (on appeal from: [2019] EWCA Civ 152).
[2] Lord Hodge and Lord Sales, with whom Lord Reed, Lady Black and Lord Kitchin agreed.
[3] Para 28.

On the facts, the Supreme Court found that the law did not impose any duty upon the defendant doctor in relation to unrelated risks which might arise in any pregnancy. The defendant was only liable for the costs which were caused by the child's haemophilia and not by the costs caused by his autism.[4]

At the time of writing, the Supreme Court's judgement in *Khan v Meadows* is new, having been handed down on 18 June 2021. It remains to be seen how the principles in *Khan v Meadows* will be applied in other areas of clinical negligence practice.

Afterword

From the viewpoint of medical practitioners, it is important to remember that, regardless of the numerous legal debates in this field, the relevant standard of care is governed by *Bolam/Bolitho* principles. The two cases set out in the medical commentary above (*Mordel* and *Shaw*) illustrate this: in *Mordel*, there were two obvious missed opportunities to achieve standard pre-natal diagnosis of Down's syndrome, whereas in *Shaw*, the Court found that the mistakes which were made could have been made even if the claimant had received a high level of specialist care: *"even experts in specialist centres miss agenesis of the corpus callosum and even when they are scanning with the benefit of clues that make them look extra hard"*. The *Bolam/Bolitho* standard of care applies whether the 1976 Act is engaged or whether the case is approached under the common law.

One interesting question for the future will be the approach which the courts may take to consent cases brought under the 1976 Act following *Montgomery*.[5] The wording of section 1(5) of the 1976 Act predates the *Montgomery* judgement by four decades. Although the legal principles are not clear, the safest approach is likely to be to assume that *Montgomery* will apply to 1976 Act cases, and to ensure that prospective parents are consented in a *Montgomery*-compliant manner in relation to unborn or prospective children as well as to themselves.

Clinical Commentary

David Howe

Introduction

The great majority of medicolegal claims brought relating to prenatal diagnosis follow the birth of a child with disabilities that were not recognised antenatally. A much smaller number of claims are brought following complications of antenatal investigations or intrauterine treatment.

Where a child with an unrecognised disability is born, the claim is made on the basis that this is a "wrongful birth". Wrongful birth claims fall into two categories:

1) Births following failed sterilisation where the child is healthy but unexpected.
2) Babies born with disabilities where the parents were not warned of these and would have chosen termination of pregnancy if they had known in advance, which is the subject of this chapter.

---

[4] Para 68–69.
[5] The issue did not arise in *Montgomery* itself, as the 1976 Act does not extend to Scotland.

Another regular cause for litigation in cases seen by fetal medicine consultants is failed management of the complications of monochorionic twins, and discussion has been included here as it is not covered in other chapters.

Good Practice Guidance

The NHS Fetal Anomaly Screening Programme (FASP) requires that all eligible pregnant women in England are offered screening to assess the risk of their baby being born with Down's, Edward's or Patau's syndrome and a number of structural fetal anomalies. Although the standards are published by Public Health England, they are applied across the United Kingdom four nations. The performance of the first trimester ultrasound, including nuchal translucency measurements, is described in the *Handbook for Ultrasound Practitioners* [1] and the standards for the second trimester anomaly scan are given in the *NHS Fetal Anomaly Screening Programme Handbook* [2]. In addition to trisomies and structural anomalies, prenatal diagnosis also includes identification of genetic syndromes where there is a relevant family history or where it is revealed by other screening such as for haemoglobinopathies.

Informing Mothers about Screening for Fetal Trisomies and Structural Anomalies

Women need to be seen promptly in early pregnancy so that they can receive information about screening in time to consider this and have their first trimester scan arranged. Their initial assessment should include a history of any genetic conditions in the family of both parents since this may require further assessment or investigation, including urgent referral for genetic advice. Good communication with primary care may be critical if they hold relevant information and failure to inform the maternity services of known issues when referring for booking is a cause of litigation. If parental haemoglobinopathy screening suggests the fetus is at risk, the mother may need to be offered invasive testing.

In order to give informed consent for screening, mothers must understand what they are being screened for, the methods offered, and the implications of the results, including the meaning of a higher or lower risk result and the limitations of the process. For screening for trisomies, information on obtaining consent is no longer included in the FASP handbook but standards were set out in the 2007 "Working Standards for Down Syndrome Screening" [3]. This emphasises that consent should be obtained and documented before any screening test and that the mother must not be pressured to feel that she must accept screening. Her decision to accept or decline screening should be recorded, and if she later withdraws consent, her decision should be respected. Information about screening tests should be given as early as possible in pregnancy and the mother should have at least 24 hours to consider the information before being asked to make any decisions. The verbal information should be supported by written information, with many units using the national booklet "Screening Tests for You and Your Baby" which is available in a number of translations. The information provided should also include discussion of the mid-pregnancy anomaly scan, its aims and limitations.

If the mother opts for first trimester combined screening, this needs to be organised in the correct gestational window (11^{+2} to 14^{+1} weeks). The scan needs to be performed competently by sonographers who regularly undergo audit of their measurements. Women who present too late for first trimester screening, or where this is technically unsuccessful due to fetal position or maternal build preventing adequate views, should be offered second trimester serum screening which can be performed from 14^{+2} to 20^{+0} weeks.

The results of screening should be documented in the maternal notes when reviewed at around 16 weeks of pregnancy. This provides an opportunity to confirm that a mother has chosen to decline screening if it has not been performed, but the discussion should avoid implying the mother was wrong to choose not to be screened.

If a high-risk screening result is received, the implications need to be explained to the mother, including the options for further testing, the information this provides and its limitations. In most cases this will involve invasive testing, with its associated risks, but mothers should also be advised about the possibility of non-invasive prenatal testing, although at the time of writing this is not available through the NHS and is still a screening rather than a diagnostic test.

Ultrasound Diagnosis of Anomalies

Although some major fetal abnormalities will be recognised during the first-trimester scan, this is not the main purpose of that visit. Most fetal anomalies will be detected during the mid-pregnancy anomaly scan carried out between 18 to 20^{+6} weeks. The standards for these scans are set out by the Fetal Anomaly Screening Programme, with regular updates since first described in 2010. The most recent guidance was published in 2018 [2]. This includes a base menu describing what structures should be seen, what measurements should be made and what images should be stored. Currently, only six images are required to be stored. For fetal cardiac examination, four planes should be examined, and the abdominal situs confirmed. FASP does not require that cardiac images or an image of situs be recorded, although many departments routinely do so and sonographers should be aware of, and follow, their local protocol.

Particular care should be taken in recording the required planes and measurements of the brain. Both the transventricular view and the transcerebellar view should include the cavum septum pellucidum (CSP). One of the causes of litigation for wrongful birth is failure to recognise agenesis of the corpus callosum (ACC). The CSP is a key landmark to identify the correct planes of the head, and is absent in fetuses with ACC but may be mimicked by other structures, including the columns of the fornices, two vertical commissures immediately below the CSP which are commonly mistaken for it [4] (Figure 5.1).

Another source of litigation is failure to identify ventriculomegaly. The threshold for distinguishing normal and abnormal ventricle diameter is fixed: a measurement ≥ 10 mm is abnormal, so in borderline cases slight variations in the placement of the calipers can cause the measurement to fall just above or just below this threshold. The consequences of undermeasurement are possibly missing a significant fetal abnormality, whereas slight overmeasurement may lead to unnecessary intervention and investigation, and, in the worst cases, causes parents such worry that their baby has brain damage that they opt for termination of pregnancy of what would have been a healthy child. The image in the FASP programme guide showing the placement of the calipers to measure the ventricular atrium is misleading, and the most complete description of how to make

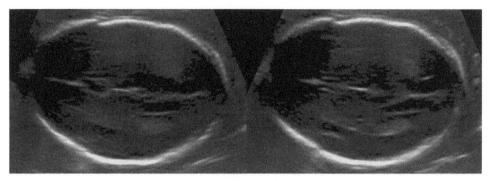

Figure 5.1 Images showing the normal CSP (left) and the columns of the fornices (right). The CSP contains no midline echo in contrast to the columns.

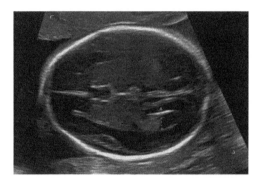

Figure 5.2 Correct placement of calipers to measure ventricular atrium diameter.

this measurement was described by Guibaud [5] in a paper proposing international standardisation of the technique (Figure 5.2).

If the required anatomical features cannot be seen at the first scan, due to technical issues such as fetal position or maternal build, a repeat scan should be organised before 23 weeks. If the second scan is still incomplete, no further scans are required but the mother should be informed that screening is incomplete and this should be documented.

Investigation of Fetal Abnormalities

If a fetal abnormality is seen or suspected, the mother should be referred promptly for further investigation and advice, often to the nearest tertiary fetal medicine unit. When seen there, the fetus will be re-examined in detail to confirm the abnormality and to look for additional anomalies which may have an important influence on prognosis. Appropriate additional investigations may be required, which may include invasive testing for chromosome or specific genetic abnormalities, viral testing and further imaging, including MRI.

In many tertiary units there is separation between examination of the fetal heart, carried out by paediatric cardiologists, and examination of the remainder of the baby, performed by fetal medicine consultants. This is a particular source of medicolegal risk. Any fetus seen in a tertiary unit should have a detailed examination of the heart as this is often a key signifier of underlying chromosome or genetic syndromes. This requires either that all fetuses referred are seen by a paediatric cardiologist, or that fetal medicine consultants are trained to examine the heart in sufficient detail. Equally, if mothers are seen by paediatric cardiologists alone, they must be able to recognise and investigate non-cardiac conditions that may present with cardiac changes, e.g. cardiomegaly in fetal anaemia, and should have a clear pathway for the management of additional obstetric issues the mother may present with, such as fetal growth restriction or maternal illness. There is no national guidance on what should be examined and recorded as part of a tertiary fetal anomaly scan, or as a fetal echocardiogram, but it would be expected that many more images are recorded than required by FASP, including images of the situs and all planes of the heart. As a suggested minimum, a tertiary level examination should include all the features described in the International Society for Ultrasound in Obstetrics and Gynecology (ISUOG) practice guidelines for the routine mid-pregnancy anomaly scans [6] and for screening the fetal heart [7].

Counselling about Anomalies

Once a fetal anomaly is identified, the parents should be informed of the diagnosis, of any uncertainty about this, and about the implications for the baby. This will include the effects or possible complications during pregnancy and the implications for the baby after birth. They also need information about relevant investigations, the information these may provide and how that may be used by the parents and any limitations of testing. For invasive tests, they need to be informed of the risks of the procedure. If the abnormality meets the legal criteria for termination of pregnancy, they need non-directive counselling about the choices open to them. They will often benefit from being signposted to relevant support groups, such as ARC (Antenatal Results and Choices (www.arc-uk.org)) and there are a number of other helpful parent groups for specific abnormalities.

Counselling will often benefit from or require involvement from relevant specialties who will be involved in the postnatal management of the child, such as paediatric surgeons, neurologists or cardiologists, who can provide more information about treatment options and the long-term implications.

Management of Monochorionic Twins

Approximately 30% of twin pregnancies are monochorionic (MC), where the fetuses share a single placenta with intertwin vascular communications. From the moment of diagnosis, such pregnancies are amongst the highest risk for fetal loss, since life-threatening complications occur in at least 15%. The two major complications are selective growth restriction (sGR) and twin oligohydramnios polyhydramnios sequence (TOPS), often colloquially called "twin-twin transfusion syndrome". A rarer form of intertwin transfusion (twin anaemia polycythaemia sequence (TAPS)) affects a much smaller number, most commonly after previous laser treatment for TOPS.

The key to reducing the complications of such pregnancies is well-organised antenatal care by clinicians who are experienced at recognising the early signs of developing problems and arrange or refer on for treatment promptly.

All multiple pregnancies should have chorionicity established at the earliest opportunity. The ultrasound features distinguishing dichorionic from monochorionic pregnancies (the "T" and "λ" membrane insertions on the placenta) are most obvious in the first trimester and become more difficult to distinguish after 14 weeks. Once identified, these pregnancies should be supervised with scans at least every two weeks from 16 weeks of pregnancy until delivery, looking for evidence of TOPS, shown by discrepant liquor volume and bladder size. The scan should be performed by a sonographer experienced at recognising the features of TOPS, including early signs such as infolding of the membranes as they collapse down towards the twin with oligohydramnios. From 20 weeks the scan should include umbilical artery Doppler assessment and the fetal size discordancy should be assessed. A difference of more than 20% in estimated fetal weight is associated with increased fetal loss rates.

Even with fortnightly ultrasound supervision, TOPS can develop rapidly between assessments. Mothers should be informed of the symptoms and advised to attend hospital promptly if concerned. Any mother with MC twins presenting with abdominal pain should be scanned to exclude TOPS before discharge: mothers should be informed of this and advised to insist on this, and staff in maternity day units, who may encounter MC twin pregnancies relatively infrequently, should be aware of the necessity to exclude the diagnosis. Women presenting with TOPS will need referral to a regional or supra-regional centre for consideration of laser therapy to divide the intertwin vessels.

The management of sGR may require balancing the conflicting needs of the two fetuses. In addition, the death of one twin results in a high risk of death or permanent neurological damage in the other, making the decisions about timing of delivery even more critical. Interpretation of Doppler findings is also more complex: there is a longer latent period between the development of abnormal UA Doppler and delivery in MC twins compared with singletons. Since these pregnancies are rare, they should normally be referred to a tertiary fetal medicine unit with expertise in their assessment and management.

Causes of Litigation

The causes of litigation in relation to prenatal diagnosis and screening include the following:

1. Screening for Down's, Edward's and Patau's syndrome and other genetic conditions

   a. Failure of General Practice to notify of relevant family genetic history when referring for antenatal care, and failure by booking midwives to take a sufficient family history.

   b. Failure to offer screening, or explain the process adequately, preventing an informed choice whether to accept or decline screening.

   c. Failure to complete screening as planned:

      - first trimester scan not booked in time;
      - inaccurate measurements of CRL or nuchal translucency on scan;
      - failure to take blood for second serum screening at the correct time, especially after failure of first trimester screening due to technical problems;
      - Failure to document when screening has been declined by parents.

2. Ultrasound diagnosis of fetal abnormalities

   a. Failure to follow national guidance from the Fetal Anomaly Screening Programme on the performance of the scan, including arranging it at the correct gestation, repeating the scan if incomplete and recording the required views and measurements.

b. Failure to identify fetal abnormalities when present.

c. Failure to advise adequately about the implications of anomalies seen and the future risks to the fetus.

d. Failure to carry out appropriate investigations when an anomaly is seen.

e. Errors at the interface between fetal medicine and fetal cardiology:

- Failure to recognise fetal cardiac abnormalities by obstetric sonographers.
- Failure to recognise or counsel about non-cardiac issues by fetal cardiologists.

3. Recognition of complications of monochorionic multiple pregnancy

a. Failure to confirm chorionicity and identify MC twins.

b. Failure to arrange scans to screen for TOPS.

c. Failure to recognise features of TOPS on scan and refer promptly for treatment.

d. Failure to arrange additional scans in mothers presenting with symptoms of TOPS.

e. Failure to recognise and respond to sGR, resulting in the death of one twin and death or permanent neurological damage in the other.

Avoidance of Litigation

1. Screening for Down's, Edward's and Patau's syndrome and other genetic conditions

a. Ensure that referral from primary care to maternity services includes relevant family and genetic history.

b. At booking the history should include family history of genetic and birth abnormalities in both parents.

c. The availability of screening tests, their purpose and how they are performed should be explained, supported be explanatory information, and the discussion documented.

d. Screening tests should be arranged at the appropriate time, with scan measurements performed competently. If first trimester screening is not possible for technical reasons, second trimester serum screening should be offered and clear arrangements made to perform this.

e. The results of screening should be reviewed and documented at the 16 weeks antenatal visit to ensure they are complete in accordance with the mother's wishes.

2. Ultrasound diagnosis of fetal abnormalities

a. The purpose of scans and their limitations should be explained before mothers undergo them.

b. The scan should be completed at the appropriate gestation and in accordance with relevant standards. For the mid-pregnancy anomaly scan this should be performed between $18-20^{+6}$ weeks gestation with the anatomy described in the Fetal Anomaly Screening Programme handbook viewed, and images and measurements taken as required.

   c. If the first scan is incomplete for technical reasons, a second attempt should be organised before 23 weeks. If that is still incomplete the mother should be informed that screening has not been completed and this should be documented.

3. Recognition of complications of monochorionic multiple pregnancy

   a. The chorionicity of all multiple pregnancies should be established and documented. This is best achieved in the first trimester.

   b. For all MC pregnancies, fortnightly scans should be performed from 16 weeks until delivery.

   c. The scans should be performed by staff able to recognise the early and established ultrasound features of twin oligohydramnios polyhydramnios sequence (TOPS), and able to make immediate referrals for further management if needed.

   d. The mothers should be advised of the symptoms of TOPS and the need to present to hospital promptly if concerned.

   e. Maternity day assessment units should be aware of the symptoms of TOPS and the need to scan promptly, before discharge, any mother with an MC multiple pregnancy presenting with relevant symptoms and to refer immediately if concerned.

   f. Any discrepancy in fetal weight should be calculated and umbilical artery Doppler assessment performed after 20 weeks. A discrepancy of >20% is associated with an increased fetal loss rate.

   g. Where there is significant sGR, particularly where the UA Doppler is abnormal, the mother should be referred to a tertiary fetal medicine unit for monitoring and decisions about the delivery, because these pregnancies are rare and the management decisions are complex.

References

1. Fetal Anomaly Screening Programme. *Fetal Anomaly Screening Programme Handbook for Ultrasound Practitioners.* Published 2015.

2. Fetal Anomaly Screening Programme. *NHS Fetal Anomaly Screening Programme Handbook.* Published 2018.

3. National Down's Syndrome Screening Programme for England. *Antenatal Screening - Working Standards for Down's Syndrome Screening.* Published 2007.

4. Callen PW, et al. Columns of the fornix, not to be mistaken for the cavum septi pellucidi on prenatal sonography. *J Ultrasound Med* 2008; 27(1): 25–31.

5. Guibaud L. Fetal cerebral ventricular measurement and ventriculomegaly: time for procedure standardization. *Ultrasound Obstet Gynecol* 2009; 34(2): 127–30.

6. Salomon LJ, et al. Practice guidelines for performance of the routine mid-trimester fetal ultrasound scan. *Ultrasound Obstet Gynecol* 2011; 37(1): 116–26.

7. Carvalho J, et al. ISUOG Practice Guidelines (updated): sonographic screening examination of the fetal heart. *Ultrasound Obstet Gynecol* 2013; 41(3): 348–59.

Obstetric Perineal Trauma

Abdul H Sultan

CASE COMMENTARY

Swati Jha

Successful Claim

Sarah Davison v Craig Leitch [2013] EWHC 3092 (QB)

The Claim

The claimant, an equity sales trader in the City of London, during the birth of her first child suffered an obstetric anal sphincter injury whilst in private obstetric care. This went undetected, leaving her with significant ongoing symptoms which caused embarrassment, inconvenience and distress, resulting in an impact on her career trajectory. It was claimed that the defendant performed a midline episiotomy which caused a third-degree tear affecting both her internal and external anal sphincter.

The Summary

The claimant had a midline episiotomy during labour. At the time this was repaired but no clear records of what was done were kept and the discharge summary merely stated "a small mid-line episiotomy extended slightly and repaired with vicryl".

She subsequently underwent a secondary overlap repair and reconstruction of her perineum. However, due to ongoing symptoms, she was unable to resume her usual work in which her gross salary had been over £200,000. The experience also took a toll on her mental well-being.

The defendant acknowledged liability for having missed the grade and severity of the tear, but denied that the loss of earnings amounted to the values claimed. The defendants made the case that it was a lifestyle choice for the claimant to not return to her usual employment as she had two more children following on from the alleged negligence. The entire case centred around quantum and its various elements including i) loss of past earnings due to the injury, ii) loss of future earnings, iii) loss of residual earning capacity (challenges in finding a suitable area of work and then employment in it), iv) loss of congenial employment (injury prevented return to any form of work in the financial sector and had severely limited the nature of any future employment) and v) multiplier applicable for loss of future and residual earnings.

The Judgement

It was judged that the performance of a mid-line episiotomy was at variance with the usual UK practice of a mediolateral episiotomy and caused the third-degree tear. There was no proper assessment post-delivery, so the severity of the tear remained undetected, and no antibiotics given. The defendant failed to inform the claimant of the injury or repair. So, liability, once accepted was never in dispute.

In determining quantum, as the claimant had three young children, it was felt that even if she had been fit, she would have moved to a less stressful role within the bank, reducing her earning capacity. Following consideration of all the facts, the final payment was £1.6 million and in excess of the offer made by the defendant or the claimant in the part 36 offer.

Unsuccessful Claim

Starkey v Rotherham NHS Foundation Trust [2007] 2 WLUK 243

The Claim

The claimant underwent a forceps delivery and an episiotomy was performed, but this extended, causing an anal sphincter injury. It was claimed that the defendant fell below a reasonable standard of care to perform an adequate examination and detect the anal sphincter injury, which in turn has led to many years of discomfort from fecal incontinence.

The Summary

The claimant went into spontaneous labour and during labour, due to features of fetal distress, was delivered by forceps with the performance of an episiotomy. The registrar who performed the delivery examined the episiotomy and the perineum and found no evidence of tears extending to the anal canal or involving the sphincter, so went on to repair the episiotomy as per usual practice. The claimant was constipated for the next few days but had diarrhoea following this and developed fecal incontinence. As a consequence, she was unable to return to work. Due to faecal incontinence, she subsequently underwent a secondary repair of the anal sphincter but the improvement only lasted for five months. In her next pregnancy she was delivered by caesarean section. Due to ongoing faecal incontinence, a claim was made. The claim was denied and it was argued that the examination and the medical knowledge were appropriate for the time. On the basis that damage to the sphincter was difficult to detect, the injury was not likely to have been obvious, even when carrying out a correct and competent examination.

The Judgement

By the standards of the time (2000), reasonable care required that a visual inspection be carried out by inserting two fingers into the vagina. It was not routine to carry out a rectal examination unless there was a suspicion of an anal sphincter injury. This was performed adequately and historical data at the time demonstrated that there had always been a significant number of situations where a tear in the external anal sphincter had not been recognised. On a balance of probability, the anal sphincter injury would not have been obvious to a clinician even when performing an examination in a competent manner. In addition, it was ruled that the fecal incontinence was not wholly due to the injury to the sphincter as there was evidence of both pudendal neuropathy and functional bowel problems unrelated to the anal sphincter injury.

Legal Commentary

Eloise Power

Sarah Davison v Craig Leitch [2013] EWHC 3092 (QB)

The underlying facts of this matter demonstrate the grave effects which can follow an episode of perineal trauma: it was accepted by both sides that the claimant had suffered significant and permanent colorectal symptoms, as well as psychiatric effects, consequent upon her injury. Bearing in mind the prevalence of perineal trauma consequent upon vaginal delivery, it is perhaps surprising that patients are not routinely consented that perineal trauma and incontinence are risks consequent upon vaginal delivery.

One point of interest in respect of the underlying facts concerns the record-keeping and communication with the patient: it is evident from the judgement that the defendant did not keep a clear record of the repair of the third-degree tear, nor did he inform the claimant about the injury or the repair which he had undertaken. *Davison v Leitch* predates the duty of candour regulations, which came into force in respect of the NHS in November 2014. Having said that, the legal provisions relating to the duty of candour drew upon pre-existing principles, and it is clear that the defendant in *Davison v Leitch* did not seek to justify his conduct at trial. If these facts were to fall for consideration today, the injury and/or repair may well be regarded as a notifiable safety incident.

The issues considered at trial before Andrews J (as she was) in *Davison v Leitch* related solely to quantum: the dispute concerned the claim for past and future earnings and for the loss of congenial employment. In practice, many disputes of this kind are resolved outside Court: the reason why *Davison v Leitch* came to trial is likely to be that Mrs Davison, the claimant, was a high earner: her pre-injury salary was £206,828 gross in her capacity as an equity sales trader in Canary Wharf.

The key question for the Court was how Mrs Davison's career would have progressed but for her injury. Prior to her injury, Mrs Davison was on course for promotion and had been marked out as someone *"who had the potential for a stellar career with the Bank."* The defendant argued that Mrs Davison's decision not to return to work was not a result of her injury but was a lifestyle choice: following the injury, Mrs Davison's husband accepted an excellent job offer in Hong Kong, Mrs Davison proceeded to have two more children. On the facts, the Court found that if it had not been for the injury, Mrs Davison would initially have obtained employment in Hong Kong at a level which was commensurate with her pre-injury career in London.

One of the interesting features of the judgement is the level of detail which the Court goes into in respect of the assumed course of Mrs Davison's hypothetical career. The Court's task was made somewhat easier by the provision of detailed witness evidence from Mrs Davison's former manager, as well as a wealth of detail about what had actually happened to her family since the date of the injury. The Court observed that *"a claim for loss of future earnings is not a claim for the loss of a chance"*. Notably, there have been certain cases where future earnings have indeed been approached on the basis of the loss of a chance, assessed in percentage terms: see, for example, *Langford v Hebran* [2001] EWCA Civ 361, where the Court had to determine whether a claimant would have become a highly succcessful kick-boxing champion or whether he would have remained as a bricklayer. However, the Court of Appeal in *Herring v Ministry of Defence* [2003]

EWCA Civ 528 held that in most situations, loss of earnings should not be approached by way of the loss of a chance but rather by *"forming a view as to the most likely future working career"* of an uninjured claimant.

A further point of interest is the distinction made by the Court between having two children and having three children. While the Court was prepared to accept that after having two children, Mrs Davison would have returned to her high-pressure job, the Court made a finding of fact that after having three children, things would be different:

> She genuinely believes that being the mother of three young boys would not have affected her enthusiasm to return to her high-pressure job. In this respect, however, I consider Mrs Davison to be unrealistic. It is true that Tier 1 banks are extremely supportive of women who wish to return to work and do their best to make it possible. Nevertheless there is a world of difference between juggling a career with two small children and trying to do so with three under the age of five. It is not impossible, but it is rare.

The finding was that Mrs Davison would have moved to a less stressful position.

This is a paradigmatic example of a situation where a Court makes findings based upon common sense/life experience. It is interesting to speculate how the same situation would have been approached if the claimant had been a father of three young children (would a Court infer that he would be more, not less, motivated to increase his earnings?) At a wider level, the issues considered in *Davison v Leitch* raise the question of whether the defendant's approach to the case contravened Equality Act provisions and whether it should be permissible for defendants (and Courts) to draw inferences to the effect that mothers are less likely to return to work than fathers.

The parties were agreed that credit would have to be given for the cost of the childcare which was needed to enable Mrs Davison to return to work. The claimant originally argued that credit should only be given in respect of a half share of these expenses, as the childcare was needed to enable both Mrs Davison and her husband to work. This point was eventually conceded, and the Court observed as follows:

> In my judgment Mr Mylonas was right to concede that in principle, the whole of that expense must be brought into account, because what matters in this context is how much had to be spent on childcare to enable Mrs Davison to go back to work (regardless of whether she and her husband paid or what they each contributed). If and to the extent that the costs of domestic help were not a necessity, in that sense, but a lifestyle choice, i.e. something that would have eased the domestic burden on Mrs Davison, they are irrelevant and the costs fall to be excluded (again, regardless of who actually paid or what they contributed).

Clearly, the exclusion of the need to give credit for "lifestyle" domestic help is likely to be of more benefit to wealthier claimants.

For completeness, a Part 36 offer refers to an offer made under the provisions of Part 36 of the Civil Procedure Rules. The purpose of Part 36 is to encourage parties to settle claims outside Court by imposing consequences in costs and other penalties upon parties who fail to do better than the Part 36 offer at trial. In *Davison*, the claimant did not merely beat the Part 36 offer made by the defendant but also beat her own Part 36 offer (which had been refused by the defendant). Accordingly, the defendant was penalised in costs, although the full consequences of Part 36 did not apply as there were various developments in the case which occurred after the offers had been made.

Starkey v Rotherham NHS Foundation Trust [2007] 2 WLUK 243

A key point of interest in this judgement is that the experts are likely to have come to a different view if the case had been determined today: based upon the RCOG Green-top Guideline No. 29 on Third- and Fourth-degree Perineal Tears Management, a rectal examination is now mandatory to rule out sphincter injury. This Guideline post-dates the events in *Starkey*, which occurred in 2000. The present edition was published in 2015, but an earlier version of the document was available by the date of the trial in Starkey in 2007. This is by no means an unusual situation: in practice, it is common for cases to reach trial years after the underlying events occur.

The judgement in *Starkey* makes clear that the Court was alert to the importance of judging the standard of care by reference to the standards of the time: the Court found as follows:

> I also have to consider the expert evidence as to what would constitute a competent examination, bearing in mind that this must be looked at as at March 2000 and not by any different standards which may currently exist.

The Court's approach in *Starkey* was correct as a matter of legal principle. The point goes back as far as the case of *Bolam* itself, in which the Court approved the statement that *"in the case of a medical man, negligence means failure to act in accordance with the standards of reasonably competent men at the time"* – subject to the point that there may be one or more perfectly proper standards.

What, then, about *Montgomery*? One of the features of *Montgomery* which typically causes confusion or concern is that the principles apply retrospectively. A distinction must be made between legal principles and matters of medical evidence, standards and literature: it is the legal principles in *Montgomery* which apply retrospectively, rather than matters of medicine which could not have been known retrospectively. In relation to *Montgomery*, many commentators have also made the point that the judgement merely put longstanding GMC guidance into effect.[1]

Clinical Commentary

Abdul H Sultan

Good Practice Guidance

Classification and Definitions

In the United Kingdom, approximately 85% of women having a vaginal delivery sustain some form of perineal trauma during vaginal delivery, and 69% of these lacerations will require to be sutured. This includes an episiotomy, which is a deliberate incision made by the midwife or doctor, and this will be discussed later.

However, prior to any suturing, a structured and comprehensive assessment needs to be performed to ensure that a third- or fourth-degree tear, collectively called Obstetric Anal Sphincter Injury (OASI), has not occurred. The new classification of perineal trauma described by Sultan in 1999 [1] has been accepted internationally (Figure 1) and published in the RCOG Green-top guidelines [2] since the first edition in July 2001.

---

[1] See, for example, *Montgomery and Informed Consent: Where Are We Now? BMJ 2017; 357: j2224.*

If the tear involves the rectal mucosa with an intact anal sphincter complex, it is, by definition, not a fourth-degree tear and should be recorded as a rectal buttonhole tear. However, although rare, a buttonhole tear can occur concomitantly with an OASI, in which case there is an intervening section of intact rectal mucosa between the two injuries. [3].

Assessment of Perineal Trauma

The following principles should be followed [2,4,5]:

- An explanation must be given to the woman as to what is planned and the reasons for the procedure. Informed consent should be obtained for vaginal and rectal examinations.
- If the examination is restricted because of pain, adequate analgesia such as inhalational or local anaesthesia must be given prior to examination.
- Ensure good lighting is available to enhance visibility.
- There must be adequate exposure of the genital structures and the perineal injury. If this is not possible, particularly when there are multiple and deep tears, then the woman should be placed in the lithotomy position.
- The initial examination must be performed gently and with sensitivity. Following a visual examination of the genitalia, the labia should be parted, and a vaginal examination should be performed to establish the full extent of all vaginal tears.
- In order to exclude an OASI or a rectal buttonhole tear, a systematic assessment of genital trauma should be performed as follows:
  - The woman should be asked to contract her anal sphincter, and if it is completely disrupted, a gap may be seen anteriorly. If the perineal skin is intact, there may be an absence of puckering on the perianal skin anteriorly. This may not be evident if the muscles are paralysed during regional or general anaesthesia.
  - A rectal examination should be performed by a trained midwife or doctor to exclude injury to the anorectal mucosa and anal sphincter. The vagina should be exposed by parting the labia with the thumb and index finger of the other hand. The index finger in the rectum should then be moved from side to side whilst elevating the anterior rectal wall so that the posterior vaginal wall can be visualised to exclude a rectal buttonhole tear.
  - Next, the woman should be asked to squeeze her anal sphincters and the injury should be confirmed by palpation.
  - Finally, by palpating the anal sphincter with the index finger in the anal canal and the thumb of the same hand placed at the vaginal outlet, the anal sphincter can be palpated by performing a pill-rolling motion and checking for continuity of the muscle ring [4]. This motion should start at the 9 o'clock position and continue until the 3 o'clock position, so that the whole anterior ring of the anal sphincter is palpated.
- The external anal sphincter (EAS) is the colour of red meat, and lies medial to an important landmark, the ischioanal fat [4,6].
- The Internal anal sphincter (IAS) is a circular smooth muscle that appears paler (similar to raw fish). Under normal circumstances, the distal end of the IAS lies a few millimetres proximal to the distal end of the EAS. However, if the EAS is relaxed

following regional or general anaesthesia, the distal end of the IAS will appear to be at a lower level. In general, if the IAS or anal epithelium is torn, the EAS will invariably be torn. It is possible to find a perineal tear extending to just inside the anal verge without disruption of the anal sphincters, but by definition this is not a fourth-degree tear.

• Advice should be sought from a more experienced healthcare professional if there is uncertainty about the nature or extent of the trauma.

• Findings of the assessment must be clearly documented, preferably including a drawing to accurately illustrate the full extent of the trauma.

First- and Second-degree Tears

First-degree tears involve the skin of the perineum but superficial skin injuries that do not involve muscle can occur on the labia and vagina. Unless the skin edges are well opposed, it is recommended that the wound should be sutured in order to improve healing. If the trauma is bilateral, the lacerations can sometimes adhere to each other and form labial adhesions which can cause difficulty during sexual intercourse, and voiding difficulties if covering the urethral orifice. If the tear is left unsutured, the midwife or doctor must discuss the implications with the woman and this should be fully documented.

Second-degree tears involve the skin and perineal muscles. The torn muscles should be sutured to avoid gaping wounds. However, prior to suturing, a rectal examination is mandatory to exclude an OASI.

Episiotomy

An episiotomy is an incision performed to enlarge the vaginal outlet to facilitate delivery of the baby. In the United Kingdom (and most parts of the world) only mediolateral episiotomies are performed, although there are some that perform lateral episiotomies, while median (midline) episiotomies are prevalent in the United States. Midline episiotomies are known to have a high risk of being associated with an OASI following extension of the incision. The mediolateral episiotomy is an incision that commences within 1 cm of the posterior fourchette of the vagina and is directed away from the anal sphincter. It has previously been taught that the angle should be at 40–60 degrees and the technique recommended was to cut from the posterior fourchette towards the ischial tuberosity. However, more recently, it has been shown that an episiotomy cut at 40 degrees during distension of the perineum by the baby's head results in a sutured angle of 22 degrees, and episiotomies cut at 60 degrees resulted in sutured angles of 45 degrees [2]. It was also found that the suture angle of the episiotomy at 45 degrees resulted in a 20-fold OASIs reduction compared to a sutured episiotomy angle of 25 degrees.

Mediolateral episiotomy should be considered in instrumental deliveries. Where episiotomy is indicated, the mediolateral technique is recommended, with careful attention to ensure that the angle is 60 degrees away from the midline when the perineum is distended [2,7]. The RCOG guidance recommends a 60-degree angled episiotomy at the time of crowning and stresses the difference between the incision angle and the sutured episiotomy angle. The guidance also asserts that sutured episiotomy angles of 40–60 degrees are more important that the incision angles of 45–60 degrees [2].

If an episiotomy is performed, the recommended technique is a mediolateral episiotomy originating at the vaginal fourchette and usually directed to the right side. The angle to the vertical axis should be between 45 and 60 degrees at the time of the episiotomy. A policy of routine episiotomy for all vaginal deliveries has not been shown to reduce OASIs. NICE recommends to "perform an episiotomy if there is a clinical need, such as instrumental birth or suspected fetal compromise".

When carrying out perineal repair, the doctor or midwife must ensure that tested effective analgesia is in place, using adequate local anaesthetic or top up of the epidural if necessary. After identifying the apex of the vaginal incision, perineal repair should be performed using a continuous non-locked suturing technique for the vaginal wall and muscle layer, followed by a subcutaneous suture to the skin. If a different suture technique is used, the reasons for departure from the recommended technique should be documented.

It is important to ensure good anatomical alignment of the wound to achieve good cosmetic results.

A thorough rectal examination should be performed after the repair to ensure that a suture has not been inadvertently inserted through the rectal mucosa. If present or in case of any doubt, the repair should be undone and the suture removed. It would be prudent to provide antibiotic cover for at least three days. If the rectal suture is not removed there is a risk of developing a rectovaginal fistula that may only form after necrosis some 7 to 10 days later.

Assisted Vaginal Birth

Assisted vaginal birth is performed by forceps or vacuum in 10–15% of pregnant women but is required in one of three nulliparous women. It should be performed by, or in the presence of, an operator who has the knowledge, skills and experience necessary to assess the woman, complete the procedure and manage any complications that arise [7]. In the absence of any contraindication to a particular instrument, the choice of instrument is operator-dependent but should involve and respect the woman's wishes.

The RCOG guideline on OASI [2] states that there is evidence that a mediolateral episiotomy should be performed with instrumental deliveries as it appears to have a protective effect on OASI. The odds ratios are as follows:

Ventouse delivery without episiotomy (OR 1.89, 95% CI 1.74–2.05)

Ventouse delivery with episiotomy (OR 0.57, 95% CI 0.51–0.63)

Forceps delivery without episiotomy (OR 6.53, 95% CI 5.57–7.64)

Forceps delivery with episiotomy (OR 1.34, 95% CI 1.21–1.49)

However, the RCOG guideline on Assisted Vaginal Delivery [7] states that "mediolateral episiotomy should be discussed with the woman as part of the preparation for assisted vaginal birth. In the absence of robust evidence to support either routine or restrictive use of episiotomy at assisted vaginal birth, the decision should be tailored to the circumstances at the time and the preferences of the woman. The evidence to support the use of mediolateral episiotomy at assisted vaginal birth in terms of preventing OASI is stronger for nulliparous women and for birth via forceps".

These guidelines lack consistency and clarity in terms of which "circumstances" should be taken into consideration in deciding whether to perform an episiotomy or not. Clearly, the preferences of the woman should be respected as with any other aspect of obstetrics, but it does imply that prior counselling must be performed in the antenatal period and the wishes of the woman should be documented. When midpelvic or rotational delivery is anticipated, the risks and benefits of assisted vaginal birth versus that of second stage caesarean section should be considered in the light of the skill of the operator. The woman should always be involved in the decision-making process, and written consent should be obtained for a trial of assisted vaginal birth in an operating theatre.

Third- and Fourth-degree Tears (Obstetric Anal Sphincter Injuries)

In the United Kingdom, the overall mean reported national rate of OASI is 2.9% (range 0–8%), and 6% (range 0–15%) of women having their first vaginal delivery will sustain an OASI. Risk factors have been identified and include first vaginal delivery, Asian ethnicity, birthweight >4kg, shoulder dystocia, occipito-posterior position, and prolonged second stage of labour [2]. Unfortunately, these risk factors are not predictive of a woman sustaining an OASI and the risk factors are not necessarily cumulative. Therefore, more importantly is the ability of the midwife and doctor to identify the full extent of the injury. As midwives perform most of the deliveries in the United Kingdom, it is more important that they develop the expertise to identify the injury so that they can escalate subsequent management to the obstetrician.

It has been shown that a number of OASIs previously believed to be "occult" (only identified by endoanal ultrasound) [8] were in fact clinically missed OASIs [9]. This led to the development of structured hands-on perineal and anal sphincter trauma courses [6] which have now been established internationally. When an OASI is diagnosed (or even suspected), the woman should be taken to the operating theatre and examined under regional anaesthesia. The consent process should include a full explanation of the intended procedure and the specific risks which should include wound breakdown, anal incontinence in up to 40% of women and the need for further sphincter surgery. A rectovaginal fistula is also another complication that occurs in less than 5% of women, but those who have sustained a fourth-degree tear are more at risk. The full extent of the injury should be established and classified as per Figure 6.1.

Repair should only be performed by a competent clinician or under supervision. When a fourth-degree tear is identified, the torn rectal mucosa should be repaired from the apex to just outside the anal verge using a continuous absorbable suture (Vicryl 3-0). The next important structure is the IAS which is adjacent and adherent to the anal mucosa. The IAS would be easily recognisable following a fourth-degree tear and should be repaired by approximation (end-to-end) repair using interrupted (preferably mattress sutures). No attempt should be made to perform an overlap repair of the IAS. The EAS should then be repaired using either the end-to-end or overlapping technique depending on the mobility of the torn ends of the muscle and operator expertise. It is important to identify and confirm that the torn ends of muscle are part of the EAS by performing the finger elevation test (insertion of the finger in the anal canal and grasping the torn ends of the muscle with Allis forceps). Elevation of the Allis forceps must be accompanied by elevation and tightening of the finger in the anal canal. This ensures that the torn superficial transverse perineal muscle is not inadvertently mistaken for the EAS [10]. It is also important that the full length of the torn EAS is exposed before suturing, as restoration of the full length of the sphincter is the best predictor of continence.

First-degree tear: Injury to perineal skin and/or vaginal mucosa

Second-degree tear: Injury to perineum involving perineal muscles but not involving the anal sphincter

Third-degree tear: Injury to perineum involving the anal sphincter complex:

Grade 3a tear: Less than 50% of external anal sphincter (EAS) thickness torn.

Grade 3b tear: More than 50% of EAS thickness torn.

Grade 3c tear: Both EAS and internal anal sphincter (IAS) torn.

Fourth-degree tear: Injury to perineum involving the anal sphincter complex (EAS and IAS) and anorectal mucosa.

Rectal Buttonhole Tear

Isolated rectal tear with or without injury to the anal sphincter (as above)

Figure 6.1 The Sultan classification of perineal trauma [1–3].

For grade 3c tears, the torn IAS should be repaired as described above. Grade 3a and partial thickness grade 3b tears should always be repaired by end-to-end approximation. An overlap repair can only be performed with full thickness EAS tears so that the two free ends can be grasped and pulled across.

The perineal muscles and skin are then sutured as described above, followed by a rectal examination.

While the rising OASI rate has been attributed to improvements in training and diagnosis, there is also emerging concern that there may be an element of overdiagnosis [10]. Hands-on workshops using models, animal tissue, and audiovisual aids have been shown to be effective in improving knowledge, recognition of the full extent of the injury, better classification, and improvements in repair techniques [11].

Post-operative Care and Follow-up after Obstetric Anal Sphincter Injuries

Intra-operative intravenous antibiotics should always be given for OASIs and depending on local protocols this can be continued orally for up to 5 days. Stool softeners such as Lactulose should be prescribed for 10 to 14 days to minimise the risk of stool impaction and wound dehiscence. Pelvic floor and anal sphincter exercises should be encouraged, preferably by a physiotherapist. It is important that debriefing by the obstetric team is conducted prior to discharge. A patient information leaflet such as the one produced by the RCOG or equivalent should be provided [12]. The patient should be made aware that if bowel action has not occurred within three days of the repair that she will need stronger laxatives.

Follow-up should be performed at a convenient time (usually 6–12 weeks postpartum) and where possible, review should be made by clinicians with a special interest in OASIs. Ideally, follow-up should be in a dedicated perineal clinic with access to endoanal ultrasonography and anal manometry, as this can aid decision-making for future deliveries. The perineal clinic can be multidisciplinary such that it allows for further debriefing and provides specialist advice at a dedicated focal point [13].

Management of Subsequent Pregnancies

There are no systematic reviews or randomised controlled trials to suggest the best method of delivery following OASIS. Although there has been one randomised control trial on the role of caesarean section in preventing anal incontinence after asymptomatic OASIs (diagnosed by endoanal ultrasound), only one fifth of the women in this study had a previous repair of an OASI [14]. There have also been concerns raised regarding the definition of defects and subsequent management [15]. The risk of sustaining a further third- or fourth-degree tear after a subsequent delivery is up to 10% [16]. The RCOG guideline states that "all women who have sustained OASIs in a previous pregnancy and who are symptomatic or have abnormal endoanal ultrasonography and/or manometry should be counselled regarding the option of elective caesarean birth" [2]. Counselling these women is essential but more importantly, they need to be given consistent advice by an obstetric perineal clinic specialist. These patients need to be informed of the following so that they can make an informed decision:

1. The risk of recurrence of an OASI in a subsequent pregnancy is between 5–10% [16] and is therefore higher than the rate expected in multiparous women (1.7%).
2. When outcome of continence status following a subsequent pregnancy is based on criteria relating to endoanal scan and manometry, there was no significant difference between caesarean and vaginal delivery [17]. Based on these criteria, 70% of women underwent a vaginal delivery after OASIs.
3. There is evidence from a large multicentre study of 2,272 primiparous women who sustained OASIs that a prophylactic mediolateral episiotomy during a subsequent vaginal delivery reduces the risk of a subsequent OASI by 80% [16].
4. There is no data on outcome of mode of delivery based on the presence or absence of symptoms of anal incontinence or findings on digital examination.
5. In the case of fourth-degree tears, it has been shown that based on RCOG the criteria, 93% of women would be counselled for a caesarean section. Therefore, in the absence of endoanal and manometry scan facilities, it would not be unreasonable to offer these women a caesarean section [18].
6. The risk of developing a repeat OASI is similar to the risk factors associated with first OASI and should be taken into consideration during counselling [2,19].
7. All women should be counselled regarding the short- and long-term effects of single and repeat caesarean sections.

Training and Competence

According to the 2019 RCOG core curriculum, the trainee must complete at least three summative OSATS (Objective Structured Assessment of Technical Skills) confirming competence by more than one assessor. At least one OSATS confirming competence should be supervised by a consultant. Competence at perineal suturing should be achieved at ST2 level (including attendance of a third-degree tear course), and OASI repair at ST4 level. The first hands-on perineal and anal sphincter trauma course was commenced in 2000 [6] and is now conducted internationally. In order to maintain consistency, there does need to be a standardisation of the curriculum and hands-on component of these courses at a national level. The difficulty in certifying competence is that a trainee may achieve competence in repairing three Grade 3a/3b tears and be signed off for OASI repair, having not done a grade 3c or fourth-degree tear repair. The trainee should therefore take the necessary precautions of supervision when performing repairs unsupervised. NICE recommends that all relevant healthcare professionals should attend training in perineal/genital assessment and repair and ensure that they maintain these skills.

Causes of Litigation

In the United Kingdom, perineal trauma was the fourth highest reason for obstetric medico-legal claims in obstetrics over a 10-year period, accounting for about 9% of claims. Of the 441 claims made for perineal trauma, 31 million pounds were paid out.

Allegations of negligence include failure to:

1. Abandon vaginal delivery and consider a caesarean section.
2. Appropriately apply delivery instruments.
3. Perform an episiotomy, particularly with forceps.
4. Perform an adequate episiotomy at the correct angle.
5. Diagnose the true extent of and appropriately classify the injury, including failure to perform a proper rectal examination.
6. Diagnose a buttonhole injury of the rectum.
7. Appropriately align the perineal repair to achieve an acceptable cosmetic result.
8. Repair conducted by doctor or midwife not certified for competence.
9. Request for timely colorectal assistance for extensive rectal injuries.
10. Repair the anal sphincter injury inadequately or not at all.
11. Perform a rectal examination after the repair to check for sutures inserted inadvertently; failure to diagnose and remove them to prevent the development of a rectovaginal fistula.
12. Provide a duty of candour, appropriate communication and adequate post-partum care.

Avoidance of Litigation

Firstly, midwives and doctors owe a duty of care and candour to pregnant women. Although it is not possible to include information on every aspect of care during the antenatal classes, issues pertaining to decisions and consent under emergency conditions must be discussed antenatally. The preferences of the woman must be documented in the birth plan together with the agreed plan with the midwife/obstetrician. Further discussion and confirmation should take place when the woman and birth partner come for delivery.

National, RCOG and local guidelines should be adhered to and any deviation should be justified and documented accordingly. Any clinician who has failed to adhere to national guidelines and does not have a reasonable explanation for his/her actions will be inviting the court to uphold the allegations of negligence [20].

A doctor or midwife who has not completed their requirements for competency should always perform the procedure under supervision. If there is any doubt about a diagnosis, a second opinion should always be sought from a senior colleague. With particular reference to diagnosis of OASIs, the steps outlined above must be followed and documented, particularly the rectal examination before and after the repair. Particular attention needs to be paid to the diagnosis of IAS injuries and clear documentation must be made regarding the fact that it was looked for. If an injury is identified, it must be repaired separately [2]. The technique of identifying the EAS and repair must be described in detail.

It is very important to ensure that there is no contradiction between the midwifery notes and the doctor's notes. Evidence of ensuring fine detail in note-keeping will be very supportive during investigations of adverse outcomes.

As part of the duty of candour, one must be frank and open with the woman (and birth partner) regarding any complications, and it is recommended that every attempt is made to see the woman the next day for debriefing. If this is not possible, inform the woman that a colleague will be seeing her.

It is important to ensure that the community midwives have been alerted about any complications and appropriate follow-up has been arranged.

References

1. Sultan, AH. Obstetric perineal injury and anal incontinence. *Clin Risk* 1999; 5: 193–6.

2. Royal College of Obstetricians and Gynaecologists. RCOG Green-top Guideline No. 29. *Management of Third- and Fourth-degree Perineal Tears Following Vaginal Delivery.* London: RCOG Press; 2015.

3. Roper, JC, Thakar, R, Sultan, AH. Isolated rectal buttonhole tears in obstetrics: case series and review of the literature. *Int Urogynecol J* 2021; 32(3): 745.

4. Sultan, AH, Thakar, R, Fenner, D. *Perineal and Anal Sphincter Trauma.* London: Springer; 2007, 13–32.

5. National Institute of Health and Care Excellence. Intrapartum Care [CG190]. London: NICE; 2014. Available at: www .nice.org.uk/guidance/cg190

6. www.perineum.net

7. Murphy, DJ, Strachan, BK, Bahl, R, *on behalf of the Royal College of Obstetricians Gynaecologists.* Assisted Vaginal Birth. *BJOG* 2020. https://doi.org/10.1111/1471-0528.16092

8. Sultan, AH, Kamm, MA, Hudson, CN, Thomas, JM, Bartram, CI. Anal sphincter disruption during vaginal delivery. *New Engl J Med* 1993; 329: 1905–11.

9. Andrews, V, Thakar, R, Sultan, AH, Jones, PW. Occult anal sphincter injuries – myth or reality? *BJOG* 2006; 113: 195–200.

10. Sioutis, D, Thakar, R, Sultan, AH. Overdiagnosis and rising rate of obstetric anal sphincter injuries (OASIS): time for reappraisal. *Ultrasound Obstet Gynecol* 2017; 50(5): 642–7.

11. Andrews, V, Thakar, R, Sultan, AH. Outcome of an obstetric anal sphincter injury can be optimised by structured training and using an evidence-based protocol. *Int Urogynecol J* 2009; 20(2): 973–8.

12. Royal College of Obstetricians and Gynaecologists. *A Third- or Fourth-degree Tear during Birth: Information for You.* London: RCOG; 2015.

13. Wan, OYK, Taithongchai, A, Veiga, SI, Sultan, AH, Thakar, R. A one-stop perineal clinic: our eleven-year experience. *Int Urogynecol J* 2020; 31(11): 2317–26.

14. Abramowitz, L, Mandelbrot, L, Bourgeois Moine, A, Tohic, AL, Carne Carnavalet C, Poujade, O, Roy, C, Tubach, F. Caesarean section in the second delivery to prevent anal incontinence after asymptomatic obstetric anal sphincter injury: the EPIC multicentre randomised trial. *BJOG* 2020. https://doi.org/10.1111/1471- 0528.16452

15. Okeahialam, NA, Wong, KW, Roper, J, Thakar, R, Sultan, AH. Cesarean section in the second delivery to prevent anal incontinence after asymptomatic obstetrical anal sphincter injury: the EPIC multicentre randomised trial. *BJOG* 2021; 128(4): 770–1.

16. D'Souza, JC, Monga, A, Tincello, DG, Sultan, AH, Thakar, R, Hillard, TC, Grigsby, S, Kibria, A, Jordan, CF, Ashmore C. Maternal outcomes in subsequent delivery after previous obstetric anal sphincter injury (OASI): a multi-centre retrospective cohort study. *Int Urogynecol J* 2020; 31(3): 627–33.

17. Jordan, PA, Naidu, M, Thakar, R, Sultan, AH. Effect of subsequent vaginal delivery on bowel symptoms and anorectal function in women who sustained a previous obstetric anal sphincter injury. *Int Urogynecol J* 2018; 29(11): 1579–88.

18. Taithongchai, A, Thakar, R, Sultan, AH. Management of subsequent pregnancies following fourth-degree obstetric anal sphincter injuries (OASIS). *Eur J Obstet Gynecol Reprod Biol* 2020; 250: 80–5.

19. Jha, S, Parker, V. Risk factors for recurrent obstetric anal sphincter injury (rOASI): a systematic review and meta-analysis. *Int Urogynecol J* 2016; 27(6): 849–57.

20. Sultan, AH, Ritchie, A, Mooney, G. Obstetric anal sphincter injuries: review of recent medico-legal aspects. *Clin Risk* 2016; 22(3–4): 57–60. https://doi.org/10.1177/1356262216676131.

Medical Disorders of Pregnancy

Kara Dent

CASE COMMENTARY

Swati Jha

Successful Claim

Cooper v Royal Berkshire NHS Foundation Trust [2015] EWHC 664 (QB)

The Claim

The claimant suffered irreversible hypoxic neurological damage five days postnatally and it was claimed this was a consequence of a cerebral venous thrombosis (CVT). It was claimed that the CVT occurred due to incorrect information regarding the mode of delivery and that she should have been advised against a vaginal birth after a previous caesarean section (CS) and also due to lack of consistent heparin postnatally which caused or contributed to the CVT.

The Summary

Mrs Cooper had her first delivery vaginally but elected to have a caesarean section in her second by choice. In her third pregnancy she opted to have a vaginal delivery after caesarean (VBAC) and there were multiple discussions about the mode of delivery as she had a previous caesarean section, including the risk of scar rupture. During the course of labour, she did suffer a uterine rupture which warranted an emergency CS but culminated in the death of the baby several weeks later.

After she was delivered, she was admitted to the ward and was prescribed heparin to prevent DVT/PE. She does not appear to have received this as prescribed, and several doses were missed. Her blood pressure was noted to be within normal range with the occasional level being raised at a diastolic >90mm Hg. Five days postnatally, she described a headache, vomiting and blood pressure was raised. Due to concerns with pre-eclampsia, a medical review was requested, but the claimant collapsed with evidence of having suffered a seizure and was in asystole. She suffered irreversible hypoxic neurological damage and never regained consciousness.

The defendant made the case that she had been adequately counselled about the risks of uterine rupture and that the cause of seizures was postpartum eclampsia (PPE) rather than a CVT. They admitted liability with regards the administration of heparin but denied that this contributed to her condition. The basis of this case therefore became establishing whether the cause of the seizure was a CVT or eclampsia. The CT scan failed to confirm a CVT, but its absence did not rule out the occurrence of the event.

The Judgement

It was admitted that the claimant suffered a seizure, leading to cardiac arrest and the resultant hypoxic brain injury caused either by a PPE or CVT. The arguments in favour of and against the diagnosis of both the PPE and the CVT were heard. Based on the occurrence of the seizure and cardiac arrest occurring five days postnatally when the patient was in a prothrombotic state and in the presence of several risk factors including uterine rupture, emergency CS, pyrexia, vomiting and immobility, a CVT was felt to be the more likely cause of events. This was contributed to by the inconsistent administration of heparin. On this basis the claimant was successful in establishing liability.

Unsuccessful Claim

Tanya Linehan v East Kent Hospitals University NHS Foundation Trust
The Claim

The claimant suffered a still birth of a term pregnancy. It was claimed that the defendant had failed to act on a diagnosis of pre-eclampsia and had they done so the baby would have been delivered alive. Failing to consider the issue of pre-eclampsia was a breach of duty and this caused further psychological harm to the claimant.

The Summary

The claimant was overweight with a BMI of 37 and pregnant with her first child. Antenatal progress was uneventful though it was noted that the baby was large and there was excess fluid around the baby as well as oedema of the legs and feet. Tests for gestational diabetes were performed twice and reported to be negative. Blood pressure readings during the antenatal period were normal. A plan was made for induction of labour postdates, as per hospital policy.

Ms Linehan presented to her GP nine days before the due induction date with swelling and headaches and was referred to hospital for further review. Blood pressure on admission to hospital was marginally raised at 150/94 but settled to 134/84, and there were 2+ protein in her urine dipstick but the protein creatinine ratio (PCR), a more reliable indicator of proteinuria, was within normal range at 21. The uric acid was noted to be raised but other parameters were normal. By the time the claimant attended hospital the headache was settled. She was therefore discharged home as pre-eclampsia was not confirmed, hence there was no indication for immediate delivery. She came back three days later with tightenings, but on this occasion no further concerns about pre-eclampsia were raised as her blood pressure was normal and there was no proteinuria.

She came back the same evening and fetal demise was diagnosed.

The Judgement

The guidelines used to establish breach of duty were the NICE Clinical Guideline Number 107, "Hypertension in pregnancy: the management of hypertensive disorders during pregnancy" (August 2010). It was agreed that hypertension is significant if there were two consecutive readings on >90mm Hg several hours apart, which was not the case in the instance of Ms Linehan. In addition, she had no significant proteinuria, hence the diagnosis of pre-eclampsia was not substantiated. Though uric acid was raised, this was not part of the criteria for the diagnosis of pre-eclampsia but was of relevance once a diagnosis was confirmed. During both hospital attendances, when the opportunity to deliver her arose prior to the stillbirth, there was no clinical indication to do so, and the clinical decisions made were reasonable in light of what was known. The claim therefore failed on breach of duty.

Legal Commentary

Eloise Power

Cooper v Royal Berkshire NHS Foundation Trust [2015] EWHC 664 (QB)

The tragic history of this case illustrates the risks that remain in pregnancy and delivery for mothers as well as for infants. The claimant, at the age of 36, underwent a vaginal birth after CS in her third pregnancy. She suffered a uterine rupture, as a result of which her baby and the placenta entered the peritoneal cavity. Sadly, the baby suffered an hypoxic injury and died shortly before his second birthday. Following the birth, the claimant remained in hospital. Five days later, she suffered a cardiac arrest. As a result, she sustained irreversible hypoxic neurological damage. The underlying events happened almost a decade before the case came to trial. During those years the claimant never regained consciousness. Proceedings were brought by her partner, who acted as her litigation friend.

The defendant admitted breach of duty in respect of the lack of post-natal provision of Heparin. It was common ground that if the cause of the cardiac arrest was a CVT, then the provision of Heparin would have been causative of the claimant's current condition. Causation was in dispute: the claimant argued that the cause of the cardiac arrest was a central venous thrombosis (CVT), whereas the defendant argued that the cause of the cardiac arrest was post-partum eclampsia (PPE).

This key question could not be answered with medical or diagnostic certainty, as the Court recognised at paragraph 80 of the judgement. The Court's task was to evaluate competing expert opinions in multiple disciplines (obstetricians and gynaecologists, obstetric physicians, neuroradiologists and neurologists) in order to arrive at a judgement on the balance of probabilities. In a careful and thorough judgement, Jeremy Baker J found that on the balance of probabilities, the cause of the cardiac arrest was a CVT, and that the claimant had accordingly succeeded in establishing liability against the defendant.

The approach which the Court took to the statistical evidence is of interest. In his conclusions, Jeremy Baker J found as follows:

> It is clear that at the outset of the trial the main focus of the defendant's case was its submissions relating to the relative incidence of the occurrence of PPE over CVTs. However, I consider that when properly analysed and due regard is had to the timing of the cardiac arrest, the evidence does not support those submissions. If any differential in favour of the incidence of PPE exists, then in my judgment it is so relatively insignificant as to carry little weight in the overall consideration of this case. In the event however, for the reasons I have set out above, I am persuaded that at 5 days post partum it is unlikely that there is any differential.

The defendant expert obstetric physician, Dr Pirie, had observed that (in general terms) the prevalence of PPE is far commoner than CVT "by an order of at least two magnitudes". However, the claimant expert obstetric physician, Dr Williams, had broken down the statistics with closer attention to the circumstances of the claimant's individual case: the claimant's risk of pre-eclampsia was 1%; of the patients with pre-eclampsia, only 1% develop eclampsia, only 20% suffer post-partum eclampsia after the first 24 hours post-partum, the majority of women with the condition have children with a poor birth weight (the weight of the claimant's baby was normal), and there is an absence of hypertension in only 20% of cases where a woman has an eclamptic seizure (the claimant's systolic blood pressure was normal). By contrast, between 25–30% of all CVTs occur in relation to pregnancy, most commonly in the post-partum period: the Court found that the incidence of peripartum and post-partum sinus thrombosis was about 12 cases per 100,000 deliveries, even though the absolute risk of CVT in the population as a whole was three to four cases per million.[1] Taken in conjunction with the radiology, the clinical presentation and the history, the Court preferred the claimant's evidence.

Use of Statistical Evidence

The judgement in *Cooper* illustrates the importance of ensuring that statistical evidence is applied in a manner which is as relevant as possible to the facts of the particular case before the Court. The broader issue of the approach which the Courts should take to statistical evidence was considered more recently by the Court of Appeal in *Schembri v Marshall* [2020] EWCA Civ 358. *Schembri v Marshall* was a fatal case involving an untreated pulmonary embolism. The key issue was whether the deceased would have survived with appropriate treatment. Giving unanimous judgement for the Court of Appeal, McCombe LJ made the following findings in relation to the use of statistical evidence:

(a) He approved the following statement from *Clerk & Lindsell on Torts*:[2] *"The assessment of causation would turn upon the detailed medical evidence, both as to the overall statistical chances of survival and the particular condition and circumstances of the patient"* [para 44].

(b) He summarised the general position as follows, citing *Clerk & Lindsell on Torts*:[3] *"Proof of causation is almost inevitably about a burden of persuasion and sometimes statistics can be highly persuasive"* [para 46].

(c) He observed that the trial judge was correct in having regard to the medical literature and the overall mortality of patients. The trial judge's approach was *"also legitimate because of the 'large number of unknowns' to which the judge referred and because the reason why the actual outcome is not known is that the admitted negligence prevented it becoming known"* [para 50–51]. This point can be compared with the approach taken in *Keefe v Isle of Man Steam Packet Co Ltd [2010] EWCA Civ 683* and applied in the context of clinical negligence and causation in *Younas v Dr Okeahialam [2019] EWHC 2502*: please see Chapter 15 for a more detailed discussion of these cases. Neither *Keefe* nor *Younas* were cited in the judgement in *Schembri v Marshall*.

(d) He found that the trial judge was right to take the *"'common sense and pragmatic view' of the 'evidence as a whole'"* [para 53].

---

[1] Para 94.
[2] Twenty-second edition, 2018, para 2–30, p75.
[3] *Supra*, para 2–30.

(e) He found that the trial judge was entitled to be satisfied that the deceased's death would have been prevented with treatment in hospital even *"without being able to prove the precise mechanism of survival to the requisite standard"* [para 56].

(f) He found that statistics had not been determinative of causation, but that *"there is a legitimate place for statistical evidence in cases of this type. The employment of that evidence by the judge in this case was closely linked by him to his assessment of the evidence as to the Deceased's own particular condition, in which her prospects of survival (on hypothetical admission to hospital) were very good indeed."* [para 56].

Although *Cooper* predates the Court of Appeal's judgement in *Schembri v Marshall*, it is clear that Jeremy Baker J's approach was similar to that which was endorsed by the Court of Appeal. The lessons which emerge from both cases are: statistical evidence has a legitimate part to play in establishing causation; statistical evidence cannot be considered in isolation from the test results, clinical presentation, history and individual characteristics of the claimant; statistical evidence will be most persuasive where it is tailored as far as possible to the particular circumstances of the claimant.

Tanya Linehan v East Kent Hospitals University NHS Foundation Trust (Unreported, 3 July 2018)
Approach to NICE Guidelines

This case is of some interest because of the approach to the NICE Guidelines taken by the expert instructed by the claimant. The key issue which fell for consideration by the Court was whether the claimant's baby should have been delivered earlier (on 1 November 2012 or the morning of 4 November 2012). It was common ground that earlier delivery would have prevented the stillbirth of the claimant's baby; the baby died at some point prior to 9 pm on 4 November 2012.

The Court considered the applicability of NICE CG 107, "Hypertension in pregnancy: the management of hypertensive disorders during pregnancy", published in August 2010. The expert instructed by the claimant accepted that pre-eclampsia could not have been diagnosed *"on a strict interpretation"* of the test set out in the Guideline [para 71]. However, he nevertheless maintained that all obstetricians would have ignored the Guideline, diagnosed pre-eclampsia and proceeded to deliver the baby. Unsurprisingly, this approach did not find favour with the Court. In the trenchant words of HHJ Robinson [underlining added]:

> 73. *Mr Duthie stated his final position clearly and unambiguously. I wrote it down and read it back to him to ensure its accuracy. He agreed that this is an accurate statement of his final position, 'all obstetricians would ignore the NICE Guidelines in this case and would diagnose pre-eclampsia and get the baby out'. I omitted to describe the body of obstetricians as reasonable, but this is what I and I am sure Mr Duthie meant.*

> 74. *I am afraid that I have been left with the clear impression that Mr Duthie has approached this case back to front. He has concluded that baby Ashton should have been delivered on 1 November 2012 and sought to justify that result by a variety of means. One of those means is the startling proposition that all, not merely some, but all reasonable obstetricians would have departed from the NICE Guidelines and made a diagnosis of pre-eclampsia and such diagnosis was clearly contraindicated by reference to the NICE Guidelines. I simply cannot accept that. . .*

> 76. *It is with regret that I conclude on this occasion Mr Duthie has lost his objective focus. In his desire, I may say understandable desire, in this tragic case to reach conclusions favourable for the claimant, he has resorted to forensic analysis upon which I am unable to place reliance."*

Further consideration is given to the use of NICE Guidelines at Chapter 9. On the one hand, it is likely to be correct to observe that the NICE Guidelines are clinical guidelines created for practical purposes and that they do not have the force of law.[4] On the other hand, it is unlikely to be persuasive to argue that NICE Guidelines should be ignored altogether – still less to go further than that and to argue that clinicians had a positive duty to ignore the Guidelines, as the claimant expert sought to do in *Linehan*.

The Court's observations emphasise the importance for experts of ensuring that they maintain objectivity, analyse breach of duty from a prospective viewpoint and approach cases in a logical manner; these issues are considered further at Chapter 3.

Damages for Breach of Duty of Candour

A further point of interest arising from the *Linehan* judgement is that the claimant sought to argue that she was entitled to damages for psychiatric injury arising from an alleged breach of the defendant's duty of candour. The allegation was that the defendant's investigation and Root Cause Analysis report were inadequate because they did not consider pre-eclampsia as a cause of the baby's death.

As the Court recognised (and as was agreed by both Counsel), the imposition of a duty of care which sounded in damages would amount to an *"incremental and novel case"*. In the absence of directly relevant authority, the Court would have to consider the general legal criteria relating to the imposition of a duty of care in novel contexts arising from *Caparo v Dickman* [1990] UKHL 2: in other words, (a) whether damage had been suffered; (b) proximity of relationship and (c) the reasonableness or otherwise of imposing a duty. Counsel for the defendant made the important point that the duty of candour was created by Regulation 20 of the Health and Social Care Act 2008 (Regulated Activities) Regulations 2014, which came into force on 6 November 2014. The 2014 Regulations do not provide for a civil remedy in damages to be provided in the event of a breach of the duty of candour.

Unfortunately, the issue did not fall to be determined as a matter of law. The Court held that the allegation failed on the facts, as the claimant had not made out that she suffered from pre-eclampsia. Further, the defendant had considered pre-eclampsia as a potential cause of death in any event. As far as the author is aware, the question of whether a free-standing right to claim damages exists for breach of the statutory duty of candour remains unanswered by the Courts.

Clinical Commentary

Kara Dent

Introduction

In recent years, the incidence of medical disorders seen in pregnancy is on the increase. This is predominantly because of increasing maternal age and also better understanding and treatment of medical conditions. This understanding allows patients with these diseases to consider the possibility of becoming pregnant, when they would have been advised against it before. The most recent MBRRACE-UK report (2016–2018) recognises

---

[4] *Sanderson v Guy's and St Thomas' NHS Foundation Trust* [2020] EWHC 20 (QB).

that two thirds of maternal deaths occurred in women with pre-existing medical disorders. Cardiac disease remains the commonest cause (23%), with neurological disorders, such as epilepsy and stroke, the third most common [1]. This highlights the need for good antenatal care of these complex conditions to reduce both maternal and fetal complications.

When assessing the stillbirths in the 2015 MBRRACE report, the commonest underlying maternal diseases found were diabetes and hypertensive disease. The assessors felt that when looking at all these cases, 60% of the stillbirths could have been prevented with better antenatal care. This report particularly highlighted the concerns of undiagnosed and untreated gestational diabetes (GDM). They recommended focusing on improving the detection and management of this pregnancy-specific disorder in order to reduce the national stillbirth rate [2].

NHS Resolution published a report on 10 years of maternity claims (from 2000–2010), looking at a total of just over 5,000 claims in all. Antenatal care accounted for 7.6% of claims, whilst antenatal investigations came to 4.5%. Together then, these show that 14.1% of successful claims were because of poor antenatal care or interpretation of antenatal investigations.

Maternal medicine is a vast subject in itself, but for the purposes of this chapter, we will concentrate on those conditions that are more commonly found in medicolegal cases: diabetes, hypertensive diseases and neurological disorders including epilepsy and stroke. Principles of good maternal obstetric care are common to all these diseases and will be outlined in the guidance.

Good Practice Guidance

Pre-existing Diabetes in Pregnancy

We have seen the prevalence of diabetes rise in the last decade, particularly in type 2 diabetics, as a consequence of increased maternal age and rising obesity rates. For the first time, type 2 diabetics are more prevalent than type 1. However, for the purpose of a pregnancy, they are treated and managed the same.

In assessing common causes of stillbirths, women with pre-existing diabetes in pregnancy are known to carry a four- to six-fold increase in stillbirths compared with a pregnancy without diabetes, and careful multi-disciplinary team (MDT) management in pregnancy is crucial to reduce this risk. Good practice would be to offer this cohort careful pre-pregnancy counselling in order to optimise blood sugar control and start them on high dose folic acid (5mg). If the HbA1c is raised at conception, there is an increased risk of congenital conditions, namely cardiac and neural tube defects. The upper limit of normal for HbA1c levels is 48 mmol/l (6.5%). HbA1c levels should be taken at booking and then again in the second and third trimesters of the pregnancy, in order to monitor diabetic control.

Once pregnant, this group are booked immediately under an MDT that comprises of a named consultant obstetrician, diabetic physician, diabetic specialist midwife, diabetic specialist nurses and dieticians. With organogenesis and development of the fetal structures and organs occurring in the first 11 weeks of the pregnancy, careful diabetic management is essential to reduce risks of congenital abnormalities.

At 12 weeks they have a dating scan and are started on low dose aspirin (75–150 mg) to reduce the risk of pre-eclampsia (PET) in pregnancy [3], as we know that diabetics are at two-fold increased risk of PET. An anomaly scan is arranged between 18–20+6 weeks as per the national Fetal Anomaly Screening Programme (FASP)recommendation. Ultrasound surveillance for growth and liquor is then four-weekly from 28 weeks gestation. These babies are at an increased risk of macrosomia with poor diabetic control or intrauterine growth restriction (associated with PET).

Delivery is advised between 37 weeks and 38 weeks plus 6 days. This is to reduce the risk of stillbirth or complications, having reached a gestation when the baby is mature enough to deliver. Maternal steroid administration is advised for fetal maturation if delivering by caesarean section (CS) (before 38+6 weeks). Babies born to diabetic mothers on insulin have an increased risk of respiratory distress syndrome due to reduced surfactant production, and steroid administration will reduce this risk by up to 50%.

Diabetic Ketoacidosis (DKA) is a serious complication of diabetes that can have consequences for both mother and baby. Pregnant diabetic women are at increased risk of DKA due to the relative or complete absence of insulin together with an increase in pregnancy hormones. The physiology of pregnancy means their bodies have a lower buffering ability so DKA can occur more quickly than we are used to seeing outside pregnancy.

These patients present feeling unwell, with nausea and vomiting, lethargy or ketotic breath (smells like pear drops). The diagnosis is made on investigation:

- Known diabetic or blood glucose >11.0 mmol/l
- Capillary blood ketone level ≥ 3 mmol/l or ++ketones or more on urinalysis
- Venous bicarbonate <15 mmol/l +/− venous PH <7.3

A life-threatening condition for the mother, DKA also carries risk for the fetus. This is thought to be due to the effects of the maternal acidosis and electrolyte imbalance with a corresponding volume depletion in the mother that may then affect placental flow.

Treatment must be immediate and requires:

1. Aggressive fluid replacement
2. Insulin infusion
3. Electrolyte correction
4. Identification and correction of cause

Common causes include hyperemesis gravidarum (vomiting in pregnancy) and infection.

Gestational Diabetes in Pregnancy

It is estimated that 16 out of a 100 woman will develop gestational diabetes (GDM) in their pregnancies. Undiagnosed, and therefore untreated, GDM carries a higher stillbirth risk than a non-diabetic pregnancy – with a raised fasting plasma glucose they are at a four-fold greater risk of stillbirth [3,4]. GDM is a condition specific to pregnancy where there is increased insulin resistance secondary to the increase in hormones such as cortisol and progesterone. The main culprit however is human placental lactogen produced by the placenta, hence its effect increases as the pregnancy continues and the placenta grows.

Careful monitoring of these pregnancies is essential to avoid macrosomia and large for gestational age (LGA) babies that are then at a higher risk of delivery complications, specifically the risk of shoulder dystocia.

Screening for GDM is done at 24–28 weeks into the pregnancy with an oral glucose tolerance test (OGTT) – most UK centres do the 75g two-hour test, with a diagnosis made if the fasting plasma glucose is 5.6 mmol/l or more or the two-hour plasma glucose level is 7.8 mmol/l or above. If they have had a previous pregnancy with GDM, this screening test is recommended sooner, after the booking visit [5]. As it is very likely they will have GDM again in the current pregnancy, it allows earlier monitoring and possible treatment. If the first test is negative, it should be repeated at the later gestation of 24–28 weeks.

The population at risk of GDM include:
- BMI above 30 kg/m^2
- Previous macrosomic baby weighing 4.5 kg or more
- Previous GDM
- Family history of diabetes in first-degree relatives
- Ethnicity: Asian/Hispanic/Black, African-Caribbean or Middle Eastern origin
- Glycosuria of 2+ on one occasion or + on two occasions
- Polyhydramnios in current pregnancy

It is essential that these at-risk women are screened appropriately to enable them to be put on the higher risk gestational diabetes pathway that includes growth surveillance with ultrasound and care provided by the MDT. Delivery in these pregnancies is recommended by 40 weeks +6 days to reduce complications.

Essential Hypertension in Pregnancy

Women planning pregnancy with a history of chronic hypertension should ideally been seen pre-conceptually. This provides an opportunity to review their medication and ensure that it is safe and non-teratogenic for pregnancy. ACE inhibitors and thiazide diuretics should be swapped for a safer alternative such as labetalol or nifedipine if possible.

At their dating scans, low-dose aspirin (75–150 mg) should be prescribed, if there are no contra-indications (such as unstable asthma) in order to lower their increased risk of pre-eclampsia. Antenatal care needs to be consultant-led with close monitoring of blood pressure, aiming for an ideal target pressure of 135/85 mm Hg [3] in order to reduce the risk of stroke. Together with epilepsy, strokes were responsible for 13% of maternal deaths in the latest MBRRACE-UK report [3]. Overview of these cases identified poor care where raised blood pressure readings were not acted upon, especially in the post-natal period. If a stroke is suspected, FAST (a validated tool used to screen for the diagnosis of a stroke) is useful. It is time-critical for treatment to be administered and effective. The tool is an acronym for Facial drooping, Arm weakness, Speech difficulties and Time – early thrombolysis is required to improve the outcome.

Hypertension in pregnancy is considered a major risk factor for small-for-gestational age fetuses and requires serial assessments for fetal size and umbilical artery dopplers from 26–28 weeks' gestation [6]. Superimposed pre-eclampsia should be screened for as below.

Pre-eclampsia

Pre-eclampsia (PET) is a pregnancy-specific disorder and a multi-organ disease, that can lead to severe complications of HELLP syndrome (haemolysis, elevated liver enzymes and low platelets) and eclampsia (fitting) if not treated and managed appropriately.

Whilst it classically presents with a triad of hypertension, oedema and proteinuria, this is not always the case. A UKOSS study of eclampsia [7] in 2005 showed that only 38% had hypertension and proteinuria preceding a fit. A high index of suspicion is therefore needed when a woman presents with one of the following signs or symptoms:

- Visual disturbances
- Headaches (frontal)
- Epigastric pain
- Hypertension
- Oedema

Investigations to help the diagnosis include a full blood count/platelets, liver function tests, renal function blood tests (U&ES) and PIGF-based testing. Protein creatinine ratio (PCR) is used to quantify significant proteinuria of over 3mg/dl.

Ultimately, the only treatment for pre-eclampsia is delivery, as the pathophysiology is due to abnormal placentation. Antihypertensive therapy is used to reduce the risk of maternal cerebrovascular accident and prolong the pregnancy if safe to do so. The fetus is at risk of intrauterine growth restriction and regular ultrasounds are required to monitor for this. The timing of delivery will be decided on maternal and/or fetal factors.

Magnesium sulfate is used to prevent seizures in unstable and symptomatic women with pre-eclampsia, given as an infusion after a loading dose of 4gm intravenously. It has the beneficial effect of also protecting the brain of a premature baby, reducing the risk of cerebral palsy. It should be considered in any threatened preterm labour below 34 weeks and a minimum of four hours infusion is needed to have the best affect. Care needs to be taken if maternal renal function is compromised. A build-up of maternal serum concentrations can lead to respiratory depression and cardiac arrest.

Epilepsy

The 2020 MBRRACE report raises the fact that more women die during or after pregnancy from epilepsy than as a result of pregnancy hypertensive disorders. The risk of death in epileptic pregnancies is 10 times higher than in pregnancies without [8]. Lack of specialist care was highlighted alongside the lack of education for this group of women. Again, pre-conceptual care is important to plan the pregnancy and provide an opportunity to review medication. Antiepileptic drugs (AEDs) work by being anti-folate and this increases the risk of neural tube defects in the fetus. This risk can be reduced by taking 5 mg folic acid, ideally pre-conceptually and throughout the first trimester. The risk of congenital defects is dependent on the type and number of anti-epileptic drugs taken. Pre-conceptual counselling is a good opportunity to reduce or change the medication if it is safe to do so and only with the input of a specialist. If unexpectedly pregnant, it is important not to stop the medication abruptly as it puts the woman at a bigger risk of seizures. Whilst evidence seems to show that Lamotrigine is the safest of the AEDs, sodium valproate has the most significant effect on neurodevelopment of the fetus. RCOG guidance on epilepsy in pregnancy recommends that all women are given verbal and written information on the risks of self-discontinuation of AEDS and the effects of seizures and AED on the fetus and on the pregnancy.

The dating scan at 12 weeks and anomaly scan at 18–20+6 weeks (FASP) are used to screen for congenital anomalies. Being at risk of having a small-for-gestational-age fetus, growth surveillance is then recommended from 28 weeks. It is vital that these patients have easy and rapid access to epilepsy specialists that are working with obstetric teams. Whilst routine serum testing for drug levels is not recommended, increased seizure activity should act as a red flag for immediate review. With the blood volume in a pregnant woman increasing by 40% over the pregnancy, dilutional effects are likely.

Causes of Litigation

1. Failure to diagnose DKA and treat this life-threatening condition promptly, reducing morbidity and mortality for mother and fetus
2. Failure to screen for and diagnose gestational diabetes in pregnancy
3. Scan surveillance not being interpreted correctly, and growth restriction not recognised or acted upon
4. Failure to diagnose pre-eclampsia so that it can be investigated and managed safely
5. Failure to recognise and treat severe hypertension in order to prevent a cerebrovascular accident
6. Failure to counsel fully any risks of a medical disorder on pregnancy or drugs used to treat the disorder being teratogenetic
7. Failure to recognise increased seizure activity and fast-tracking access to specialists to review medication

Avoidance of Litigation

1. A) Any known diabetic woman seen unwell in pregnancy should have blood sugar monitoring and ketones checked for on admission, to rule out DKA.

   B) Treatment of DKA has to be immediate, with aggressive fluid resuscitation, insulin infusion and correction of electrolyte imbalance whilst identifying and treating the cause.

2. A) If glycosuria is seen 1+ on two occasions or 2+ on one occasion, an oral glucose tolerance test (OGTT) should be indicated to rule out GDM.

   B) A careful history must be taken on booking in a pregnancy, to identify risk factors for GDM and an OGGT to be arranged.

3. Medical disorders associated with growth restriction or acceleration need careful ultrasound monitoring and interpretation of growth patterns, together with liquor and doppler measurements.

4. If a pregnant woman presents with any of the signs or symptoms of PET, the appropriate investigations need to be done to diagnose the condition. This can be more difficult to spot if there is an underlying diabetic nephropathy/ hypertension.

5. A sustained systolic blood pressure of 140 mmHg or higher OR diastolic blood pressure of 90mm Hg or higher should trigger antihypertensive treatment with a target BP of 135/85 mmHg. Possible causes of hypertension should be screened for to rule out PET.

6. A) In diabetic pregnancies, the mother should have careful counselling and education on how poor blood sugar control can cause congenital anomalies, affect growth of the fetus and increase the risk of stillbirth and delivery complications such as shoulder dystocia.

B) Counselling in epilepsy needs to be clear and supportive. Whilst AEDs have possible teratogenic effects on the fetus, increased seizures will put the fetus and mother at a greater risk. Administration of folic acid 5mg will reduce the effects of the drugs. The lowest effective dosages of medication are to be aimed for to further reduce possible effects.

7. Timely reviews of increased seizure activity in pregnancy are vital to review drug dosages and management options. These should be a red flag and serum drug levels can be checked to ensure they are within a therapeutic range.

References

1. MBRRACE-UK. Saving Lives, Improving Mothers' Care 2020: Lessons to inform maternity care from the UK and Ireland Confidential Enquiries in Maternal Death and Morbidity 2016–2018.

2. Draper, E, Kurinczuk, J, Kenyon S, on behalf of MBRRACE-UK. MBRRACE-UK 2015 Perinatal Confidential Enquiry into term, normally formed antepartum stillbirth. Leicester; 2015.

3. National Institute for Health and Care Excellence. Hypertension in pregnancy: diagnosis and management. NICE guideline NG 133. Published 25 June 2019. Available at: www.nice.org.uk/guidance/ng133

4. Stacey, T, Tennant, PWG, McCowan, LME et al. Gestational diabetes and the risk of late stillbirth: a case-control study from England, UK. *BJOG* 2019; 126: 973–82.

5. National Institute for Health and Care Excellence. Diabetes in pregnancy: management from preconception to the postnatal period. NICE guideline NG 3. Published 25 February 2015. Available at: www.nice.org.uk/guidance/ng3

6. Royal College of Obstetricians and Gynaecologists. The investigation and management of the small-for gestational-age fetus. Green-top Guideline No. 31. Second edition, published February 2013.

7. Knight, M on behalf of UKOSS. Eclampsia in the United Kingdom 2005. *BJOG* 2007; 114: 1072–8.

8. Royal College of Obstetricians and Gynaecologists. Epilepsy in pregnancy. Green-top Guideline No. 68. Published June 2016.

Fetal Growth Restriction and Unexplained Stillbirth

Emma Ferriman

CASE COMMENTARY

Swati Jha

Successful Claim

GM v Royal Cornwall Hospitals NHS Trust (2019)

The Claim

The claimant, a 38-year-old, suffered a stillbirth while under the care of the defendant trust. She claimed that it was negligent in failing to recognise that the baby was not growing normally and in failing to carry out a growth scan in spite of hospital attendances for reduced fetal movements and. Had this been performed it would have been identified that there was reduced liquor and the baby was small and a delivery expedited earlier preventing the still birth. She claimed for damages on the grounds of suffering psychiatric injury and also suffered a loss of self-confidence and was unable to return to work.

The Summary

This was her first pregnancy. She was considered low risk hence was scheduled for midwifery-led care. At term she attended hospital and it was found that the symphyiso-fundal height (SFH) was reduced and there had been a 2 cm drop since the last assessment two weeks earlier. She also reported reduced movements. She attended hospital again a week later (41+2 weeks) and again reported reduced movements. The SFH was not measured, recorded or plotted on the growth chart. She was reassured everything was alright and sent home.

She attended in early labour, a day before her scheduled induction of labour and fetal demise confirmed. She went on to deliver a stillborn baby two days later.

She went on to suffer nightmares and flashbacks, was unable to focus and struggled to complete everyday tasks. She became obsessive about developing an infection, as she had originally been told this was how her daughter had died and it was something she did or caused. In her next pregnancy she developed an obsessive-compulsive disorder (OCD) which impacted on her family life. She found her motivation was significantly impaired and her ability to function psychologically was also significantly impaired. She was therefore unable to work due to her OCD, as it was too time consuming and distressing to be able to function in activities of daily living. If she did return to work this would be at a lower level/part-time. The OCD caused tiredness and significantly impaired her concentration and self-confidence. There was some recovery following cognitive behaviour therapy, but it was felt this would never return to the pre-morbid levels.

The Judgement

If the tailing off of the baby's growth had been identified at the visit at term and the reduced movements acted on, an ultrasound scan would have been performed. This would have identified the reduced growth and liquor and an induction of labour would have been expedited and the baby would have been born alive. This would have prevented the ongoing psychological problems, and the case was settled in favour of the claimant on a global basis.

In a similar case of RH v James Paget University Hospitals NHS Foundation trust (2020), a baby was born with no signs of life and the claimant was successful in her claim for psychological injury.

Unsuccessful Claim

Wild & Wild v Southend University Hospitals NHS Foundation Trust [2014] EWHC 4053 (QB)

The Claim

Mr and Mrs Wild were informed of the in-utero demise of the pregnancy which resulted in the stillbirth of their first child. It was claimed that the trauma of these events caused psychological damages to Mr Wild as a secondary victim following the stillbirth and delivery of his child by his wife. It was claimed that the psychiatric illness was both recognisable and reasonably foreseeable and should therefore be compensated for. The defendant denied this claim.

The Summary

Mrs Wild delivered a stillborn baby at 40 weeks gestation and it was claimed that this was a consequence of the negligence in the recording of the baby's growth. Had this been adequately monitored, fetal compromise would have been detected earlier and delivery achieved before the stillbirth. This included a claim for psychological trauma. This was conceded by the defendants and pay-out arranged. However, when Mr Wild, as the secondary victim, claimed that the events surrounding the diagnosis of the stillbirth and subsequent delivery were a shocking event which had violently agitated him, causing him to suffer a recognisable psychiatric illness including pathological grief and depressive episode, this was denied by the defendant. The defendant made the case that the mother and fetus are one legal person, so a father could not succeed in the case of fetal demise as this could not be considered a death as the fetus never obtained life.

The Judgement

For a secondary victim to succeed in a claim, several criteria would need to be fulfilled. The first two were fulfilled in this case and included a relationship to the primary victim (Mrs Wild) either marital or parental and the events being a sudden and unexpected shock. However, the other criteria were not fulfilled for this claim to succeed. This required the secondary victim (Mr Wild) to be present at the time of the event, rather than be a witness to the manifestation of the negligence.

Whereas it was admitted that Mr Wild experienced sufficient shock to have foreseeably caused psychiatric illness, it was successfully denied that this was negligent.

Legal Commentary

Eloise Power

GM v Royal Cornwall Hospitals NHS Trust

The case report in relation to GM's matter is sadly typical of many stillbirth cases. Following the stillbirth of GM's baby at full term, the claimant suffered psychiatric injury (obsessive-compulsive disorder, with a particular focus on infection). The majority of the damages sought in the case related to the consequences of the claimant's psychiatric injury.

In relation to psychiatric injury, the law as it stands makes a distinction between "primary victims" and "secondary victims". Primary victims are those who have suffered physical injury themselves, or alternatively those who have not suffered physical injury, but where physical injury was sufficiently foreseeable.[1] Where a primary victim has suffered a psychiatric injury as a result of negligence, damages are recoverable (subject to the normal principles of establishing breach of duty and causation). The definition of secondary victims and the many additional hurdles which they have to overcome in order to recover damages, are considered below.

The courts have generally been prepared to accept that mothers of stillborn babies are primary victims. It is becoming increasingly clear from the case law that this is based upon the principle that prior to birth, the fetus and the mother are indivisible, and hence that an injury to the fetus is an injury to the mother. In *Wells & Smith v University Hospital Southampton NHS Foundation Trust* [2015] EWHC 2376 (QB), Dingemans J held as follows [para 83]:

> *In my judgment Mrs Wells was a primary victim. This is because the negligence (if it had been established) would have occurred when Layla and Mrs Wells were still one. That meant that Layla would (albeit unknown to Mrs Wells) have aspirated the meconium, which later caused her death, when Mrs Wells and Layla were one person. This aspiration of the meconium caused Layla's death and caused the adjustment order suffered by Mrs Wells. Although some of the distinctions in this area of law are arbitrary it does seem to me that in such circumstances Mrs Wells is a primary victim.*

A similar approach was taken to the position of the mother by Michael Kent QC, sitting as a Deputy High Court Judge in *Wild* [para 21]. It is notable that in both *Wells* and *Wild*, a clear distinction was drawn between the position of the mother and the father; this is discussed in more detail below.

In *YAH v Medway NHS Foundation Trust* [2018] EWHC 2964 (QB), Whipple J held that it is *"settled law that a baby is part of its mother until birth; there is, up to that point, a single legal person"*.[2] Taking the principle a step further, Whipple J proceeded to hold that *"it is important to be clear that the claimant did not cease to be a primary victim at the moment XAS was born. The fact that the claimant's psychiatric damage became*

---

[1] *Page v Smith* [1996] 1 AC 155 (*per* Lord Bridge of Harwich, p432).
[2] Para 21.

manifest later in time, after XAS was born, does not change the claimant's status. She was and is a primary victim, in so far as she suffered personal injury caused by negligence which occurred before XAS was born".[3]

In *Zeromska-Smith v United Lincolnshire Hospitals NHS Trust* [2019] EWHC 980 (QB), Martin Spencer J held that the mother of a stillborn baby was a primary victim and not a secondary victim. He observed as follows: *"Although the baby, if born alive, has its own set of rights derived from the Congenital Disabilities (Civil Liability) Act 1976, those rights do not derogate from the right of the mother to sue as a primary victim."*[4] He observed that primary victims do not have to satisfy the control mechanisms for secondary victims, and went a step further: *"In consequence, if the Claimant has suffered injury, including mental injury, as a primary victim it is unnecessary for her to show that what she has suffered amounted at the relevant time to a formal classified psychiatric injury. In particular, although damages cannot be recovered for 'normal' bereavement, in my judgment damages can be recovered for 'abnormal' bereavement or a pathological grief disorder and it matters not whether this amounts to a formal psychiatric diagnosis within ICD-10 or DSM-5".*[5]

In practice, it will readily be seen that it is considerably more straightforward for claims arising out of stillbirth to be brought on behalf of mothers/birthing parents rather than fathers/non-birthing parents.

It is important for lawyers and experts to be aware of the potential for other types of damage arising out of stillbirth besides psychiatric injury and associated losses. The present author recently settled a stillbirth claim involving a serious gynaecological injury consequent upon stillbirth: the claimant developed sepsis which resulted in Asherman's syndrome, which in turn caused infertility and the requirement for high-value fertility treatment. In addition, she suffered a serious psychiatric injury.

Wild & Wild v Southend University Hospitals NHS Foundation Trust [2014] EWHC 4053 (QB)

The judgement in *Wild* underlines the stark difference between the principles governing psychiatric injury suffered by primary and secondary victims. The mother of the stillborn child was held to be a primary victim, and her claim succeeded. The claim of the father failed.

The concept of secondary victimhood derives from the well-known principles, also described as "control mechanisms", set out by Lord Oliver in the case of *Alcock v Chief Constable of South Yorkshire Police* [1992] 1 AC 310 [p20–1]:

> *First, that in each case there was a marital or parental relationship between the plaintiff and the primary victim,*[6] *secondly, that the injury for which damages were claimed arose from the sudden and unexpected shock to the plaintiff's nervous system, thirdly, that the plaintiff in each case was*

---

[3] Para 24.

[4] Para 96.

[5] Para 97.

[6] This was expanded to "close ties of love and affection" in the case of *White v Chief Constable of South Yorkshire and others* [1999] 2 AC 455. In that case, claims brought by police officers who actively witnessed the Hillsborough disaster failed on the basis of the lack of close ties of love and affection.

either personally present at the scene of the accident or was in the more or less immediate vicinity and witnessed the aftermath shortly afterwards, and, fourthly, that the injury suffered arose from witnessing the death of, extreme danger to, or injury and discomfort suffered by the primary victim. Lastly, in each case there was not only an element of physical proximity to the event but a close temporal connection between the event and the plaintiff's perception of it combined with a close relationship of affection between the plaintiff and the primary victim.

It must, I think, be from these elements that the essential requirement of proximity is to be deduced, to which has to be added the reasonable foreseeability on the part of the defendant that in that combination of circumstances there was a real risk of injury of the type sustained by the particular plaintiff as a result of his or her concern for the primary victim.

In relation to the concept of "shock", Lord Ackner observed as follows [p10–11]:

"Shock", in the context of this cause of action, involves the sudden appreciation by sight or sound of a horrifying event, which violently agitates the mind. It has yet to include psychiatric illness caused by the accumulation over a period of time of more gradual assaults on the nervous system.

For this reason, claims of this nature are often described as "nervous shock" claims.

The control mechanisms set out above establish high hurdles which must be overcome before secondary victim claims can succeed. *Alcock* concerned psychiatric injury suffered by relatives and friends of victims of the Hillsborough tragedy. The majority of the claimants had viewed footage of the tragedy on television rather than being present at the scene. Four claimants were present at the football ground but were not in the area where the disaster occurred. One claimant lost both of his brothers. All of the claims failed.

The *Alcock* control mechanisms have been considered by the courts in various clinical negligence matters. In the case of *North Glamorgan NHS Trust v Walters* [2002] EWCA Civ 1792, a mother succeeded in a nervous shock claim after witnessing the final 36 hours of her infant son's life (the baby was aged 10 months at the time, so there was no proper basis upon which she could have been regarded as a primary victim).

In recent years, many secondary-victim claims have failed. In *Taylor v A Novo (UK) Limited* [2013] EWCA Civ 194, the Court of Appeal considered a case where a mother suffered injury in a workplace accident. As a result of the initial injury, the mother sustained a deep vein thrombosis and pulmonary emboli and died unexpectedly at home, some 21 days after the accident. Her daughter witnessed the death, but not the accident. She suffered a psychiatric injury. The Master of the Rolls, giving judgement for the unanimous Court of Appeal, held that the accident, rather than the death, should be treated as the relevant "event" [para 32]:

A paradigm example of the kind of case in which a claimant can recover damages as a secondary victim is one involving an accident which (i) more or less immediately causes injury or death to a primary victim and (ii) is witnessed by the claimant. In such a case, the relevant event is the accident. It is not a later consequence of the accident... Ms Taylor would have been able to recover damages as a secondary victim if she had suffered shock and psychiatric illness as a result of seeing her mother's accident. She cannot recover damages for the shock and illness that she suffered as a result of seeing her mother's death three weeks after the accident.

Needless to say, the distinction made in *Taylor v Novo* between the originating event and its consequences has made it still harder for claimants to satisfy the control mechanisms.

In *Liverpool Women's Hospital NHS Foundation Trust v Ronayne* [2015] EWCA Civ 588, a claimant suffered a psychiatric injury after seeing his wife in a poor condition following surgery. The Court of Appeal held that there was no *"sudden appreciation of an event"*; instead, there was a gradual realisation on the part of the claimant that his wife's life was in danger. Further, the appearance of his wife was held not to be horrifying by objective standards: the Court observed that *"what is required in order to found liability is something which is exceptional in nature"* (para 41). Unsurprisingly, the claim failed.

Turning to the case of *Wild*, the approach of the Court to the father's claim is of interest. Having accepted that the mother was a primary victim (as to which, please see above), the Court proceeded to consider the position of the father:

> Even though the alleged secondary victim's shock-induced psychiatric illness may be more to do with his concern for the unborn child than for the mother, nevertheless his shock is a consequence of the injury or threatened injury to the mother in that her foetus is damaged or destroyed by the relevant negligent act. Therefore I do not accept the proposition (which would create a form of legal "black hole") that a father could never succeed in an Alcock-type secondary victim claim in a still-birth case, if it is not accompanied by his witnessing at the same time the actual or threatened death or serious injury to the mother. It seems to me that, because of the treatment of foetus and mother as one legal person, this type of case is analogous to a case such as that of Froggatt v. Chesterfield & Derbyshire NHS Trust, (unreported 13 December 2002 Forbes J) where a negligent diagnosis of cancer led to an unnecessary right-sided mastectomy. The operation caused a physical injury to the Claimant's wife just as, by the negligence in this case, the Defendant caused the loss of Mrs Wild's child in utero [para 22, underlining added].

The analogy drawn by the Court between a cancer and a fetus may well be seen as somewhat unfortunate. However, this approach at least made it clear that a father/partner could potentially recover even where the parent giving birth has not suffered a serious injury – subject to satisfying the stringent control mechanisms.

The father's claim in Wild ultimately failed by application of the control mechanisms and by application of the decision in *Taylor v Novo*. On the facts, the Court found that

> Mr Wild was experiencing a growing and acute anxiety which started when the second midwife failed to find a heartbeat. This developed to the point at which, simply because of the behaviour (and no doubt body language) of the clinical staff and the words of the doctor 'I concur', he had a correct realisation that the baby had died. But none of that, in my judgment, equates to actually witnessing horrific events leading to a death or serious injury. That what Mr Wild experienced was capable of and did generate sufficient shock to have foreseeably caused psychiatric illness is not in dispute. But the authorities show that the control mechanisms often have the effect of excluding such cases [para 47, underlining added].

The Court rejected the submission made by Counsel for the claimant to the effect that distinguishing between the psychiatric injury suffered by fathers and mothers arising out of virtually the same set of circumstances imports a gender bias, holding that

> given the acceptance that there is an arbitrary line drawn between classes of claimants in these cases, it does not seem to me that the fact that cases similar to the one before me might never be able to succeed can be a ground for extending or modifying the control mechanisms in nervous shock cases, particularly when the subject has been so comprehensively travelled over by the higher courts.[7]

---

[7] Para 50.

Ultimately, the Court concluded that the father's claim must fail, accepting that – in accordance with Lord Oliver's observations in Alcock – "the law in this area is not wholly logical".

Many commentators have drawn attention to the lack of logic and often arbitrary line-drawing which have resulted from the Alcock judgement. At the time of writing, there is a possibility that the law in this area may be on the move. Two cases are being appealed to the Court of Appeal: *Paul v The Royal Wolverhampton NHS Trust* [2020] EWHC 1415 (QB) and *Polmear v Royal Cornwall Hospitals NHS Trust* [2021] EWHC 196 (QB). *Paul* involves a heart attack and death occurring 14.5 months after an incident of clinical negligence. *Polmear* involves the death of a child occurring five or seven months after a negligent failure to diagnose pulmonary veno-occlusive disease. In *Polmear*, Master Cook granted permission to appeal against his own decision in which he declined to strike out the claim, as he accepted that the contrary view was properly arguable and had reasonable prospects of success. He found that the appeal raised an important point of principle:

> namely the circumstances in which the control mechanism of proximity can be satisfied by a Claimant bringing a claim for damages as a secondary victim, when the negligence complained of preceded the sudden shocking event giving rise to the psychiatric injury for which compensation is sought, and what constitutes the relevant event for the purposes of establishing proximity.

It remains to be seen what approach the Court of Appeal will take to these cases; under the circumstances, a number of other secondary victim claims have been stayed, and the law in this area should be regarded as potentially in flux.

Clinical Commentary

Emma Ferriman

When assessing a small baby, the essence of management depends on the underlying cause. The trick is to establish whether the baby is constitutionally small with a normal growth process or whether it is growth restricted, implying a pathological restriction of its genetic growth potential. Definitions of small-for-gestational-age (SGA) babies vary, leading to difficulties in data interpretation with regard to outcome. The RCOG defines SGA as a baby with an estimated fetal weight (EFW) or abdominal circumference (AC) measurement less than the tenth centile and severe SGA as an EFW or AC less than the third centile. The likelihood of fetal growth restriction (FGR) is higher in severe SGA babies and as a result these babies are more likely to have an underlying pathological process present with evidence of fetal compromise including reduced amniotic fluid volumes and abnormal Dopplers. FGR may be placentally mediated or not. In those babies with poor placental function, this usually manifests later in the pregnancy with asymmetric growth restriction with preservation of the head circumference (HC) and femur length (FL) and an AC measurement < tenth centile. In non-placentally mediated growth restriction this is likely to have an earlier onset and lead to a symmetrically small baby with all measurements < tenth centile. Possible causes include chromosomal abnormality, genetic conditions or congenital fetal infections. Approximately 30% of SGA babies will be growth restricted and therefore at risk of adverse outcome. It is even more difficult to recognise those babies above the tenth centile with reducing growth velocity in the late third trimester who are also at risk of adverse outcome.

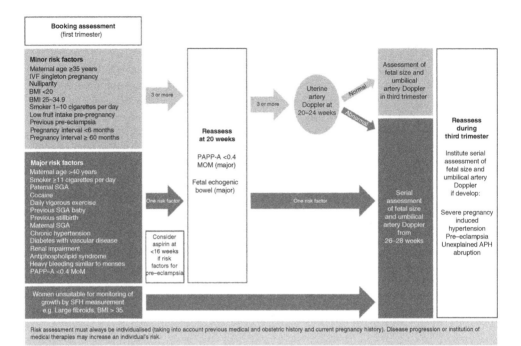

Figure 8.1 The Royal College of Obstetricians and Gynaecologists screening algorithm for the small-for-gestational-age baby.

All pregnant women should be screened for risk factors for fetal growth restriction. For low-risk women there should be serial assessment of the symphysis fundal height (SFH) from 24 weeks gestation. The RCOG recommends plotting serial SFH measurements on a customised growth chart rather than a population-based chart with customisation for maternal height, weight, parity and ethnic group. For those identified as high-risk, serial ultrasound assessment is advised from 26–28 weeks. The algorithm suggested by the RCOG is used in many units across the United Kingdom as detailed in Figure 8.1. Once a baby is identified as being SGA, it is important to follow national guidance for management, which in the United Kingdom is based on the RCOG green-top guidelines [1] and elsewhere will follow the ISUOG guidance [2]. The cause of the SGA should be investigated, and this will involve a detailed structural survey looking for associated abnormalities, a discussion regarding karyotyping in severe SGA with associated abnormalities or in those detected at less than 23 weeks and screening for congenital cytomegalovirus (CMV) and toxoplasmosis infection in severe SGA. In addition, consideration should be given to testing for syphilis and malaria in high-risk populations. Low-dose aspirin may have a small effect in preventing SGA in women at risk of pre-eclampsia and should be considered in high-risk women at or before 16 weeks gestation. Other interventions such as smoking cessation and steroid and magnesium sulphate administration for women at risk of early delivery should also be employed. Surveillance will involve serial growth scans and assessment of liquor volume and fetal Dopplers; the aim being to prolong the pregnancy for as long as possible whilst avoiding stillbirth. There is a fine balance between performing appropriate investigations and surveillance

Table 8.1. Characteristics of early versus late onset fetal growth restriction

Table 1 Main clinical characteristics of early- and late-onset fetal growth restriction (FGR)		
Characteristic	*Early-onset FGR*	*Late-onset FGR*
Main clinical challenge	**Management**	**Detection**
Prevalence	30%	70%
Gestational age at manifestation	<32 weeks	≥32 weeks
Ultrasound findings	Fetus may be very small	Fetus not necessarily very small
Doppler velocimetry	Spectrum of Doppler alterations that involves umbilical artery, middle cerebral artery and ductus venosus	Cerebral blood-flow redistribution
Biophysical profile	May be abnormal	May be abnormal
Hypertensive disorders of pregnancy	Frequent	Not frequent
Placental histopathological findings	Poor placental implantation, spiral artery abnormalities, maternal vascular malperfusion	Less specific placental findings, mainly altered diffusion
Perinatal mortality	High	Low
Maternal cardiovascular hemodynamic status	Low cardiac output, high peripheral vascular resistance	Less marked maternal cardiovascular findings

ISUOG Practice guidelines: diagnosis and management of the small for gestational age fetus and fetal growth restriction 2020.

leading to the avoidance of adverse outcome such as stillbirth or neonatal death, whilst avoiding over medicalisation of the pregnancy.

The International Society of Ultrasound in Obstetrics and Gynaecology (ISUOG) describes two phenotypes for FGR which are shown in Table 8.1. The distinction between early and late onset FGR is usually based on diagnosis before or after 32–34 weeks gestation. The definitions for early and late onset FGR will vary between different guidelines and author groups. The RCOG does not make the distinction between the two groups and recommends a universal pathway for management of these babies. ISUOG make the distinction between the two entities and tailor management accordingly.

The fundamental factor in the management of the SGA and FGR baby is when to deliver. Delivery too early may result in neonatal morbidity and mortality and too late may result in stillbirth or a baby with neurological injury. The first randomised controlled trial regarding the timing of delivery in FGR was the growth restriction intervention trial (GRIT), which evaluated the effect of immediate delivery versus expectant management when the clinicians were uncertain with regards to the timing of delivery.

The mean time to delivery was 4.9 days compared to 0.9 days and there was no significant difference in neurological outcome at two years of age [3,4]. The TRUFFLE study is the largest randomised trial on timing of delivery in early onset FGR based on three randomisation arms: early ductus venosus (DV) Doppler changes (PI > 95th centile, late DV Doppler changes (a-wave at or below baseline) and a reduced fetal heart rate short term variation (STV) based on computerised cardiotocograph (cCTG). In addition, in all three arms, safety net criteria were applied as an absolute indication for delivery. The protocol recommended delivery if there was reversed end diastolic flow (EDF) in the umbilical artery (UA) after 30 weeks and absent EDF in UA after 32 weeks. Overall, the TRUFFLE study showed evidence that timing of delivery based on DV with cCTG safety netting improved neurodevelopmental outcome at two years in survivors [5].

Stillbirth is defined in the United Kingdom as the death of a baby before birth after 24 completed weeks of gestation. In the 2012 NHS Litigation Authority report, which looked at 10 years of maternity claims from 2000 to 2010, there were 251 claims for stillbirth, accounting for 4.93% of the total claims and costing £15,712,695 [6]. Confidential enquiries into normally formed antepartum stillbirths identified deficient care contributing to outcome in 60%, rising to 80%, in intrapartum stillbirths. Risk factors include FGR, maternal medical co-morbidities including diabetes and hypertension, cigarette smoking and maternal perception of reduced fetal movements. Over the years there have been many classifications suggested to identify possible causes of stillbirth. The commonest classification system was that proposed by Wigglesworth et al in 1986 [7] but numerous classification systems have been proposed since then. Using this system, up to 66.2% of stillbirths are unexplained. More recent systems propose that this system misses a significant proportion of babies affected by FGR which are a potentially avoidable cause of stillbirth.

In 2019 the stillbirth rate in the United Kingdom was 3.8/1000 (2,763 stillborn babies), a fall from 5.1/1000 in 2010. Stillbirth has a devastating effect on parents and families and a major effect on the health economics in maternity services. In 2014, the Secretary of State for Health stated a commitment to reduce the stillbirth rate by 50% by 2025 and by 20% in 2020. Figure 8.2 shows the stillbirth rate against the linear trend required to meet the target by 2025. In response to this, the RCOG launched Each Baby Counts in 2014, a five-year quality improvement initiative. The scheme required all United Kingdom maternity units to report all cases of intrapartum stillbirth, early neonatal death and severe brain injury occurring during term labour. The key recommendations were a robust review of incidents by a multidisciplinary team, communication with parents that a review was occurring with an invitation for participation, the importance of an external panel member and an approach focusing on systematic rather than individual level actions and recommendations. The final progress report was published in 2021 and analysed babies delivered in 2018. There were 651,587 births at term of which 1,145 babies were eligible and 687 were fully reported. One-hundred-and-twenty-one (11%) of these were intrapartum stillbirths. Parents were asked to contribute to investigations in 70% of cases. Seventy-four per cent of cases showed that with different care the outcome may have changed. The report concluded that the project had raised the profile of maternity safety [8].

In parallel with Each Baby Counts, NHS England introduced a care bundle for reducing stillbirth rates, Saving Babies' Lives Care Bundle (SBLCB). The first version was introduced in 2016 [9]. A care bundle is not a new strategy in healthcare. It brings

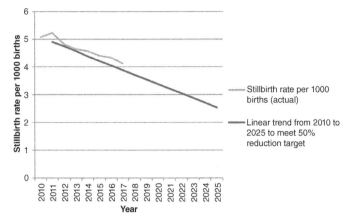

Figure 8.2 The stillbirth rate against the linear trend required to meet the Secretary of State for Health's target by 2025.

together a small number of focused interventions designed to effect an improvement on a particular disease, treatment or aspect of care. When implemented as a package, evidence shows that greater benefits are achieved at a faster rate than if these improvements were implemented in isolation. The first version of the care bundle consisted of four elements:

1. Reducing smoking in pregnancy by performing carbon monoxide testing on all pregnant women at booking to identify smokers and those exposed to smoking. This enables referral to smoking cessation programmes. There is strong evidence that reducing smoking in pregnancy reduces the risk of stillbirth [10].

2. Risk assessment and surveillance for FGR by using an algorithm to aid decision-making on classification of risk and corresponding pregnancy surveillance. For women at high risk, serial growth scans in the third trimester are recommended, and for low-risk women, serial measurement of symphysis fundal height (SFH) from 24 weeks gestation. All SGA babies should be audited to determine the false positive and false negative rates for detection. FGR is accepted as being the greatest risk factor for stillbirth [11,12]. Controversy still exists regarding the use of customised growth charts.

3. Raising awareness of reduced fetal movement. The confidential enquiries into stillbirths have consistently described a relationship between episodes of reduced fetal movement and the incidence of stillbirth. All pregnant women should be provided with an information leaflet on fetal movement from 24 weeks and fetal movements should be discussed at each subsequent visit. The AFFIRM study 2018 evaluated the use of a care package for pregnant women and clinicians to increase women's awareness of early reporting for reduced fetal movements and to standardise management in these women including ultrasound assessment with fetal biometry, liquor volume and umbilical artery (UA) Doppler after presentation with reduced fetal movements after 26 weeks, and to offer induction to those women with recurrent reduced fetal movements after 37 weeks. The package failed to show a reduction in the stillbirth rate over the study period, but the package did result in an increased number of inductions and caesarean sections. The pathway did however reduce the number of SGA babies born after 40 weeks gestation [10]. Management of

women with reduced fetal movements should be standardised according to the RCOG green-top guideline [13].

4. Effective fetal monitoring in labour. All staff who care for women in labour are required to take an annual training and competency in CTG interpretation and fetal heart auscultation. In addition, a buddy system should be in place for CTG review with a pathway for escalation. The INFANT study in 2017 was a randomised controlled trial which evaluated the role of cCTG in women undergoing continuous fetal monitoring in labour. This showed no improvement in clinical outcomes for mothers and babies [14].

In 2016, NHS England commissioned a retrospective evaluation of the SBLCB (Saving Babies' Lives Project impact and results evaluation (SPIRE)) involving extensive consultation with stakeholders and participating Trusts. Data was collected from 19 NHS Trusts over nine clinical networks. The report showed that all elements of the SBLCB were implemented to a degree across the early adopter trusts. Recommendations on cigarette smoking were almost universally adopted, allowing referral to smoking cessation services. Structured screening for SGA babies resulted in an increase in the antenatally detected SGA babies from 33.8% to 53.7%. Most pregnant women were given information on fetal movements and monitored movements accordingly. A buddy system was in place in most units to improve CTG interpretation. During the time period there was a statistically significant reduction in the stillbirth rate in the early adopter Trusts of 20%. However, the reduction could not be solely attributed to the SBLCB, due to variations in the timings and implementation of the various elements across the adopter Trusts. Over the time period there were 116 fewer stillbirths in participating Trusts and 1,106 fewer stillbirths across England between April 2015 and April 2017. The SBLCB had a significant service impact, with a 25.7% increase in the number of ultrasound scans. There was also an increased rate of induction of labour (19.4%) and emergency caesarean sections (9.5%) as would be expected as a consequence of the increased detection rate of SGA babies. It was also noted there was an increase in the number of elective caesarean sections, although this cannot be explained by the SBLCB, which does not advocate elective caesarean section. The key messages for clinicians were heightened awareness of the SBLCB and to consider how its recommendations could be implemented in their own practice. Clinicians also needed to reflect upon the increased rates of caesarean section and preterm birth and how (if at all) they relate to implementation of the bundle. There should be a multidisciplinary approach to health promotion messages such as smoking cessation and reduced fetal movements and finally to be aware of process and outcome measures within their own maternity unit. Overall, the cost implication in the 19 Trusts was £29 million [15,16].

Following the 2016 SPIRE evaluation, the second version of the care bundle was published in 2019, which aimed to provide detailed information for care providers and commissioners of maternity healthcare on how to reduce perinatal mortality. The second version (SBLCB 2) [17] brings together five key elements recognised as evidence-based or best practice. The four key elements from the first care bundle remain, with the addition of a focus on reduction in preterm birth rates. This occurred in response to the Department of Health's paper Safer Maternity Care, published in 2017. There was a commitment to reduce the preterm birth rate from 8% to 6% in three key areas: prediction using a risk assessment algorithm to stratify women into risk groups, prevention with aspirin in relevant groups, smoking cessation, appropriate management of multiple pregnancy and a clinician with an interest in preterm birth to provide transcervical ultrasound and cervical cerclage and finally preparation for those women who are going to deliver preterm with optimisation of the delivery.

Seventy per cent of stillbirths occur before term and nearly 40% are in the extreme prematurity group less than 28 weeks. The SBLCB2 developed the themes from version 1, with a focus on continuous improvement. The care bundle promotes the principles of offering women choice and a personalised care plan with a drive for continuity of care and targets BAME groups and those living in deprived areas. Women should receive high-quality information pre-pregnancy and during the pregnancy and Trusts are encouraged to implement NICE guidance relating to antenatal, intrapartum and post-natal care. Stillbirth has a devasting effect on parents and their families and it is imperative that there should be best practice in the event of such an occurrence. One such suggested best practice pathway was developed by the Greater Manchester and Eastern Cheshire Clinical Network [18]. One of the key elements of SBLCB2 is offering early delivery for women at risk of stillbirth, but it is important that this initiative is targeted at high-risk groups. Babies born at 37–38 weeks are twice as likely to be admitted to a neonatal unit than babies born at later gestations. Concerns have also been raised about longer-term outcomes for these babies, in particular with regard to brain development. At 39 weeks and beyond, induction of labour is not associated with an increased rate of caesarean section, instrumental vaginal delivery, fetal morbidity or neonatal unit admission and therefore delivery before this gestation needs careful consideration by a senior clinician.

From 1st April 2018, the Healthcare Safety Investigation Branch (HSIB) became responsible for all patient safety investigations into maternity incidents occurring in the NHS. HSIB uses the criteria first adopted in the RCOG Each Baby Counts project. The pregnancy is greater than 37 completed weeks and fulfils one of three criteria:

1. Intrapartum stillbirth. The baby was active at the start of labour and was born with no signs of life.
2. Early neonatal death (death within 0–6 days)
3. Severe brain injury in the first seven days of life (grade 111 hypoxic ischaemic encephalopathy (HIE), active therapeutic cooling, reduced central tone, comatose and seizures).

The Healthcare Safety Investigation Branch replaces the local investigation into these cases, although the relevant Trust is still responsible for the Duty of Candour. HSIB enables an independent investigation process, with independent assessments and recommendations. It has been operational in all 130 Trusts in England since March 2019. There are 14 teams of investigators. In 2019 there were 1,168 referrals, of which 867 cases went on to full investigation. Through this process there is the continued commitment to investigate these cases in an independent manner and provide ongoing learning for the relevant Trusts in a structured, non-judgemental approach. The individualised reports are shared with the family, the Trust and healthcare professionals involved in the incident and the aim is for completion within six months of the incident. HSIB publish national learning reports describing common themes arising from both the national investigations and maternity investigations programme, which inform future HSIB reports. The latest independent HSIB report [19] identified a number of themes:

1. Early recognition of risk, particularly in women who are categorised as low risk at booking, where risk factors change during the pregnancy, for example women with recurrent episodes of reduced fetal movements.
2. Safety of intrapartum care, with variation of the advice given to women experiencing symptoms of early labour.
3. Appropriate escalation for senior review, but also allowing health professional autonomy in the process.
4. Handovers between healthcare professionals varied with essential information being lost.
5. Larger babies are at risk of birth injury, brain injury and shoulder dystocia.
6. Neonatal collapse following maternal skin to skin.
7. Group B streptococcus (GBS) – not all mothers were provided with the relevant information provided by the RCOG for GBS carriage.
8. Cultural considerations, in particular with regard to the maternal mortality rates for Black and Asian women who are at significant risk when compared to white women.

The perinatal mortality review (PNMR) tool was established to support an objective, robust and standardised review of stillbirth, to provide answers for bereaved parents as to why their baby died. Its secondary aim is to facilitate local and national learning to improve care and prevent future deaths. Its first annual report was published in 2019 and provides data on 1,500 reviewed cases. Since its launch, 6,300 reviews have been started or completed and all Trusts and Health Care Boards across England, Wales and Scotland have engaged. It is estimated that 88% of eligible perinatal death cases have been reviewed, comprising 90% of stillbirths and late miscarriages and 83% of neonatal deaths. In over 90% of cases there was at least one issue identified with care, with an average of four issues per death. In 60% of cases the overall grading of care indicated that there were no issues with care that would have affected outcome. In 25% of cases there were issues with care identified but these would not have affected the overall outcome. There were only a small number of cases where the grading showed different care would have affected outcome: 13% related to pregnancy care, 10% related to labour and delivery and 9% related to neonatal care. This report highlights that in the majority of cases deaths occurred despite an appropriate standard of care [20].

Good Practice Guide

With regard to the management of the SGA or growth restricted baby, care should be focused on early identification of those women at an increased risk of a small baby using either the algorithm proposed by the RCOG or the modified algorithm recommended in SBLCB1. Low-risk women should have SFH measurements taken from 24 weeks and plotted on a customised growth chart [1,2]. Women who have a single measurement less than the tenth centile or serial measurements demonstrating static or slow growth should be referred for an ultrasound assessment. If growth is deemed normal at this assessment they can revert to the low-risk pathway. If growth indicates SGA, they will move to the high-risk pathway of serial ultrasound assessments. For those women in whom SFH measurements are deemed inaccurate (body mass index (BMI) > 35, large fibroids or polyhydramnios) serial assessment with ultrasound should be employed.

In high-risk women, there should be fetal growth measurements every two to three weeks, with assessment of the umbilical artery (UA) Dopplers. When UA Dopplers are normal, these should be repeated every 14 days. In the severe SGA baby, Dopplers are indicated more frequently. For abnormal UA (pulsatility or resistance index $> +2$ standard deviations above the mean for gestational age), the RCOG recommend repeating UA Dopplers twice weekly where there is positive EDF and daily where there is absent/reversed EDF where delivery is not indicated. Assessment of liquor volume should be based on either a single deepest vertical pool (sDVP) measurement or an amniotic fluid index (AFI). The RCOG recommends using a sDVP as a measurement of <2 cms as the lower limit of normal because when compared to an AFI of <5 cms, the AFI resulted in more inductions of labour for oligohydramnios without an improvement in perinatal outcome.

The use of middle cerebral artery (MCA) Doppler and DV Dopplers are helpful in the timing of delivery in the SGA baby. The MCA shows cerebral vasodilatation and a "brain sparing" effect in chronic hypoxia but has limited accuracy in predicting acid-aemia and adverse outcome in preterm babies and should not be used to time delivery. The DV Doppler reflects atrial pressure-volume changes during the cardiac cycle. As FGR worsens, the DV velocity reduces in the a-wave due to the increased pre and after loads as well as increased end diastolic pressure resulting from the direct effects of hypoxia and acidaemia. DV Dopplers therefore have a moderate predictive value for acidaemia and adverse outcome and are recommended for surveillance in the preterm SGA baby with abnormal UA Dopplers to time delivery.

The crucial stage in the management of these babies is the timing of delivery. This should balance the risks of early delivery with continuation in utero and the risks of death and organ damage due to tissue hypoperfusion. In the preterm infant where there is reversed or absent EDF in the UA prior to 32 weeks, delivery is indicated when the DV Dopplers become abnormal, provided the baby is viable and following steroid and magnesium sulphate administration. Even when DV Dopplers are normal, the RCOG recommends delivery by 32 weeks, with consideration between 30–32 weeks. If the MCA Doppler is abnormal, delivery should be recommended no later than 37 weeks. For the late onset SGA baby detected after 32 weeks with an abnormal UA Doppler, delivery is indicated no later than 37 weeks. In the SGA baby, detected after 32 weeks, delivery with normal UA Dopplers the RCOG recommend a senior obstetrician being involved in the decision-making process. Delivery should be offered at 37 weeks. With regards mode of delivery, caesarean section should be recommended when there is absent/reversed EDF in the UA Doppler. In the SGA baby with normal UA Dopplers or with a raised UA PI but positive EDF, induction of labour can be discussed but women should be aware of the increased rates of caesarean section. Continuous fetal monitoring should occur in labour and therefore early admission is also recommended.

In women for whom stillbirth is diagnosed, good practice should follow the RCOG guidance for late fetal death and stillbirth [22]. The diagnosis is made by ultrasound and ideally a senior second opinion should provide confirmation. Information should be given to mothers when they are accompanied and supported by partners, family members or friends. Discussions should aim to support maternal or parental choice and written information should also be provided. Parents should be offered investi-gations to determine the cause of death, including a post-mortem examination and cytogenetic evaluation which may provide information on the recurrence risk in a future pregnancy. However, investigation results should be interpreted with care, as an abnormal test result is not always directly related to the fetal death. Parents should be advised that in up to 50% of stillbirths no cause of death will be found. The timing and mode of delivery should take into account the mother's preferences as well as any medical conditions and her previous intrapartum history. Women should be advised regarding urgent delivery if there is sepsis, placental abruption or pre-eclampsia. Vaginal birth is the recommended mode of delivery for most women, but caesarean section will need to be considered for some. Women should deliver in an environment that provides appropriate facilities for emergency care. Following delivery, bereavement officers should coordinate postnatal services and provide bereavement support and follow-up. The parents should be offered a postnatal debrief to assess psychological well-being and, if necessary, referral to other support services, to discuss the results of any investigations performed and to make a care pathway for a possible future pregnancy. A comprehensive pathway for the management of women with stillbirth is proposed by the Greater Manchester and Eastern Cheshire Clinical Network [19].

Reasons for Litigation

Reasons for litigation may include:

- A failure to follow National and local guidelines
- Poor risk assessment for women at risk of an SGA baby
- Failure to assign women to an appropriate care pathway
- Once SGA or FGR are detected, a failure to perform appropriate investigation, including identification of fetal anomalies, abnormal karyotype and fetal infection
- Failure to provide adequate antenatal surveillance with regular growth, liquor and Doppler assessments
- Failure to refer to a fetal medicine specialist in complex cases such as severe early onset FGR
- Deficiencies relating to modifying risk factors within the pregnancy, particularly with regard to smoking and reduced fetal movements
- Lack of senior obstetric input in high-risk cases
- Failure to offer delivery in a timely manner
- Failure to refer to neonatal services in a timely manner
- Poor documentation

Avoidance of Litigation

This group of patients are subject to many controversies in management which will differ from clinician to clinician. Where there are a number of potential management strategies, the various options should be fully documented, including the potential risks and benefits of each course of action. Management should also take into consideration the parental wishes which can be especially challenging in such cases where the clinician considers that delivery should be delayed and the parents wish to expedite delivery to remove any possible risk of stillbirth. Given that the majority of Trusts in England are adopting the recommendations of the SBLCBs adherence to these guidelines would indicate best practice and deviation from these recommendations will be subject to criticism and ultimately litigation in the event of an adverse outcome.

The RCOG guidance is clear in that any baby less than the tenth centile should be delivered at 37 weeks. For those women who decline delivery, there should be a clearly documented discussion surrounding the rationale for delivery including the associated perinatal morbidity and mortality. Following these discussions, if delivery is still declined, there should be a clear management plan of fetal surveillance with senior review. This will allow the early identification of any deterioration in the fetal condition. Prolongation of a pregnancy beyond 37 weeks in a baby growing below the tenth centile would represent substandard care. Babies growing on the tenth centile with normal liquor and Dopplers can justifiably be offered induction or delivery at 39 weeks. When comparing delivery at 37 weeks to delivery at 39 weeks there are significantly increased rates of admission to the neonatal unit and emerging evidence that delivery at 37 weeks may also have a negative impact on long-term brain development when compared to delivery at 39 weeks.

When FGR presents at a very early stage, <23 weeks, this may present a number of controversies. The detection of a very small baby at this gestation suggests other causes of fetal growth restriction and in these cases, it is imperative to make an early referral to a fetal medicine specialist. A detailed anomaly scan should be carried out, looking for the presence of other fetal abnormalities. FGR in conjunction with other abnormalities may fulfil the criteria for karyotype, microarray or targeted exome sequencing. Investigation may also include a specialist fetal cardiology scan or magnetic resonance imaging (MRI). Discussions should occur around fetal karyotyping and potential underlying genetic or syndromal causes. The management should be multi-disciplinary and may involve neonatologists, paediatric neurologists and clinical geneticists. In these scenarios, counselling needs to be honest and comprehensive in order to help parents make very difficult decisions. These discussions may involve late termination of pregnancy or continuing with a pregnancy that is likely to have a poor outcome. It is imperative that counselling is fully understood by the parents. This is particularly important for couples for whom English is not their first language. Every effort should be made to obtain face to face impartial translators who can explain often very complex conditions and scenarios. Failure to counsel appropriately may lead to potential litigation for wrongful birth.

Stillbirth accounted for nearly 5% of all NHS litigation authority claims in their 10-year review. It is a highly emotive and painful topic for parents. Clinicians need to pay particular attention to the known risk factors of FGR, smoking, reduced fetal movements and preterm birth. Once identified, any of these factors warrant careful investigation and a detailed, individual management plan to ensure optimum management overseen by a senior obstetrician. Continuity of care is particularly important in these cases. Issues arise where there are multiple clinicians with differing opinions which leads to fragmented and contradictory care. It is these situations that parents are particularly likely to express dissatisfaction with care and seek legal redress.

References

1. Royal College of Obstetricians and Gynaecologists (RCOG). Green-top Guideline No.31. The Investigation and Management of the Small-for-Gestational-Age fetus. Second edition, published February 2013. Minor revisions published in January 2014. Available at: www.rcog.org.uk/globalassets/documents/guidelines/gtg_31.pdf

2. Lees, CC, Stampalija, T, Baschat, AA, da Silva Costa, F, Ferrazzi, E, Figueras, F,

Hecher, K, Kingdom, J, Poon, LC, Salomon, LJ, Unterscheider, J. ISUOG Practice Guidelines: diagnosis and management of small for gestational age fetus and fetal growth restriction. *Ultrasound Obstet Gynecol* 2020; 56: 298–312. https://doi.org/10.1002/uog.22134

3. Growth Restriction Intervention Trial (GRIT) Study Group. A randomised trial of timed delivery for the compromised preterm fetus: short term outcomes and Bayesian interpretation. *BJOG* 2003; 110 (1): 27–32.

4. Growth Restriction Intervention Trial (GRIT) Study Group. Infant wellbeing at 2 years of age in the Growth Restriction Intervention Trial (GRIT): multicentred randomised controlled trial. *Lancet* 2004; 364(9433): 513–20.

5. Lees, C, Marlow, N, Arabin, B, Bilardo, CM, Brezinka, C, Derks, JB, Duvekot, J, Frusca, T, Diemert, A, Ferrazzi, E, Ganzevoort, W, Hecher, K, Martinelli, P, Ostermayer, E, Papageorghiou, AT, Schlembach, D, Schneider, KT, Thilaganathan, B, Todros, T, van Wassenaer-Leemhuis, A, Valcamonico, A, Visser, GH, Wolf H. TRUFFLE Group. Perinatal morbidity and mortality in early-onset fetal growth restriction: cohort outcomes of the trial of randomized umbilical and fetal flow in Europe (TRUFFLE). *Ultrasound Obstet Gynecol* 2013; 42: 400–8. Available at: https://fetalmedicine.org/var/material/publication_pdf/sga_management/Bilardo_et_al-2017-Ultrasound_in_Obstetrics__Gynecology.pdf

6. NHS Litigation Authority. Ten years of maternity claims. An analysis of NHS Litigation Authority Data. 2012. Available at: https://resolution.nhs.uk/wp-content/uploads/2018/11/Ten-years-of-Maternity-Claims-Final-Report-final-2.pdf

7. Hey EN, LLoyd DJ, Wigglesworth JS. Classifying perinatal death: fetal and neonatal factors. *Br J Obstet Gynaecol* 1986; 93: 1213–23.

8. Royal College of Obstetricians and Gynaecologists (RCOG). Each Baby Counts. 2020 final progress report. March 2021. Available at: www.rcog.org.uk/globalassets/documents/guidelines/research–audit/each-baby-counts/ebc-2020-final-progress-report.pdf

9. O'Connor D. On behalf of NHS England. Saving Babies' Lives care bundle. A care bundle for reducing stillbirth. 21 March 2016. Available at: www.england.nhs.uk/wp-content/uploads/2016/03/saving-babies-lives-car-bundl.pdf

10. Takawira, CM, Ahankari A, Coleman, T, Lewis, S. Maternal smoking and the risk of still birth: systematic review and meta-analysis. *BMC Public Health* 2015; 15: 239. https://doi:10.1186/s12889-015-1552-5. Available at: www.biomedcentral.com/1471-2458/15/239

11. Gardosi, J, Madurasinghe, V, Williams, M, Malik, A, Francis, F. Maternal and fetal risk factors for stillbirth: population based study. *BMJ*: f108. Available at: www.bmj.com/content/346/bmj.f108

12. MBRRACE-UK. Perinatal Confidential Enquiry Term, singleton, normally-formed, antepartum stillbirth. Published 2015.

13. Norman, JE, Heazell, AE, Rodriguez, A, Weir, CJ, Stock, SJ, Calderwood, CJ, Burley, SC, Frøen, JF, Geary, M, Breathnach, F, Hunter A. Awareness of fetal movements and care package to reduce fetal mortality (AFFIRM): a stepped wedge, cluster-randomised trial. *Lancet* 2018; 392(10158): 1629–38. Available at: www.thelancet.com/action/showPdf?pii=S0140-6736%2818%2931543-5

14. Royal College of Obstetricians and Gynaecologists (RCOG). Green-top Guideline No. 57. Reduced Fetal Movement. 2011. Available at: www.rcog.org.uk/globalassets/documents/guidelines/gtg_57.pdf

15. Brocklehurst, P, Field, DJ, Juszczak, E, Kenyon, S, Linsell, L, Newburn, M, Plachcinski, R, Quigley, M, Schroeder, L, Steer, P. The INFANT trial. *Lancet* 2017; 390(10089): 28. Available at: www.thelancet.com/pdfs/journals/lancet/PIIS0140-6736(17)30568-8.pdf

16. Widdows, K, Roberts, SA, Camacho, EM, Heazell, AEP. Evaluation of the implementation of the Saving Babies' Lives Care Bundle in early adopter NHS Trusts in England. Maternal and Fetal Health Research Centre, University of Manchester, Manchester, UK. 2018.

17. Widdows, K, Roberts, SA, Camacho, EM, Heazell, AEP. Stillbirth rates, service outcomes and costs of implementing NHS England's Saving Babies' Lives care bundle in maternity units in England: a cohort study. *PLoS ONE* 2021; 16(4): e0250150. https://doi.org/10.1371/journal .pone.0250150

18. NHS England. Saving Babies' Lives Version Two. A care bundle for reducing perinatal mortality. March 2019. Available at: www.england.nhs.uk/wp-content/uploads/2019/07/saving-babies-lives-care-bundle-version-two-v5.pdf

19. Greater Manchester and Eastern Cheshire Clinical Network. Management of Stillbirth. Integrated Care Pathway. March 2018. Available at: https:// healthinnovationmanchester.com/wp-content/uploads/2018/10/NW-Stillbirth-ICP-V3-March-2018.pdf

20. Healthcare Safety Investigation Branch (HSIB). Summary of Themes Arising from the HSIB Maternity Programme. March 2020. Available at: www.hsib.org .uk/documents/224/hsib-national-learning-report-summary-themes-maternity-programme.pdf

21. National Perinatal Mortality Review Tool (PMRT). Learning from Standardised Reviews When Babies Die. First annual report. October 2019. Available at: www .hqip.org.uk/wp-content/uploads/2019/ 10/Ref-181-PMRT-first-annual-report-FINAL.pdf

22. Royal College of Obstetricians and Gynaecologists (RCOG). Green-top Guideline No.55. Late Intrauterine Fetal Death and Stillbirth. October 2010. Available at: www.rcog.org.uk/ globalassets/documents/guidelines/gtg_ 55.pdf

Fetal Monitoring and the Challenges of Identifying the Fetus at Risk of Intrapartum Hypoxia

Emma Ferriman

CASE COMMENTARY
Swati Jha

Successful Claim

NKX v Barts Health NHS Trust

The Claim

The claimant was the second child of his mother who had delivered her first pregnancy by caesarean section (CS). It was claimed that the mother was not adequately counselled about the risk of uterine rupture in the antenatal period, if she opted for a vaginal delivery, and subsequently, when she went into labour, was not informed of the desirability of continuous fetal monitoring or of the risks inherent to intermittent auscultation (IA).

The Summary

The mother attended antenatal clinic and was identified as being a candidate for a vaginal birth after caesarean section (VBAC). She was advised of the small but real risk of uterine rupture. She had two further appointments, to discuss the pros and cons of a VBAC versus a CS, and wished to proceed with a vaginal delivery. At these appointments she was informed of the 1:200 risk of uterine rupture. If rupture occurred this could lead to an hypoxic Ischaemic encephalopathy (HIE), which could lead to brain damage, and the purpose of continuous CTG monitoring was to give early warning in the event that a rupture occurred or was about to occur and an emergency CS could be performed. She wanted a water birth and was informed of the options for fetal monitoring in labour, which included wireless continuous fetal monitoring (CFM) or IA. She was also informed that IA was not recommended by the hospital or the RCOG in women with a previous CS, but there was no detailed discussion of the differences between a CFM and IA. In addition, the mother made the case that she did not appreciate that HIE meant the baby suffered from brain damage.

When she attended in labour, she went into the birthing pool and the baby was monitored by intermittent auscultation. The counselling regarding the added risks with IA were not repeated once she had gone into labour and she was not informed that in view of the labour suite being so busy on that night, she could not be guaranteed close monitoring. Also, wireless CFM was not available.

During the course of established labour and in the second stage IA was performed less frequently than would be recommended. When a fetal deceleration was identified with scar tenderness, a category 1 CS was promptly performed and delivery achieved within 20 minutes of the decision. At delivery the baby was in a poor condition and HIE diagnosed with a poor prognosis.

The Judgement

Whereas the claimant failed to establish that she did not receive adequate counselling during the antenatal period, it was deemed that the claimant's mother had not fixated on the idea of IA as opposed to CFM. Had this been rediscussed and had she been given adequate information in labour, she would have opted for CFM. The birth plan should have been revisited and discussed again. It was also accepted that once the second stage of labour was established the frequency of IA should have been every five minutes and failure to do so was below a reasonable standard of care. Though the rupture is still likely to have caused a neurodisability, this would have been mild rather than severe.

Unsuccessful Claim

Tasmin v Barts NHS Trust [2015] EWHC 3135 (QB)

The Claim

The claimant was born with HIE following an emergency CS performed for bradycardia in the first stage of labour. It was initially alleged that if the decision to perform the CS had been made earlier the bradycardia would not have ensued and the HIE would have been preventable. It was also claimed that the parents had expressed a wish for a CS which was turned down. It was also alleged that a fetal blood sampling should have been advised in view of the decelerations on the trace suggesting the baby was distressed, and there was a breach of duty in failing to recognise this.

The Summary

This was the claimant's mother's first pregnancy which was uneventful and she was induced at 41 weeks due to liquor and growth being borderline. Following an artificial rupture of the membranes (ARM) and clear liquor noted. She was commenced on continuous fetal monitoring and syntocinon started when progress did not occur spontaneously. A few hours into labour some decelerations were noted, a medical review sought and the syntocinon stopped. The cervix was only 4 cm dilated but no further action was deemed necessary at this point. After restarting the syntocinon and following concerns about a malpresentation, she was reviewed again and was noted to have occasional decelerations and 6–7 cm dilated. However, following a sudden bradycardia, a decision to perform a category 1 CS was made. The interval from decision to delivery was 20 minutes.

The Judgement

It was denied that the parents requested a CS during labour. It was admitted that there had been a pathological trace which required fetal blood sampling (FBS) and the syntocinon should not have been recommended before fetal well-being was established. However, this breach was not the cause of the adverse outcome. On a balance of probability, the result of the FBS taken before the sudden bradycardia would have been normal, hence labour would still have proceeded, leading to the same consequences. This was based on the fact that at birth the cord gases were still within normal ranges (ph 7.23 and BE was 5.4).

In a similar case of LT v NHS Lothian Health Board, a case was made and the Montgomery ruling quoted as it was against the patient's wishes to continue with labour. This was turned down in favour of the defendant's case, which was that a claimant in labour on a delivery suite had given consent to be in labour.

Legal Commentary

Eloise Power

The cases in this area, which involve issues such as misinterpretation of the cardiotoco-graph (CTG); failure to take appropriate actions or refer to medical staff upon an abnormal CTG; failure to monitor the fetus adequately and inappropriate use of synto-cinon,[1] include some of the most tragic and high-value matters in the field of clinical negligence. The consequences of such claims include cerebral palsy, quadriplegia, hemi-plegia, developmental problems and death of a baby or child.[2]

In the 10-year period covered by the 2010 study *"Ten Years of Maternity Claims: An Analysis of NHS Litigation Authority Data"*, 300 claims involving alleged CTG misinter-pretation were reported to the NHS Litigation Authority (predecessor body to NHS Resolution). The total value of the CTG misinterpretation claims was estimated to be in the region of 466 million pounds,[3] as of the date of the report. It seems likely that the present total value would be higher.

NKX v Bart's Health NHS Trust [2020] EWHC 828 (QB)

Although these cases stand out due to the tragic consequences and high quantum of damages, the legal principles governing this area are essentially the same as those governing other areas of clinical negligence law. In the successful recent case of *NKX v Bart's Health NHS Trust*, there was no dispute between the parties as to the relevant law: as to consent, the principles in *Montgomery* were applied; as to breach of duty, *Bolam* and related case law were applied, and the Court held that the claimant was required to prove, on a balance of probabilities, the causal significance of any proved breach of duty (para 10). None of this is controversial in any way. It is clear from the detailed and careful judgement that this was a case which stood or fell upon the evidence, rather than any issue of legal principle.

In the course of the judgement of Simeon Maskrey QC, sitting as a Deputy Judge of the High Court in *NKX*, the Court accepted the evidence of both sides' midwifery experts that *"the birth plan requires reconsideration during the course of the pregnancy and in particular when the mother goes into labour."* On the facts, the Court held that repeated counselling and re-assessment during labour

---

[1] Figure 12, "Ten Years of Maternity Claims: An Analysis of NHS Litigation Authority Data", NHS LA 2010.
[2] Para 2.2, "Ten Years of Maternity Claims", supra.
[3] Para 2.1, "Ten Years of Maternity Claims", supra.

should have set out the risks inherent in not having CFM but should also have emphasised that staff could not guarantee the close monitoring by a midwife that the parents had expected because the unit was so busy, that CFM simply could not happen in the pool because there was no available wireless CTG monitor, and that there may have been no staff available who had experience of caring for a VBAC mother who was not continuously monitored [para 75].

The Court held that the mother would have opted for CFM if she had been adequately consented, and that the baby would have suffered a mild rather than a severe neurodisability.

The Court's approach amounts to an interesting and helpful application of *Montgomery* principles to real world conditions: the implication is that the *Montgomery* duty extends to giving warnings about resource issues on the ground such as lack of equipment or inadequate staffing levels, as well as medical risks and benefits.

Tasmin v Barts Health NHS Trust [2015] EWHC 3135 (QB)

In *Tasmin v Barts Health NHS Trust*, the claimant's case essentially failed on the facts. Jay J found that the parents did not express a preference for a CS and that, although the treating obstetrician should have recommended a fetal blood sample in the light of a pathological CTG, the result would have been reassuring. The claimant was unable to persuade the Court that a CS should have been offered as an alternative to a fetal blood sample, nor that a CS should have been offered after the fetal blood sample would have been taken. The risk to the fetus was held to be negligible. Applying *Montgomery*:

> A risk of 1:1000 is an immaterial risk for the purposes of paragraph 87 of Montgomery. The Supreme Court eschewed characterising the risk in percentage terms, but it was doing so in the context of defining the borderline between materiality and immateriality. Here, I am quite satisfied that the relevant risk was so low that it was below that borderline. I am not to be understood as saying exactly where the threshold should be defined [para 115].

The judgement in *Tasmin v Barts Health* is also of interest because of the following observations on consent in relation to the process of childbirth (the judgement in *Tasmin* postdates the Supreme Court's judgement in *Montgomery*):

> In my view, it is impossible to decouple the issue of parental preference from that of professional advice. Whatever the strength of their feeling, these parents, as would any reasonable parents, clearly wanted to listen to medical opinion and to take it into account.
>
> It goes without saying that the parents' initial preference was for a natural birth, and in my view that must represent the default position. However, everyone agrees that childbirth is an extremely dynamic process, and events can occur which cause mothers to change their mind. Further, Mrs Nahar had no previous experience (para 40–41).

In relation to consenting the patient *during* the process of labour, the Court expressed approval (obiter) towards the following evidence given by the defendant's expert witness (para 102–103):

> Labour is a dynamic process and for obvious reasons the context is highly charged. In general, he agreed with the proposition that options and alternatives should be offered. When a woman is in labour, the plan self-evidently is to proceed if possible to natural birth. If, at every clinical encounter, he raised the options of FBS or CS, it becomes very impractical to have a running theme of how one manages the case. In answer to a direct request for CS, a reasonable obstetrician

would be mandated to discuss the risks but would have to accede to parental choice, unless seriously inappropriate...

Obstetrically, we look prospectively. With a pathological CTG, there is a risk of hypoxia which might lead to acidosis, and a severity of acidosis which might lead to delivery. The risk of a serious outcome is extremely low... Labour is a dynamic process. You can't have a lengthy discussion as the risks are changing. The way I describe the risk of a pathological trace – there are abnormalities in the FHR which might be a feature of concern for the baby. The likelihood of that is relatively modest at this stage. CTG is not diagnostic; it highlights babies who might [sic]. I recommend an FBS to obtain appropriate information to make a decision about the next course of action.

These extracts demonstrate recognition on the part of the Court of the need to strike a difficult balance between the right of mothers to change their minds and the practical difficulties around having lengthy consenting discussions during the rapidly changing events of labour. By way of comparison, the conclusion reached by the Scottish Court of Session in *LT v NHS Lothian Health Board* [2018] CSOH 29 was that where material new information arises, there is a duty to discuss the implications with the patient:

We would see Professor Murphy's reference to "intervening" as meaning departing or considering departing from the plan to proceed to spontaneous delivery. That would require discussion because it implies new information (the emergence of risk) and a new risk/benefit balance. However, if there was no question of departing from the previously agreed plan (because there was no clinical reason to consider so doing) there was no decision to be made and no need to discuss matters with the patient; her consent to what she had previously agreed was, as Professor Murphy put it, "inherent".

On the facts of *LT*, there was no duty upon the midwife to interpret the CTG trace as suspicious, let alone pathological, and the claim accordingly failed. However, it is clear that the Court of Session found that where new material information arises, this would trigger a fresh consenting discussion with the patient during labour.

Use of NICE Guidelines

An important legal and evidential issue in this area concerns the status of the NICE Guidelines concerning the use of electronic fetal monitoring in labour. In *Sanderson v Guy's and St Thomas' NHS Foundation Trust* [2020] EWHC 20 (QB), Lambert J heard detailed evidence as to the May 2001 NICE Guidelines, "The Use of Electronic Fetal Monitoring". Mr Tufnell, the expert instructed on behalf of the defendant, made the comment that the Guidelines were *"not as precise in every description as you might wish to make them forensically"* [para 56]. After hearing lengthy arguments as to what the Guidelines meant, the Court observed as follows (para 78):

Putting it shortly therefore, the Guidelines on their face appear to advocate two contradictory management options in response to a single prolonged deceleration lasting longer than 3 minutes: conservative measures where possible or feasible (expressly including fetal blood sampling) and a few short paragraphs later urgent delivery (fetal blood sampling being contraindicated). On the critical question for my determination, the Guidelines point in two, entirely different, management directions.

The Court made the following comments: *"Although no doubt a useful resource, I accept Mr Tuffnell's evidence that the Guidelines are a practical tool to be used in conjunction with clinical judgement."* Given the contradiction within the Guidelines which the Court had identified, it is difficult to see what other conclusion could have been reached. The claimant's case, which was based upon one of the possible interpretations of the Guidelines, failed on the evidence.

Although the Sanderson case came to trial in 2020, the underlying events were historic, having occurred in 2002. The 2001 Guidelines have now been superseded by the information provided in NICE CG 190, *"Intrapartum Care for Healthy Women and Babies"*, which includes recommendations for monitoring during labour and interpretation of the CTG trace. If nothing else, the judgement in *Sanderson* emphasises the need for clear and unambiguous drafting of clinical guidelines, particularly where these guidelines are to be applied in dynamic and rapidly changing settings.

Clinical Commentary

Emma Ferriman

In a review of the NHS Litigation Authority data in 2012, maternity claims represented the highest value and the second highest number of clinical negligence claims. From 1 April 2000 to 31 March 2010, there were 5,087 claims with a total value of £3.1 billion. There were 300 claims involving cardiotocograph (CTG) interpretation in labour. In addition, allegations regarding CTG interpretation were also associated with claims categorised as management of labour and an outcome resulting in cerebral palsy. The estimated total value of these claims was £466 million [1]. In the NHS litigation authority 2015/2016 report, although the number of claims remained fairly constant, the value of maternity cerebral palsy/brain damage claims continued to increase [2]. The estimated cost for obstetric claims in 2019/2020 is £718.7 million [3]. In the 2017 NHS Resolution report on five years of cerebral palsy claims, errors with CTG monitoring were the commonest theme [4]. Sixty-four per cent of claims involved errors with CTG monitoring and 91% involved CTG interpretation. The three commonest root causes identified were a failure by numerous individuals to act on a CTG (Reason's Swiss cheese model of accident causation) [5], failure to recognise the change from low to high risk and commence continuous CTG monitoring, and the uninterpretable CTG that was not acted upon [4].

In the Royal College of Obstetricians and Gynaecologists (RCOG) Each Baby Counts report, there were 556 babies for whom different care could have changed outcome. There were 409 cases where fetal monitoring was identified as a critical contributory factor [6]. There were a number of key recommendations from the report. Firstly, for all women to have a formal risk assessment when admitted in labour, irrespective of the place of birth, to determine the most appropriate method of fetal monitoring. Secondly, to follow the NICE guidance on switching from intermittent auscultation (IA) to continuous monitoring [10] and finally for healthcare professionals to be aware of the transition between the various stages of labour.

The aim of antenatal and intrapartum fetal surveillance is to identify those babies at risk of hypoxia. The CTG is a well-established method of confirming fetal well-being and screening for hypoxia in a high risk labour where continuous monitoring is required [8,9]. However, there is no clear evidence that the CTG improves perinatal outcomes. A 2017 Cochrane review of continuous CTG as a form of electronic fetal monitoring for fetal assessment in labour concluded that although continuous CTG does reduce the rate of neonatal seizures, there are no clear differences between cerebral palsy or infant mortality. Overall, continuous CTG was associated with higher rates of obstetric intervention such as CS and operative delivery [7].

NICE does not recommend the use of continuous CTG in low-risk women in established labour [10]. For these women, IA is recommended. IA should be carried out immediately following a contraction for at least one minute, at least every 15 minutes in the first stage of labour and at least every five minutes in the second stage of labour. Accelerations and decelerations should be recorded and the maternal pulse taken hourly to differentiate between maternal and fetal heart rates. Factors prompting increased auscultation are a rising baseline heart rate or decelerations. In this situation, NICE recommends auscultation over three consecutive contractions in the first instance whilst assessing the woman's whole clinical picture including maternal hydration, position, observations and the frequency and strength of contractions. If a rising baseline or the presence of decelerations is confirmed, then a continuous CTG should be commenced. In low-risk settings the woman should be transferred to a consultant-led area if it is safe to do so. NICE have a number of criteria for the commencement of continuous CTG [10] and these were further adapted in the Each Baby Counts report [6] (see Figure 9.1).

For those high-risk women requiring continuous CTG it is imperative that healthcare professionals follow prescribed methods of interpretation relying on pattern recognition.

Maternal assessment	Fetal assessment
Pulse > 120 bpm on 2 occasions 20 minutes apart	Any abnormal presentation including cord presentation
Single reading of either raised diastolic BP > 110 mmHg or systolic BP > 160 mmHg	Reduced fetal movements in last 24 hours
Raised diastolic BP of ≥ 90 mmHg or raised systolic BP ≥ 140 mmHg on ≥ 2 occasions 30 minutes apart	Deceleration in fetal heart rate heard on IA
2+ protein on urinalysis and a raised single reading of either diastolic BP ≥ 90 mmHg or systolic BP ≥ 140 mmHg	Suspected fetal growth restriction or macrosomia
Single temperature 38°C or 37.5°C on 2 consecutive readings 1 hour apart	Suspected polyhydramnios or anhydramnios
Vaginal blood loss other than a show	Fetal abnormality
Rupture of membranes > 24 hours before the onset of established labour	Fetal heart rate < 110 bpm or > 160 bpm
Presence of significant meconium	
Pain that differs from pain normally associated with contrcations	
Any antenatal risk factor that indicates a need for consultant-led care	
Confirmed delay in 1st or 2nd stage of labour	
Regional anaesthesia	
Obstetric emergency including antepartum haemorrhage, cord prolapse, postpartum haemorrhage, maternal seizure or collapse or a need for advanced neonatal resuscitation	

Figure 9.1 Main indications for continuous CTG
(adapted from the NICE guideline on intrapartum care for healthy women and babies).

However, the CTG should never be interpreted in isolation. The condition of the woman and the baby should be assessed regularly throughout labour. Any decisions made should not be made on the basis of the CTG alone but following a global overview of the pregnancy. These should include previous pregnancy history and complications, antenatal risk factor, for example fetal growth and well-being and maternal medical history as well as the stage of labour, the progress in labour, contraction frequency and duration. Maternal observations should be taken into account as well as fetal factors such as movements and amniotic fluid. The clinician should assess the whole clinical picture before making management decisions.

The basic principles of CTG interpretation rely on the assessment of four factors:

1. Baseline rate – where there is a stable baseline of between 110–160 bpm and normal variability, the risk of fetal acidosis is low.
2. Baseline variability between 5 bpm and 25 bpm.
3. Presence/absence of decelerations and their duration and characteristics.
4. The presence/absence of accelerations – if there are accelerations even in the presence of reduced variability this is generally a sign of a healthy baby.

Contraction frequency and duration should also be taken into consideration. Both NICE [10] and FIGO [11] rely on these principles and recommend that the CTG is characterised as either normal, suspicious or pathological (see Figure 9.2).

When there is a requirement for continuous monitoring in labour, the CTG should be assessed and categorised hourly. If a CTG is deemed suspicious, there should be investigation and correction of any known causes such as hypotension or uterine hyperstimulation. Conservative measures should be commenced to include changing maternal position, starting intravenous fluids and stopping syntocinon. In women where hyperstimulation is suspected, terbutaline may be given. Escalation should occur to a senior obstetrician or midwife and there should be a documented plan for CTG review. For those traces categorised as pathological, there should be a review by a senior obstetrician and senior midwife. Underlying causes should be corrected and an acute event such as cord prolapse, placental abruption or uterine rupture excluded. Where conservative measures have failed to improve a CTG, consideration should be given to a fetal blood sample or urgent delivery [10].

It should be remembered that although the general principles of fetal monitoring are the same, CTG interpretation is different for women who are not in labour. Again, there is no clear evidence that antenatal CTG improves perinatal outcome, however a Cochrane review in 2015 to assess the effectiveness of antenatal CTG (both computerised and non-computerised) in improving outcomes for mothers and babies during pregnancy showed that when comparing computerised versus non-computerised CTG, there was a five-fold reduction in perinatal mortality. However, there was no significant difference identified in potentially preventable deaths, CSs or Apgar scores less than seven at five minutes [12]. Computerised CTG analysis provides an objective CTG interpretation and shows robust numeric facts rather than an individual clinician's opinion. The Dawes Redman analysis has a database of over 100,000 CTG traces and uses numeric data in relation to clinical outcome. It is not however a substitute for clinical judgement and the final assessment of any antenatal scenario should be made using evidence from the entire clinical picture, with the computerised CTG providing just one element of that picture. The computerised CTG gives a numeric value for short-

Description	Feature		
	Baseline (beats/minute)	Baseline variability (beats/minute)	Decelerations
Normal/reassuring	100–160	5 or more	None or early
Non-reassuring	161–180	less than 5 for 30–90 minutes	Variable decelerations: • dropping from baseline by 60 beats/minute or less and taking 60 seconds or less to recover, • present for over 90 minutes • occurring with over 50% of contractions OR Variable decelerations: • dropping from baseline by more than 60 beats/minute or taking over 60 seconds to recover • present for up to 30 minutes • occurring with over 50% of contractions OR Late decelerations: • present for up to 30 minutes • occurring with over 50% of contractions
Abnormal	Above 180 or below 100	Less than 5 for over 90 minutes	Non-reassuring variable decelerations (see row above): • still observed 30 minutes after starting conservative measures • occurring with over 50% of contractions OR Late decelerations • present for over 30 minutes • do not improve with conservative measures • occurring with over 50% of contractions OR Bradycardia or a single prolonged deceleration lasting 3 minutes or more

Figure 9.2 The NICE guidance for CTG classification.
Adapted from the NICE guideline on intrapartum care for healthy women and babies.

term variation (STV) which is an important index for fetal well-being. A low STV is commonly associated with growth-restricted babies. A value of <4 is low, <3 is abnormal and <2 is grossly abnormal. Care should be taken when assessing STV as it can only be determined numerically when the CTG has been in place for 60 minutes [13]. With the advent of the computerised CTG it could be used in intrapartum care but a large randomised controlled trial, the INFANT study, failed to show any evidence that computerised CTG reduced the risk of poor outcomes for babies or the risks of developmental delay at the age of two years when compared to CTG alone [14].

The aims of fetal monitoring are to detect those babies at risk of hypoxic damage and to deliver them before damage occurs. The majority of litigation in this area surrounds the diagnosis of an hypoxic brain injury and the development of cerebral palsy. A successful claim must establish that the hypoxic insult occurred in the intrapartum period and that earlier delivery would have avoided the injury. Establishing causation is an issue that was first addressed in 1999 by an international consensus statement. A template was proposed for defining a causal relation between intrapartum events and cerebral palsy [15]. Essential criteria were defined as a metabolic acidosis cord pH of <7 or a base deficit of ≥ 12 mmol/l, early onset or severe encephalopathy in infants ≥ 34 weeks and spastic quadriplegic or dyskinetic cerebral palsy [16]. In 2003, a second consensus statement was produced in which a fourth criteria was added, the exclusion of other identifiable aetiologies such as trauma, coagulation defects, infections or genetic conditions. Criteria were also added which were suggestive of an intrapartum timing; a sentinel event, sudden fetal bradycardia, Apgar scores 0–3 at >5 minutes, multi-organ involvement at <72 hours of age and evidence on early imaging [17]. In 2014, the third consensus statement was issued, driven by the recognition that a broader perspective was required and that there was still no definitive test to identify a baby with neonatal encephalopathy attributable to an acute intrapartum event. The consensus proposed five causal pathways in the development of cerebral palsy in term infants [17].

In 2017, NHS Resolution formally recognised the trauma and distress parents with a baby diagnosed with a severe brain injury were experiencing. Following on from the recommendations of the Each Baby Counts report, they introduced the Early Notification Scheme (ENS), a national programme for the reporting of infants born with a potential severe brain injury following a term labour [3]. From April 2017, all acute maternity trusts were required to notify NHS Resolution within 30 days of all babies born at ≥ 37 weeks following labour that had a potentially severe brain injury diagnosed in the first seven days of life, based on either a diagnosis of grade III hypoxic ischaemic encephalopathy, or where active therapeutic cooling had been employed or where the baby had decreased central tone, was comatose and demonstrated seizure activity. The scheme aims to support the government strategy to halve the rate of stillbirth, neonatal death and brain injury and improve the safety of maternity care while responding to the needs of families where clinical negligence is identified. From April 2017 to March 2018 there were 746 qualifying cases and the commonest theme (70%) identified was issues with fetal monitoring. Issues recognised were delay in acting on a pathological CTG or an abnormal fetal heart rate, delayed escalation and incorrect classification. The report concluded that human factors were as important for good care as the correct classification of the CTG itself. Problems with fetal monitoring persist as the major contributory factor in poor birth outcomes, despite national initiatives and guidance to improve interpretation of CTGs [10] and national recommendations for training and competence [8,9]. The current approaches to CTG training and competency are inconsistent countrywide and there is no data to inform competency or training with any accuracy. What is clear is that CTG interpretation is not just about training and competency; interpreting and reacting to a CTG is a complex process involving individuals from multiple disciplines over time, usually in highly pressured environments. It is therefore unsurprising that the technical innovations to improve individual competency have not yet impacted on the prevention of adverse outcomes [3].

Good Practice Guidance

Problems with CTG interpretation are not new. The confidential enquiry into stillbirths and deaths in infancy (CESDI) in 1997 found that there was suboptimal care in 75% of the babies identified and most of the issues were related to CTG monitoring. There were failures to initiate a CTG, failure to ensure good-quality monitoring, poor interpretation and failure to escalate to senior colleagues. Recommendations were to ensure a robust and regular programme of CTG training for all staff, to employ simple guidelines to aid interpretation and to ensure recognised channels for communication when a CTG is abnormal [18]. The findings of the Each Baby Counts report in 2015 [6] identified similar themes to those nearly 20 years before. Effective fetal monitoring in labour forms part of the Saving Babies Lives Care Bundles [8,9]. The aims are not only to reduce rates of stillbirth but to reduce the morbidity associated with fetal brain injury and cerebral palsy. Hospital trusts must demonstrate that all staff caring for women in labour are competent in CTG interpretation, that they use a buddy system approach and escalate accordingly. A standardised risk-assessment tool should be used at the start of labour and each hospital should have a fetal monitoring lead [9]. There should also be a review of all adverse outcomes or near misses. The healthcare safety and investigation branch (HSIB) has a maternity investigation programme which undertakes independent maternity safety investigations to identify common themes and instigate change. It utilises a standard approach to maternity service investigation without attributing blame or liability. All babies born at $\geq$37 weeks whether intrapartum stillbirth, neonatal death or severe hypoxic brain injury should be reported for investigation.

Causes of Litigation

Litigation surrounding CTG interpretation has a number of recurring themes. These include:

- Misinterpretation of CTG traces.
- Inappropriate or delayed response to an abnormal trace.
- Poor quality CTG recordings leading to a failure to provide accurate interpretation.
- Failing to take a global view of the patient and basing management entirely on a CTG trace alone.
- Failing to provide regular CTG reviews.
- Not involving senior staff when a CTG becomes abnormal or is difficult to interpret.
- Failing to recognise changes in the clinical scenario.
- Inappropriate use of oxytocin.
- Human factors surrounding communication and team-working.
- Poor documentation in labour.

Avoidance of Litigation

There will never be a complete avoidance of litigation in this area because CTG interpretation is not just about technical competence issues. It involves the interplay of many factors including technical, clinical and human to ensure prompt recognition of abnormal traces and a timely response to avoid hypoxic damage. Some strategies that may reduce the risk of litigation are:

- Education and training for all qualified staff involved in caring for women in labour. This training should be mandatory and annual competence is required. This may be addressed via individual e-learning training packages, attendance at local or national courses or local reviews at morbidity and mortality meetings.
- The use of a buddy system, whereby all CTGs are reviewed hourly by two practitioners and categorised accordingly. Where there is a difference in opinion, escalation to a senior obstetrician should occur.

- The use of CTG stickers to assess and categorise a CTG hourly, based on documented criteria.
- Appropriate pathways for escalation.
- Accurate documentation of all events occurring in labour, for example vaginal examinations, the presence or absence of meconium, vaginal bleeding and the commencement of oxytocin.
- Maintaining a situational awareness at all times during labour and not focusing solely on the CTG trace. Key management decisions should not be based on the CTG alone.
- Ensuring a high quality CTG trace is maintained to aid interpretation. Where the trace is of poor quality, employing strategies to address this, such as changing maternal position, ensuring monitoring equipment is working effectively or, where there are challenges to external monitoring, resorting to internal monitoring.

All CTG tracings should be stored (ideally electronically) for a period of 21 years. This will become more feasible as trusts move away from paper records and use an electronic patient record. Paper CTG traces rapidly deteriorate with time and become increasingly difficult for expert interpretation in litigation cases.

References

1. NHS Litigation Authority. Ten years of maternity claims. An analysis of NHS Litigation Authority Data. Published 2012.

2. NHS Litigation Authority. Annual report and accounts. 2015/2016.

3. NHS Resolution. The early notification scheme progress report: collaboration and improved experience for families. An overview of the scheme to date together with thematic analysis of a cohort of cases from year 1 of the scheme 2017–2018. September 2019.

4. Magro, M. NHS Resolution. Five years of cerebral palsy claims. A thematic review of NHS Resolution data. September 2017.

5. Reason, J. Human error: models and management. *BMJ* 2000; 18(320): 768–70.

6. Royal College of Obstetricians and Gynaecologists (RCOG). Each Baby Counts. October 2017.

7. Alfirevic, Z, Devane, D, Gyte, GML, Cuthbert, A. Continuous cardiotocography (CTG) as a form of electronic fetal monitoring (EFM) for fetal assessment during labour. *Cochrane Database Syst Rev* 2017, Issue 2. https://

doi.org/10.1002/14651858.CD006066.pub3

8. National Health Service (NHS). Saving Babies Lives Care Bundle Version 1. March 2016.

9. National Health Service (NHS). Saving Babies Lives Care Bundle Version 2. March 2019.

10. National Institute for Health and Care Excellence (NICE). Intrapartum Care for Healthy Women and Babies. Clinical guideline. Published: 3 December 2014.

11. Ayres-de-Campos, D, Spong, CY, Chandraharan, E, for the FIGO Intrapartum Fetal Monitoring Expert Consensus Panel. FIGO consensus guidelines on intrapartum fetal monitoring: cardiotocography. *Int J Gynecol Obstet* 2015; 131: 13–24.

12. Grivell, RM, Alfirevic, Z, Gyte, GM, Devane, D. Antenatal cardiotocography for fetal assessment. *Cochrane Database Syst Rev* 2015(9).

13. Redman, CW, Moulden, M. Avoiding CTG misinterpretation: a review of the latest Dawes-Redman CTG analysis. *Br J Midwifery* 2014; 22(1): 2–5.

14. INFANT Collaborative Group. Computerised interpretation of fetal heart

rate during labour (INFANT): a randomised controlled trial. *Lancet* 2017; 389(10080): 1719–29.

15. MacLennan, A. A template for defining a causal relation between acute intrapartum events and cerebral palsy: international consensus statement. *BMJ* 1999; 319 (7216): 1054–9.

16. Hankins, GD, Speer, M. Defining the pathogenesis and pathophysiology of neonatal encephalopathy and cerebral palsy. *Obstet Gynaecol* 2003; 102(3): 628–36.

17. American Academy of Pediatrics. Neonatal encephalopathy and neurologic outcome: second edition report of the American College of Obstetricians and Gynecologists' Task Force on Neonatal Encephalopathy. *Pediatrics* 2014; 133(5): e1482–8.

18. Maternal and Child Health Research Consortium. Confidential Enquiry into Stillbirths and Deaths in Infancy: 4th Annual Report, 1 January–31 December 1995. London: Maternal and Child Health Research Consortium; 1997.

Chapter 1

Shoulder Dystocia

Tim Draycott

CASE COMMENTARY

Swati Jha

Successful Claim

CD (AP) V Lanarkshire Acute Hospitals NHS Trust

The Claim

C sustained a severe brachial plexus injury which resulted in him being left with a permanent disability in spite of corrective surgery.

It was claimed that the accoucheur failed in their duty to diagnose this was an obstetric emergency and diagnose shoulder dystocia, failed to call for help, failed to follow the hospital protocol for the management of the shoulder dystocia, used excessive traction in the delivery of the head and failed to keep or delegate adequate note keeping of the timings and manoeuvres and subsequently write up the notes retrospectively.

The Summary

C was a 4.2 kg baby born to a 100 kg mother. The second stage of labour was 21 minutes with good advance of the head and gave no reason for prediction of the shoulder dystocia occurring at delivery. At birth C was in the left occipito-anterior (LOA) position and the cord was around the neck, hence was cut and clamped prior to delivery. The delivery was initially being conducted by the student midwife, who made two attempts to deliver the baby, then handed over to the supervising midwife. The only documentation relating to the delivery states, "Shoulder dystocia to a moderate degree – shoulders delivered on fourth pull with egs abducted after manual rotation."

The time between the delivery of the head to the shoulders was two minutes, and four pulls were required to achieve this. The usual mnemonic used for management of this obstetric emergency is the HELPERR which works through the various manoeuvres in order of invasiveness and success. Whereas the accoucheur stated that all the manoeuvres were undertaken, with the McRoberts being performed first, but denied using manual rotation although it was documented in the records, and stated her documentation was incorrect from the time of delivery. Several other contradictions were noted in the witness statement.

The Judgement

The shoulder affected was the right shoulder which was the anterior shoulder. The injury was caused by the failure to recognise this to be an emergency and follow due protocol for delivery. The excessive traction was the only way of explaining the severe and permanent injury to the anterior shoulder and there was a clear breach of duty resulting in the causation of the permanent disability which C now faces. The sum agreed as quantum in this case was £725,000 and subject to the addition of interest at the rate of 4% per annum from 30 January 2015 to the date of decree.

Courtney Ellen Webb v Liverpool Women's NHS Foundation Trust is another case of a successful claim, however this was a claim that succeeded on the basis of an omission to perform a caesarean section (CS) early in a very slowly progressing labour. The partogram showed minimal progress during the first stage and the need for a CS much earlier on in the labour. Even though the subsequent management of the vaginal delivery was felt to be non-negligent, the claim succeeded on the grounds that had a CS been performed earlier in the labour, an obstetric brachial plexus injury (OBPI) would have been avoided.

Unsuccessful Claim

Beggs v Medway NHS Trust
The Claim

Jack Beggs was born in July 2002 and suffered an injury to his right shoulder at birth, resulting in an OBPI. His mother brought a claim against Medway NHS Trust. It was alleged that the injury was caused by the negligent manner of the delivery. This resulted in a permanent disability in spite of corrective surgery, resulting in limited use of the right hand and arm with significant shortening of the right arm compared to the left arm. It was claimed that inadequate and excessive traction on the head in order to deliver the shoulders resulted in injury to the anterior shoulder with the consequent injury.

The Summary

This was Mrs Beggs' second pregnancy and the first had been a difficult delivery too, with a mild shoulder dystocia according to her records.

In this labour, she had a long second stage. Jack was a big baby weighing 10lbs 2ozs at delivery at term plus two days. The medical records prior to the birth stated the head was in the right occipito posterior position, making the right shoulder, which was injured during the delivery, the posterior shoulder. Whereas Mrs Beggs initially could not recollect which way Jack's head was when he delivered, she subsequently stated that she had remembered seeing the right cheek and right ear first on delivery thereby making the right shoulder anterior. This was over five years after the delivery, whereas the records were completed within minutes of the events being described. The notes were of good quality and were felt to be an accurate record. There were no concerns following initial delivery of the head but due to delay, the patient's legs were put into McRoberts position and suprapubic pressure applied. This was followed by immediate delivery of the shoulders and the total time between the delivery of the head and shoulders was two minutes, hence the impression was of mild shoulder dystocia.

There were several inconsistencies in Mrs Beggs' statement when compared to the records.

The Judgement

During delivery of the fetus, the anterior and posterior shoulders experience impedance at various points in the birth canal. The posterior shoulder is the lower shoulder and has to pass the mother's sacral promontory, and if there is obstruction at this stage it is the maternal uterine propulsive efforts which propel the baby past this point. Following the delivery of the head however, the anterior shoulder still has to deliver past the symphysis pubis, and at this point excessive traction on the head, while allowing delivery of the fetus, can cause brachial plexus injury.

Similar non-negligent outcomes were seen in other cases of OBPI involving the posterior shoulder in Croft v Heart of England NHS Foundation Trust [2012] EWHC 1470 (QB), Sardar v NHS Commissioning Board [2014] EWHC 38 (QB) and Watts v Secretary of State for Health [2016] EWHC 2835.

Legal Commentary

Eloise Power

Webb v Liverpool Women's NHS Foundation Trust [2015] EWHC 133 (QB)

"A Common Emergency": How Should the Standard of Care Be Interpreted in a Crisis?

In *Webb*, one of the key witnesses used the striking phrase *"a common emergency"* to describe shoulder dystocia in the context of work on a busy delivery suite [para 191]. The Court accordingly faced the important task of considering how the *Bolam/Bolitho* standard of care should be interpreted in an emergency situation. This issue is likely to be relevant to many if not all shoulder dystocia cases as well as other obstetric/gynaeco-logical emergencies.

The approach taken by HHJ Saffman is of some interest as a matter of principle. In finding for the claimant that the decision made by an obstetrician not to proceed to a CS lacked logical force and was negligent, he made a distinction between *"split-second"* decisions and decisions taken *"in terms of minutes"*, holding that *"in this case there was no split second in which a decision had to be made to avert a crisis"* [para 192]. He observed that this distinction took the case out of the *"agony of the moment scenario"*, and that this factor, together with the lack of logic, meant that the doctor's decision at 13.50 was not merely a wrong judgement call but was negligent.

A more detailed analysis of the approach which a Court should take in crisis/emergency situations is found in the first instance case of *Mulholland v Medway NHS Foundation Trust* [2015] EWHC 268, a matter which concerned allegations of negligence against staff working in an Accident and Emergency department. Giving judgement for the defendant, Green J held that doctors in Accident and Emergency *"take decisions at short notice in a pressurised environment"* and held that *"in my judgment the standard of care owed by an A&E doctor must be calibrated in a manner reflecting reality"* [para 101]. It is arguable that similar considerations should apply to obstetricians working on emergency cases in a pressurised delivery suite.

Although the issues raised by the case of *Mulholland* and similar cases have been the subject of considerable interest among practitioners, the principles adopted in *Mulholland* and in *Webb* have not as yet been considered by a higher court. It is accordingly unclear whether the distinction made in *Webb* between *"split second"* decisions and decisions taken *"in terms of minutes"* would be upheld. As things stand, it would be wise for practitioners and experts to be aware of the approach taken in these first instance cases, but to be alert for any further developments in the case law.

Drawing Adverse Inferences from the Absence of a Witness

An interesting feature of the *Webb* judgement was that the defendant did not call a vital witness: the obstetric registrar who made the decision not to proceed to a CS at 13.50 pm on the day of delivery. This was the decision which was ultimately found to be negligent by the Court.

HHJ Saffman applied the leading authority in this area: *Wisniewski v Central Manchester Health Authority* [1998] Lloyds Reports Med 223, and directed himself to the relevant principles: adverse inferences may be drawn from the absence of a witness who might be expected to have material evidence to give on an issue, but this is subject to the caveat that no adverse inference should be drawn if the reason for the witness's absence is satisfactory. Further, the detrimental effect of the witness's absence may be reduced or modified if the reason for absence is partially satisfactory. On the facts, the Court held that at worst, the detrimental effect of the registrar's absence had been reduced or modified.

Notwithstanding this finding, it is evident that the registrar's absence played a part in the judge's approach to negligence in this case. He held that *"Even if it is inappropriate to draw adverse inferences from her absence, it is difficult to draw any positive conclusions about her treatment in the absence of any evidence from her"* [para 189].

This judgement serves as a reminder that parties to litigation should take all necessary steps to call witnesses who might be expected to have material evidence to give on the issues in the case.

CD v Lanarkshire Acute Hospitals NHS Trust [2017] CSIH 30

This Scottish appellate judgement serves as a salient reminder of the role of the appellate court in relation to challenges to a trial judge's finding of facts.

Essentially, the Court of Session was invited to find that a trial judge had erred in preferring the account given by the pursuer (claimant)'s witnesses over the defender (defendant)'s key witness, a midwife. The trial judge's reasons had included the following: there were significant and material differences between the midwife's contemporaneous records and her later evidence; the midwife's evidence was contradicted by evidence given by another midwife, and the midwife's evidence had changed as the case progressed, culminating in new material being provided in the witness box. Under the circumstances, it is perhaps unsurprising that the trial judge had preferred the evidence of the pursuer's witnesses. (See Chapter 3 for a more detailed discussion of the legal principles in relation to credibility, contemporaneous records and witness evidence).

In dismissing the defender's appeal, the Court of Session applied the principles which were re-emphasised by the Supreme Court in *McGraddie v McGraddie* 2014 SC (UKSC) 12 and which ultimately derive from earlier House of Lords case law: a judge's conclusions on matters of primary fact should be overturned only in those rare cases where it is plain that a mistake has been made, and that deference to the trier of fact is the rule, not the exception.

The Court of Session briefly considered the statistical evidence which had been adduced on behalf of the pursuer, observing as follows: *"While not sufficient on its own, there is no question but that it [the statistical evidence] is wholly consistent with the injury having been caused by the use of excessive force to overcome shoulder dystocia"* [para 31]. The approach to be taken to statistical evidence will be considered in more detail at Chapter 7.

Beggs v Medway NHS Trust [2008] EWHC 2888 (QB)

Beggs was essentially a fact-based judgement involving a clear conflict of evidence as between the infant's mother and the midwife responsible for the delivery. HHJ Hawkesworth QC placed weight upon the fact that the mother's account had changed in a significant respect: at the time of the index events, she had not remembered seeing her baby's ear and cheek as his head was delivered, whereas close to trial, some 5.5 years after the birth, she stated that she recollected seeing the ear and cheek. The Court preferred the evidence of the midwife and found that the mother's evidence was not accurate or reliable (see Chapter 3 for a discussion of the legal principles relating to credibility, contemporaneous records and witness evidence). The claimant did not come up to proof that the injury was caused by excessive traction, and judgement was for the defendant.

Clinical Commentary

Tim Draycott

Good Practice Guidance

Introduction

Shoulder dystocia is an unpredictable obstetric emergency that requires a multi-professional maternity team to efficiently and effectively execute a standard algorithm of release manoeuvres [1]. Accurate execution of these release manoeuvres has been associated with reductions in neonatal injury, particularly fractures and brachial plexus injuries [2–5]. Future research and care priorities should be directed at preventing neonatal hypoxic injury and maternal trauma [6].

Antenatal

The rate of shoulder dystocia is increasing in reported series across the world [7]. There are many recognised associations between shoulder dystocia (SD) and antenatal/intrapartum causes including fetal size [1]. However, it is common ground across all national guidelines that none of them have sufficient clinical utility for prediction [8] and therefore SD remains unpredictable and consequently unpreventable.

The Montgomery judgement applies to all pregnancies; all women should be able to discuss their options for mode of birth with a balanced discussion of the risks and benefits of each.

There is an increased recurrence risk of SD after previous SD and this is recognised in the contemporaneous national guidance [1] that recommends shared decision-making for mode of birth.

There is an increase in the rate of SD for women with gestational diabetes and large infants [9]. There has been a recent report from the Healthcare Safety Investigation Board based on 10 babies that were recognised to weigh more than 4kg but did not have any documented discussion about their options. This represents, approximately, 0.1% of the infants whose birth was complicated by SD in England and Wales per annum and therefore is not representative.

The RCOG has already published patient information for elective CS [10] and there is a shared decision-making tool for Induction of Labour at term from the Cochrane group for suspected large (EFW >4kg at term) for gestational age infants [11]. These data should be shared with women with support for their choices.

Intrapartum Care/Management of Shoulder Dystocia

Management of the Shoulder Dystocia

A reduction in injury rates has been associated with an increase in correctly managed births complicated by SD [2–5]. It is important to demonstrate that the correct manoeuvres were performed, ideally in the order of the RCOG algorithm.

A lorry and low bridge is a useful analogy for SD [12] and also can be used to explain the anatomical effect of the release manoeuvres:

SD is analogous to a lorry driving under a low bridge: the baby's head is the cab of the lorry and the shoulders are the cargo area of the lorry whilst the bridge is the mother's pelvis. The head is delivered (cab gets through the bridge) and the shoulders are obstructed by the mother's pelvis (the canopy or cargo area of the lorry gets stuck up against the bridge as the bridge is too low).

Pulling alone will not resolve the SD. It is easy to understand or visualise that attempting to tow the lorry through the bridge after it has got stuck, by pulling on the cab, would damage the top of the lorry cargo area and/or the bridge. The anterior arm is analogous to the top of the lorry at this point.

McRoberts' manoeuvre pushes the forward leaning bridge backwards, making the arch more vertical, thereby increasing the apparent height of the arch of the bridge without changing the actual diameter of the arch.

Supra-pubic pressure is like pressing on the lorry canopy to press it under the extra space provided by McRoberts'.

Or the posterior arm can be delivered. The posterior arm accounts for approximately 10% of the height of the baby/lorry. Delivering the posterior arm is like taking the wheels off the lorry – it would reduce in height and could be rolled under the low arch.

McRoberts' Manoeuvre

Best practice recommendations for the management of SD have led to the development of standard protocols, which require McRoberts' as a first-line manoeuvre. McRoberts' positioning is currently recognised as the single most effective intervention, relieving up to 39% of SDs [13].

Lithotomy is not the same as McRobert's and the legs should be actively removed from the lithotomy supports.

To perform McRobert's manoeuvre accurately requires one person to manage the delivery and two to abduct and flex the hips into the McRoberts' position and possibly another to apply suprapubic pressure. Where there are less than three birth attendants it is unlikely that the manoeuvres can be executed properly.

Suprapubic Pressure

McRoberts' is often combined with suprapubic pressure (Rubins' I) and the success rate improves to 54%. Suprapubic pressure (SPP) was also originally described in isolation and therefore the sequential use of these movements would be acceptable.

Effective SPP requires rotation of the pelvis cephalad and this can be confirmed by elevation of the maternal buttocks off the bed [12,14].

Internal Rotational Manoeuvres

If these initial manoeuvres are unsuccessful, the next step is an internal manoeuvre to rotate the fetal shoulders into an oblique angle or deliver the posterior arm, depending upon clinical circumstances and individual experience.

The eponymous internal rotational manoeuvres, Woods' Screw and Rubins II, can be very confusing and difficult to execute properly [15], but their use has been associated with reduced rates of permanent brachial plexus injury [16].

McRoberts' alone is not as effective as previously thought. In Hong Kong, McRoberts' alone was only effective in 25.8% of SDs [17]. A recent paper describes an increase in the performance of SPP (27.8% to 60.3%) and internal manoeuvres from 14.5% of SDs to 47.8% in association with a 100% reduction in brachial plexus injury and a reduction in the head–body delivery interval [16].

Moreover, earlier recourse to internal manoeuvres was associated with a reduction in the head–body delivery interval (HBDI) [16].

Alternative Management Options

In addition to the standard manoeuvres recommended by National Societies [8] – described above – a number of other manoeuvres have been described for consideration, including the "Carit manoeuvre" [18], "shoulder shrug" [19]. However, the published series are extremely small and there are insufficient data to recommend their use without additional evidence. Furthermore, the use of "digital hooking" of the anterior axilla [20] does not seem biologically plausible because direct access to the anterior axilla is extremely difficult, if not impossible.

Axillary traction on the posterior axilla using either a finger [3] or "sling traction" with a neonatal feeding tube [21] has been described. Positive results have been described for digitally applied axillary traction in small series for sling traction [22,23]. However, a more recent report described a very serious complication caused by the sling: a neonatal degloving injury of the posterior neonatal arm that required surgery for repair [21]. Digital axillary traction appears safe and effective in a large series and has been proposed as an option as an internal manoeuvre [3], although there is a theoretical increased risk of humeral fracture.

In the largest published series of SD training [2], none of these manoeuvres were required and it seems pragmatic that training should focus on the standard release manoeuvres with possible inclusion of digital axillary traction where other release man-oeuvres have not been successful. "Sling traction" should be avoided, except in extremis.

Different Settings

The management of SD should be consistent across all settings and there is a five-fold increase in the risk of neonatal admission after SD outside hospital obstetric units [24].

Effective performance of the standard release manoeuvres is required for best care in all settings, including water births. There are published descriptions of asking women to stand and/or stand with one leg on the side of the pool when SD has been diagnosed during a water birth. This may put the woman at risk of slipping and moreover no release manoeuvres can be performed in that position. Therefore, help should be called, and the woman asked to leave the pool so that she can be cared for safely and effectively. Thereafter the standard release manoeuvres can be used, including all fours [1] where required.

Neonatal

Shoulder dystocia has an associated neonatal hypoxic morbidity, but it is rare and appears to be related to the duration of the HBDI. In a recent series from Hong Kong, the risk of hypoxic ischemic encephalopathy (HIE) for HBDI <5 minutes was 0.5%, compared with 23.5% for HBDI >5 minutes (P <0.001) [25]. Moreover, there was a drop in pH of 0.01 per minute HBDI [25].

Both HSIB and NHS Resolution have published small series of infants with hypoxic brain injuries following SD with a median head–body delivery interval of seven minutes and it is likely that more effective execution of the release manoeuvres would have reduced this [1,26], thereby reducing the risk of hypoxic brain injury. There definitely does not appear to be an advantage in waiting 30 seconds for each of the release manoeuvres, which is likely to increase the HBDI and risk of hypoxic injury without improving success rates.

Neonatal Management

A recent neonatal review of infants born with encephalopathy after shoulder dystocia [27] identified that there was often a discrepancy between umbilical cord gases and neonatal condition that may be related to poor sampling and/or cord compression at the SD. There was a recommendation to continue to robustly sample umbilical cord gases and neonatologists should not be reassured by apparently normal gases.

Furthermore, the authors [27] recognised the North American literature that proposed that hypovolaemia can be a significant factor for infants after SD. The practical points proposed include resuscitation in combination with deferred cord clamping and earlier use of volume replacement and this will be included in the next iteration of the RCOG SD guideline.

Training for Shoulder Dystocia

The current RCOG SD guideline, published in 2012 [1], recommended:

> Shoulder dystocia training associated with improvements in clinical management and neonatal outcomes was multi-professional, with manoeuvres demonstrated and practiced on a high-fidelity mannequin. Teaching used the RCOG algorithm rather than staff being taught mnemonics (e.g. HELPERR) or eponyms (e.g. Rubin's and Woods' screw).

This recommendation appears to be the same today: all staff should be trained locally, annually and provided with the opportunity to practice all the manoeuvres required to release the shoulders using a high-fidelity model.

Effective training for SD is extremely cost effective, with cost savings of >£1 million per QUALY saved [28].

Causation of Injury

Brachial Plexus Injury

Medical theories and expert opinions about the causal relationships between birth, management of SD and neonatal brachial plexus injuries have ebbed and flowed over the last two decades. Opinions have ranged from *res ipsa loquitur*, through the more recent propulsion theories to recent data that suggest that a substantial majority of brachial plexus injuries related to SD can be prevented with accurate management of the SD following RCOG national guidance [29].

Until recently, all obstetric brachial plexus injuries (OBPI), including Erb's palsy, were deemed the fault of the accoucheur, who must have applied excessive traction during difficult delivery of the shoulders: *res ipsa loquitor.* However, over the past two decades there have been increasing reports of OBPI in the absence of reported/coded SD or excessive traction.

Recent data from both sides of the Atlantic has demonstrated no permanent BPI at all after SD for >17,000 consecutive births (now 28,000 births), or 562 births complicated by SD [2].

There were seven temporary injuries in the same cohort, and this suggests that whilst propulsion-based injuries may exist, they are likely to be a temporary neuropraxis, rather than a permanent injury. This fits with the single traction-related causation theories and mechanisms of injury proposed by neurosurgeons who will only usually see infants with more serious injuries. This improvement has been replicated, albeit with smaller numbers, in the United States [30,31], and most recently in Sweden [32]. Furthermore, there was substandard care identified in >50% of births with a poor outcome in a recent Norwegian series [26].

The literature on causation of obstetric brachial plexus palsy has influenced recent judicial decisions regarding the causation of OBPI. Based on this literature and case law, a template was proposed to provide guidance for those assessing issues of causation in clinical negligence claims [33].

This template has been updated [34] in the light of new published data, and now concludes:

> Whilst we are not yet in the territory of res ipsa loquitur, the recent literature demonstrates that a small subset of brachial plexus injuries, permanent injuries to an anterior arm after shoulder dystocia, are almost completely preventable with reasonable care.

Based on this literature and case law, a template was proposed to provide guidance for those assessing issues of causation in clinical negligence claims [33].

Causes of Litigation

1. Pre-emptive birth before the SD
   a. Antenatal – Montgomery consistent discussion of options, including induction of labour (IOL) and elective caesarean section (ELCS)
      i. Management of suspected fetal macrosomia
      ii. Management of previous SD
      iii. Other requests for delivery by elective CS
   b. Intrapartum
      i. Failure to deliver by CS for failure to progress or fetal distress
2. Management of SD
   a. BPI of >1 nerve root to an anterior shoulder after SD is most often avoidable

b. Common care failings

   i. Excessive traction: direction, force and nature of the force

   ii. Insufficient team members to perform

   iii. Inaccurate execution of manoeuvres

   iv. Use of fundal pressure

   v. Prolonged head–body delivery interval

c. No record of annual, local training for SD

d. Poor records

3. Neonatal care

a. Failure to call neonatal team for birth

Avoidance of Litigation

1. Document discussion of options provided antenatally
2. Signpost to Cochrane shared decision-making tool for IOL and RCOG leaflet for CS
3. Manage SD following RCOG algorithm
4. Annual, local SD multi-professional training for all staff, possibly including models with force monitoring capabilities.
5. Employ RCOG documentation sheet
6. Consider neonatal volume replacement early during resuscitation post-SD.

References

1. Crofts, J, Fox, R, Draycott, T. Shoulder Dystocia. *Greentop Guidelines*. London: RCOG; 2012, p1–18.

2. Crofts, JF, et al. Prevention of brachial plexus injury – 12 years of shoulder dystocia training: an interrupted time-series study. *BJOG* 2016; 123(1): 111–18.

3. Ansell, L, et al. Axillary traction: an effective method of resolving shoulder dystocia. *Aust N Z J Obstet Gynaecol* 2019; 59(5): 627–33.

4. Weiner, CP, et al. Multi-professional training for obstetric emergencies in a US hospital over a 7-year interval: an observational study. *J Perinatol* 2016; 36 (1): 19–24.

5. Gurewitsch Allen, ED, et al. Improving shoulder dystocia management and outcomes with a targeted quality assurance program. *Am J Perinatol* 2017; 34(11): 1088–96.

6. Mendez-Figueroa, H, et al. Shoulder dystocia and composite adverse outcomes for the maternal-neonatal dyad. *Am J Obstet Gynecol MFM* 2021: 100359.

7. Hansen, A, Chauhan, SP. Shoulder dystocia: definitions and incidence. *Semin Perinatol* 2014; 38(4): 184–8.

8. Chauhan, SP, et al. Shoulder dystocia: comparison of the ACOG practice bulletin with another national guideline. *Am J Perinatol* 2010; 27(2): 129–36.

9. Nesbitt, TS, Gilbert, WM, Herrchen, B. Shoulder dystocia and associated risk factors with macrosomic infants born in California. *Am J Obstet Gynecol* 1998; 179(2): 476–80.

10. Royal College of Obstetricians and Gynaecologists (RCOG). Choosing to Have a Caesarean Section. London: RCOG; 2015, p1–6.

11. Boulvain, M, et al. Induction of labour at or near term for suspected fetal macrosomia. *Cochrane Database Syst Rev* (Online) 2016; (5): CD000938.

12. PROMPT Editorial Board. *Trainers Manual*. PROMPT 3 ed. P.E. Board. Vol. 3. Cambridge: Cambridge University Press; 2017, p128.

13. Draycott, T, Fox, R, Montague, I. Shoulder Dystocia. Greentop Guideline 42. London: RCOG; 2005, p1–13.

14. Lok, ZL, Cheng, YK, Leung, TY. Predictive factors for the success of McRoberts' manoeuvre and suprapubic pressure in relieving shoulder dystocia: a cross-sectional study. *BMC Pregnancy Childbirth* 2016; 16(1): 334.

15. Crofts, JF, et al. Observations from 450 shoulder dystocia simulations: lessons for skills training. *Obstet Gynecol* 2008; 112(4): 906–12.

16. Crofts, J, et al. Prevention of brachial plexus injury – 12 years of shoulder dystocia training: an interrupted time-series study. *BJOG* 2016; 123(1): 111–18.

17. Leung, TY, et al. Comparison of perinatal outcomes of shoulder dystocia alleviated by different type and sequence of manoeuvres: a retrospective review. *BJOG* 2011; 118(8): 985–90.

18. Gei, AF, et al. The Carit maneuver: a novel approach for the relief of shoulder dystocia – A case series. *AJP Rep* 2020; 10 (2): e133–e138.

19. Sancetta, R, Khanzada, H, Leante, R. Shoulder shrug maneuver to facilitate delivery during shoulder dystocia. *Obstet Gynecol* 2019; 133(6): 1178–81.

20. Habek, D. Severe refractory bilateral shoulder dystocia released with digital hooking (Bourgeois-Siegemundin) manoeuvre. *J Obstet Gynaecol* 2019; 39 (4): 581.

21. McCarter, AR, Theiler, RN, Rivera-Chiauzzi, EY. Circumferential shoulder laceration after posterior axilla sling traction: a case report of severe shoulder dystocia. *BMC Pregnancy Childbirth* 2021; 21(1): 45.

22. Taddei, E, et al. Posterior axilla sling traction and rotation: a case report of an alternative for intractable shoulder dystocia. *J Obstet Gynaecol* 2017; 37(3): 387–9.

23. Cluver, CA, Hofmeyr, GJ. Posterior axilla sling traction for shoulder dystocia: case review and a new method of shoulder rotation with the sling. *Am J Obstet Gynecol* 2015; 212(6): 784 e1–7.

24. Rowe, R, et al. Neonatal admission and mortality in babies born in UK alongside midwifery units: a national population-based case-control study using the UK Midwifery Study System (UKMidSS). *Arch Dis Child Fetal Neonatal Ed* 2021; 106(2): 194–203.

25. Leung, TY, et al. Head-to-body delivery interval and risk of fetal acidosis and hypoxic ischaemic encephalopathy in shoulder dystocia: a retrospective review. *BJOG* 2011; 118(4): 474–9.

26. Johansen, LT, et al. How common is substandard obstetric care in adverse events of birth asphyxia, shoulder dystocia and postpartum hemorrhage? Findings from an external inspection of Norwegian maternity units. *Acta Obstet Gynecol Scand* 2021; 100(1): 139–46.

27. Battin, MR, et al. Shoulder dystocia, umbilical cord blood gases and neonatal encephalopathy. *Aust N Z J Obstet Gynaecol* 2021; 61(4): 604–6.

28. Yau, CWH, et al. A model-based cost-utility analysis of multi-professional simulation training in obstetric emergencies. *PLoS ONE* 2021; 16(3): e0249031.

29. Draycott, T, Montague, I, Fox, R. Shoulder Dystocia. RCOG Guideline 42. London: Royal College of Obstetricians & Gynaecologists; 2005.

30. Weiner, C, Samuelson, L, Collins, L. Five-year experience with PROMPT (PRactical Obstetric Multidisciplinary Training) reveals sustained and progressive improvements in obstetric outcomes. . *Am J Obstet Gynecol* 210(1): S40.

31. Grunebaum, A, Chervenak, F, Skupski, D. Effect of a comprehensive obstetric patient safety program on compensation payments and sentinel events. *Am J Obstet Gynecol* 2011; 204(2): 97–105.

32. Dahlberg, J, et al. Ten years of simulation-based shoulder dystocia training – impact

on obstetric outcome, clinical management, staff confidence, and the pedagogical practice – a time series study. *BMC Pregnancy and Childbirth* 2018; 18 (1): 1021–8.

33. Draycott, T, et al. A template for reviewing the strength of evidence for obstetric brachial plexus injury in clinical negligence claims. *Clin Risk*, 2008; 14(3): 96–100.

34. Draycott, T, et al. Causation of permanent brachial plexus injuries to the anterior arm after shoulder dystocia – literature review. *J Patient Saf Risk Manag* 2019; 24(2): 76–80.

11

Obstetric Haemorrhage and Retained Products of Conception

Andrew Farkas

CASE COMMENTARY

Swati Jha

Successful Claim

Cross v Cambridge University Hospitals NHS Foundation Trust (2016)

The Claim

The claimant gave birth in hospital and following delivery of the baby the placenta and membranes were delivered by controlled cord traction. There was a placental cotyledon missing at the time of delivery of the placenta and it was claimed that a failure to act sooner resulted in a massive obstetric haemorrhage, resulting in shock and need for blood transfusions. This caused a prolonged inpatient stay for recovery and she experienced a severe adjustment disorder.

The Summary

Following the delivery, it was recorded that the placenta ana membranes were slightly ragged and that a piece of placental cotyledon may be missing. Neither the registrar on call for the delivery suite nor the midwife in charge were informed of this. The claimant continued to bleed heavily and after the passage of several large blood clots the management of postpartum haemorrhage was instituted. No doctor was asked to review the patient. The claimant went into shock following the steady ongoing blood loss. She was diagnosed to have suffered a significant postpartum haemorrhage (PPH), and as a consequence of the retained placenta was taken to theatres where a cotyledon of placenta was delivered. The claimant lost half her blood volume and had a prolonged recovery due to a failure to act sooner. She went on to suffer symptoms of anxiety, intrusive thoughts, nightmares, avoidance and hyperarousal following her recovery.

The Judgement

The case was settled out of court. The PPH and the massive obstetric haemorrhage were a consequence of failing to act sooner and this resulted in the adjustment disorder. This persisted in a severe form for three months and in a mild to moderate form after this. It was believed that approximately six months after commencing the recommended treatment for the adjustment disorder, the symptoms would improve. Total damages for £21,000 were approved and of this £17,000 was for pain suffering and loss of amenity (PSLA).

In the case of PQ v Royal Free London NHS Foundation Trust [2020] EWHC 1676 (QB), during the artificial rupture of membranes (ARM) to facilitate the induction of labour, there were blood vessels traversing the cervical opening (vasa previa). This resulted in a calamitous bleed leading to cerebral palsy. This led to a successful claim on the grounds that the CTG was sufficiently suspicious to have warranted a caesarean section (CS) without performing an ARM, which would have prevented the bleed.

Unsuccessful Claim

MC, JC (A Child Proceeding by his Mother and Litigation Friend MC) v Birmingham Women's NHS Foundation Trust [2016] EWHC 1334 (QB)
The Claim
The claimant (MC) was a 40-year-old who suffered massive obstetric haemorrhage during labour, leading to an assisted delivery by ventouse, birth of a baby with cerebral palsy and a hysterectomy. It was claimed that the substandard advice and subsequent poor care led to the aforementioned injuries which were avoidable.

The Summary
MC was offered an induction of labour at term due to developing pre-eclampsia and her care during induction was felt to be in keeping with the NICE guidance (CG70 on Induction of Labour and CG55 on Intrapartum Care). Due to the severity of the pain, the claimant did not permit an initial vaginal examination but when this was finally performed, she was quite far on in labour and was noted to be 9 cm dilated and therefore well into established labour. When the CTG was applied it was suspicious but not pathological and an assisted delivery was performed but due to massive bleeding following on from this, and in spite of all reasonable attempts to stop the bleeding, a hysterectomy had to be performed.

The Judgement
The decision to offer an induction of labour and early management of the induction process was deemed appropriate. The cause of hypoxia was felt to be a late and acute abruption of the placenta which explained why there was no meconium in the liquor, the cord gasses were indicative of an acute event and the massive obstetric haemorrhage was consistent with an abruption. As all care had been consistent with reasonable practice the claim was dismissed.

In the case of Welds v Yorkshire Ambulance Service NHS Trust (2016), where a 33-week parturient had a massive obstetric haemorrhage at home, there was no culpable delay in transferring her to hospital or the subsequent delivery, but the baby suffered severe brain injury.

In the case of Tait v Tayside Health Board [2017] CSOH 18, the claim regarding failing to identify a piece of retained placenta following delivery which resulted in a secondary post- partum haemorrhage.

In the case of Shah v North West London Hospital NHS Trust [2013] EWHC 4088 (QB), a large retroperitoneal haematoma and free blood were found in the abdomen isolated to a tear of the right common iliac artery (3 cm below the aortic bifurcation) which resulted in the death of the claimant's wife two weeks postnatally. The claim was dismissed on causation.

Legal Commentary

Eloise Power

Cross v Cambridge University Hospitals NHS Foundation Trust (Unreported)

Obstetric haemorrhage is an emergency by its very nature, and many of the cases in this area turn on the issue of the appropriate response in a crisis situation. Some cases, such as *Welds v Yorkshire Ambulance Service NHS Trust and another* [2016] EWHC 3325, centre upon the care provided by emergency providers (in *Welds*, an ambulance crew) as well as or instead of the care provided by midwives and obstetricians. The issue of how the standard of care should be interpreted in an emergency is dealt with in more detail in the legal commentary at Chapter 10, which contains a discussion of the case of *Mulholland v Medway NHS Foundation Trust* [2015] EWHC 268.

The case of *Cross v Cambridge University Hospitals NHS Foundation Trust* involved a primary postpartum haemorrhage consequent upon a retained cotyledon lobe of placenta. The claimant alleged negligence based upon a failure of communication: a midwife had recorded that a piece of the placenta might have been missing and that the placenta and membranes were slightly ragged, but the obstetric registrar and the delivery suite co-ordinator were not informed of the suspicion of a retained placenta and inadequate observations were thereafter carried out. This is a typical example of a situation where poor communication gives rise to a clinical negligence claim.

Fortunately, the claimant was taken to theatre in time and survived, but lost more than half of her total volume of blood and suffered a psychiatric injury (a severe adjustment disorder). Liability was denied, but the claim was settled at a total of £21,000; unlike the other cases considered in this chapter, the value of the claim was relatively modest because of the claimant's good prognosis. For further consideration of claims for psychiatric injury, please see the legal commentary at Chapter 8.

MC, JC (A Child Proceeding by his Mother and Litigation Friend MC) v Birmingham Women's NHS Foundation Trust [2016] EWHC 1334 (QB)

This case is notable for the brevity and lucidity of the judgement handed down by Turner J. The Court heard lengthy evidence and arguments upon *"very many disputed areas both of primary fact and secondary inference"* [para 13]. Turner J applied appellate authority which favoured giving shorter, clearer judgements,[1] and held that his aim in giving judgement was

> to give reasoned decisions on those issues of fact which I consider to be central but without dealing with every peripheral issue the resolution of which would not in any event impact upon my essential findings or on the outcome of the substantive claims [para 14].

---

[1] Schiemann LJ's judgement in *Customs and Excise Commissioners v A* [2003] Fam 55, cited at para 13.

The Court accordingly identified three central issues for resolution:

(i) Did M give informed consent to undergo induction? (ii) Was M adequately cared for following induction? (iii) If not, would adequate care have prevented the injuries which M and J sustained?

The claimants' case on the first issue failed. The Court rejected the mother's evidence to the effect that she was not told about pre-eclampsia or the associated risks. One record stated: *"Discussed in depth induction of labour process. M consents to being induced."* The Court found that it was reasonable for the defendant to have recommended induction and that the mother gave her informed consent to the induction process. In rejecting the mother's evidence, the Court found that the events of the night in question were horrific with life-changing consequences: *"It is easy to understand how, over time, 'I should not have consented' can become 'I would not have consented'"* [para 31].

The claimants' case on the second issue also failed. They had argued that the mother should have been offered continuous CTG monitoring. This position was not supported by any national or local guidelines. The Court found as follows:

I do not doubt the genuineness of Mr T's views but his inability to identify any literature or contemporaneous guidelines to support his call for continuous CTG, in circumstances nowhere else recommended, left him exposed to the charge that he was introducing a level of subjectivity which was ill-suited to represent a reliable standard by which to judge the actions of the hospital staff [para 52].

Unsurprisingly, the Court preferred the approach of the defendant expert, who applied national and local guidelines in support of her position that there were no material failings in respect of the care afforded to the mother. For further discussion of the use of guidelines in clinical negligence, please see the "Legal Commentary" at Chapter 9, which contains discussion of the case of *Sanderson v Guy's and St Thomas' NHS Foundation Trust* [2020] EWHC 20 (QB). In Sanderson, Lambert J held that "the Guidelines are a practical tool to be used in conjunction with clinical judgment". On the facts in Sanderson, the relevant NICE Guidelines contained an internal contradiction which caused some difficulties for the experts and the Court. The case of MC and JC is more typical, in that the local and national Guidelines seem to have been clear and relevant and were accordingly given considerable weight by Turner J.

In relation to the third issue, the Court held that the claimants' case would have failed on causation in any event. The key issue on causation was the cause of the process which led to the baby's hypoxia and the mother's bleed. The claimants' expert contended that the cause of the mother's severe bleeding after the birth was the failure of the exhausted uterus to contract, and the cause of the baby's hypoxia was a chronic one caused by a persisting pattern of strong contractions. The defendant's expert argued that the most likely explanation was a sudden and complete rupture of the placenta. The Court was placed in a difficult position, as neither expert referred to any medical literature or studies in support of their views [para 92 (i)]. The Court also observed as follows:

The opinions of the experts on this aspect of causation continued to develop up to a very late stage and, in some respects, even during the course of trial itself... Without seeking to attribute or allocate blame, there was a distinct flavour of improvisation in the way in which these arguments were articulated by both expert obstetricians which did little to strengthen my confidence in the resilience of the hypotheses upon which they were based [para 92 (ii)].

These factors prevented the Court from *"being able to make a rational or logical choice between the stark alternatives"* [para 93], with the result that the claimants failed to discharge their burden of proof on the issue.

Turner J's judgement highlights (a) the importance of clarity, particularly where the factual and evidential issues are complicated; (b) the need for clear identification of the central issues; (c) the importance of good preparation, which includes sourcing of relevant literature and full consideration of the key medical issues. The judgement also emphasises the need for caution in situations where experts and lawyers depart from relevant local and national guidelines. Where treating clinicians have complied with all relevant guidelines, it will generally be more difficult to prove that they have been *Bolam* negligent; such guidelines are not binding on the Court, but will often be given significant weight. Where experts regard it as appropriate to depart from relevant guidelines on a particular issue, it is vital to justify the position carefully and support it by reference to medical literature and studies.

Clinical Commentary

Andrew Farkas

Introduction

Antepartum haemorrhage (APH) is defined as bleeding from or into the genital tract, occurring from 24+0 weeks of pregnancy and prior to the birth of the baby. The most important causes of APH are placenta praevia and placental abruption. APH complicates 3–5% of pregnancies. Although the recent Confidential Enquiries into Maternal Deaths (MBRRACE) in the United Kingdom showed that obstetric haemorrhage had fallen to the seventh commonest cause of death [1], it remains the most common cause of maternal death worldwide. Maternal deaths represent the tip of the iceberg as there is also substantial morbidity [2]. Up to one fifth of very pre-term babies are born in association with APH, and the known association of APH with cerebral palsy can be explained by pre-term delivery [3].

Post-partum haemorrhage (PPH) is defined as the loss of 500 ml or more of blood from the genital tract after birth. Within 24 hours of the birth it is termed primary PPH, and secondary from 24 hours to 12 weeks post-natally. The RCOG guideline on Prevention and Management of Post-partum Haemorrhage terms a minor PPH as 500–1000 ml and major as >1000 ml [4]. Generally, a loss of >1000 ml at caesarean section is regarded as constituting a PPH.

Major risk factors for PPH include previous PPH, multiple pregnancy, fetal macrosomia and failure to progress in the second stage of labour. A prolonged third stage of labour and retained placenta are strongly associated with PPH. Placenta praevia and placental accreta spectrum (PAS) will be considered separately. Perineal trauma from episiotomy and lacerations is also a significant risk factor.

Retained products of conception (RPOC) is a common cause of both primary and secondary PPH. It may be associated with sepsis as well as bleeding. There is considerable variation in practice concerning diagnosis and clinical management. Retained products of conception is a frequent issue of medico-legal litigation as highlighted by NHS Resolution [5].

Good Practice Guidance

Antepartum Haemorrhage

The most important causes of antepartum haemorrhage (APH) are placental abruption and placenta praevia. Other defined causes of APH include cervical ectropion and, rarely, cervical cancer. APH associated with spontaneous or iatrogenic rupture of the fetal membranes may be associated with ruptured vasa praevia, where fetal vessels run through the free placental membranes. Many cases of APH are unexplained. Pregnancies complicated by unexplained APH are at increased risk of adverse maternal and perinatal outcomes.

Investigations which should be performed when women present with APH include:

Maternal

- Full blood count and coagulation profile
- Group and save or crossmatched blood
- Kleihauer test in Rhesus negative women to quantify the dose of Anti-D immunoglobulin required against feto-maternal haemorrhage
- Ultrasound scan, though sensitivity of ultrasound for the detection of retroplacental clot is poor [6]

Fetal

- CTG monitoring
- Kleihauer test to quantify feto-maternal haemorrhage

Placental Abruption

Placental abruption describes the separation of the placenta from the uterine wall. The most predictive risk factor is abruption in a previous pregnancy. Other risk factors include those associated with poor placentation: pre-eclampsia, fetal growth restriction, smoking and substance misuse. In revealed placental abruption, bleeding is evident vaginally. In a concealed abruption, blood remains between the placenta and uterus and is not seen vaginally.

Clinical presentation of abruption is classically of continuous pain. Fetal movements may be reduced. Vaginal bleeding may be evident. On abdominal palpation the uterus is often tender and irritable. A "woody" feel to the uterus indicates a significant abruption.

Ultrasound assessment of the size of the retro-placental bleed is difficult and often unreliable, and a bleed may not be seen on ultrasound scan until there is already other evidence of fetal compromise or even death. Placental abruption may also be associated with maternal complications of obstetric haemorrhage. A significant fall in haemoglobin coupled with the clinical picture also suggests abruption, but by this time there are usually other indicators of fetal compromise on the CTG trace or maternal cardiovascular changes.

A small placental abruption may be managed expectantly. Antenatal steroids are given to promote fetal lung maturity if delivery is thought likely to occur. However, women with a significant bleed thought to be from abruption will require delivery. This may be vaginal if fetal welfare remains satisfactory. Alternatively, caesarean section may be required, usually for CTG abnormalities. Complications of placental abruption include fetal death, in which case vaginal delivery should be achieved if possible.

Disseminated intravascular coagulation may exacerbate bleeding, requiring close liaison with the haematologist and obstetric anaesthetist.

Placenta Praevia and Placental Accreta Spectrum

Placenta praevia is defined as a placenta involving the lower segment of the uterus, which does not develop until 28 weeks gestation. Minor placenta praevia (grades I and II) involves the lower segment but does not cover the cervix. Grades III and IV are major placenta praevia and either partially or wholly cover the cervical os. A low-lying placenta is diagnosed at fetal anomaly scan at 20 weeks gestation in around 5% of women. The estimated incidence of placenta praevia at term is 1:200 pregnancies. The discrepancy arises due to the development of the lower segment in the third trimester of pregnancy.

The classical presentation of placenta praevia is with recurrent episodes of painless vaginal bleeding. Many cases of placenta praevia are asymptomatic, in so much as there is no bleeding during the antenatal course. Placenta praevia is identified on ultrasound scan. It is appropriate for such women to be managed at home after being informed of the risks of pre-term delivery and obstetric haemorrhage. Delivery by a planned elective caesarean section is usually undertaken at 36 to 37 weeks gestation.

Women with vaginal bleeding are admitted to hospital and usually advised to remain in hospital if they have repeated episodes of bleeding. Depending on the severity and frequency of blood loss, delivery is usually planned for women with episodes of bleeding between 34 and 36 weeks gestation, following a course of antenatal steroids to promote fetal lung maturity. In women with an asymptomatic third trimester low-lying placenta, the mode of delivery should be based on clinical background and the woman's preferences, and supplemented by ultrasound findings, including the position of the fetal head relative to the leading edge of the placenta on transvaginal scan (TVS) [7]. There is a place for vaginal delivery, particularly in women with a placental edge >20 mm from the internal os, but even when less. Clinically, descent of the fetal head beyond the leading edge of the placenta is associated with an increased likelihood of vaginal delivery. Anterior placenta is also more favourable.

Women having a caesarean section for placenta praevia are at increased risk of blood loss. Pre-operatively, they should be warned of the possible need for blood transfusion and hysterectomy. The risk of caesarean hysterectomy in all women, including the more complicated cases of placenta accrete spectrum (PAS) is cited as 11:100 in the RCOG Consent Advice [8]. Two to four units of blood should be crossmatched, cell salvage is recommended and rapid infusion and fluid warming devices should be immediately available. Delivery should be performed or supervised by a senior obstetrician (usually a consultant) and senior anaesthetist (usually a consultant). Regional anaesthesia is considered safe and is usually preferred to general anaesthesia in caesarean delivery in women with placenta praevia. However, the risk of bleeding is greater in women with anterior placenta praevia and they should be warned of the risk of conversion to general anaesthesia if necessary.

Placenta accreta spectrum (PAS), also known as abnormally invasive placenta (AIP), describes abnormal adherence to, or invasion of the placenta into the uterus:

- Placenta accreta – abnormal adherence of the placenta to the uterus
- Placenta increta – invasion of placental villi into the myometrium
- Placenta percreta – villous tissue perforates through the uterine wall and may invade into surrounding pelvic organs such as the bladder.

Other terms, including abnormally invasive placenta and morbidly adherent placenta, are also used to describe these conditions.

The overwhelmingly common predisposing factors for PAS are placenta praevia in association with a previous caesarean section. Instrumentation of the uterus for other reasons such as evacuation of retained products of conception or assisted reproductive technology (ART) are also risk factors. The rise in caesarean section rate has caused an increase in the prevalence of PAS, estimates of which range between 1:300 and 1:2000 pregnancies [7]. PAS in a subsequent pregnancy is more common following delivery by elective caesarean section than by emergency caesarean section [9] and women need to be informed of this when electing to have caesarean section for non-stringent and non-clinical reasons such as maternal choice.

Placenta accreta spectrum is identified initially on ultrasound scanning. A low-lying placenta at the time of the 20-week anomaly scan in a woman with a previous caesarean section should lead to a repeat scan at 28 weeks gestation (some units prefer 32 weeks). MRI scanning is increasingly used to confirm the diagnosis of PAS and define its extent more precisely [10]. Women diagnosed with PAS should be cared for by a multi-disciplinary team in a specialist centre with expertise in diagnosing and managing invasive placentation. The team includes diagnostic radiology, obstetrics, obstetric anaesthesia, interventional radiology and access to specialties including urology, vascular surgery and general surgery. Appropriate laboratory specialties with the availability of blood and blood products and intensive care facilities are also required.

Elective caesarean hysterectomy is the generally preferred management, planned between 35 and 36 weeks gestation. This involves major surgery with significant blood loss. There is limited evidence to support uterus preserving surgery. There is a high risk of peri-partum and secondary complications, including infection and the need for secondary hysterectomy. Interventional radiology (IR) is used in a number of centres to reduce per-operative haemorrhage. Catheters are placed in either the iliac vessels or the aorta. However, the evidence base to support their use is controversial and there are no criteria for their use. They carry their own complications including lower limb ischemia.

Post-partum Haemorrhage

Post-partum haemorrhage (PPH) can be primary or secondary. Primary PPH is the loss of more than 500 ml of blood within the first 24 hours of delivery. Secondary PPH is abnormal or heavy vaginal bleeding between 24 hours and 12 weeks after birth. The key to managing primary PPH is prediction, recognition and treatment.

The risk factors for PPH are listed in the NICE guidelines on intrapartum care (see Table 11.1). These risk factors can also be considered in terms of four "Ts"; tissue, thrombin, tone and trauma [11]. Anaemia in pregnancy should be corrected antenatally. Anticipation of potential PPH is important. Women with risk factors should deliver in hospital where blood products are available if necessary.

Recognition of PPH is vital. Visual estimation often underestimates blood loss [12]. More accurate methods including blood collection drapes and weighing swabs may be used. Clinical assessment of hypovolaemia, including pulse and blood pressure measurements, are basic but vital clinical tools.

The most important intervention in reducing the rate of PPH is active management of the third stage of labour. This includes the use of uterotonics, usually Syntometrine,

Table 11.1. Risk factors for post-partum haemorrhage

Antenatal risk factors

- Previous retained placenta and post-partum haemorrhage
- Maternal haemoglobin level below 85 g/l at onset of labour
- BMI >35 kg m^2
- Multiparity (parity four or more)
- Antepartum haemorrhage
- Overdistension of the uterus (for example multiple pregnancy, polyhydramnios or macrosomia)
- Existing uterine abnormalities
- Low-lying placenta
- Maternal age ≥35 years

Risk factors in labour

- Induction of labour
- Prolonged first, second or third stage of labour
- Oxytocin use (may be an association rather than causative)
- Precipitate labour
- Operative birth or caesarean section

and controlled cord traction (CCT) to expedite delivery of the placenta, with the aim of reducing blood loss. The standard oxytocic agent, given by intramuscular injection with delivery of the anterior shoulder, is Syntometrine, a combination of 500 mcg ergometrine and 5 IU of oxytocin. Ergometrine has a slightly more prolonged effect than oxytocin and may cause nausea.

Many studies have demonstrated the value of active management of the third stage in labour. These are summarised in the Cochrane systematic review [13] showing reduction in the average risk of maternal primary haemorrhage >1000 ml at the time of birth with active compared to passive management following birth; (average risk ratio [RR] 0.34, 95% confidence interval) [CI] 0.14–0.87) and maternal haemoglobin <90 g/l) (average RR 0.50, 95% CI 0.30–0.83).

Other uterotonics given in the management of PPH include prostaglandin analogues such as carboprost (Hemabate) and misoprostol which can be given orally, sublingually, vaginally or rectally. Other medication used to promote clotting and reduce blood loss includes tranexamic acid.

Estimated blood loss (EBL) at delivery or at caesarean section is often underestimated. Resuscitation procedures for minor PPH (500 to 1000 ml) and major PPH (>1000 ml) are included in the RCOG Guidelines [4]. Integral to these are adequate fluid replacement and availability of blood products, including red blood cells, fresh frozen plasma, platelet concentrate and cryoprecipitate as necessary.

Cases of major PPH are usually managed in conjunction with the obstetric anaesthetist. With a PPH >1500 ml the RCOG Guidelines indicate the need for consultant obstetric involvement. Most obstetric units activate a major/massive obstetric haemorrhage pathway following a PPH >1500 ml.

The commonest cause of primary PPH is uterine atony. It is important to confirm that the placenta and membranes are delivered and complete. The following measures should then be instituted:

- Palpate the uterine fundus and rub up a contraction
- Ensure that the bladder is empty
- Pharmacological measures: an oxytocic infusion [40 IU and 500 ml saline] with additional oxytocin or ergometrine as necessary
- Carboprost and misoprostol as necessary

Bleeding at and after caesarean section may be caused by uterine atony, but also by failure to adequately identify and repair the uterine incision and any extension. Caesarean section at full cervical dilatation is a risk factor.

Surgical Measures

If bleeding continues, consideration must be given to other sources such as perineal trauma or a cervical tear. Where possible, any perineal trauma should be sutured promptly. Transfer to theatre is necessary if there is ongoing bleeding. Initially, uterine exploration should be undertaken to exclude the presence of retained products of conception or if there is a suspicion of absent placental membranous tissue. This also facilitates evacuation of blood and clot from the uterus, cervix and vagina, so allowing uterine contraction.

Uterine balloon tamponade with a large balloon catheter inflated with fluid is popular. Bakri or Rusch [14] balloons are generally used. Balloon tamponade applies pressure to the placental bed, but is counter intuitive as it prevents contraction of the post-partum uterus. A different strategy is the use of a B-Lynch haemostatic brace suture [15], which can be used in combination with a balloon catheter. This requires a laparotomy and is particularly useful when the abdomen has already been opened for a caesarean section. Hysterectomy may be required on rare occasions and should not be delayed until the woman is in extremis. This raises issues around the surgical experience of the obstetrician and their ability to perform post-partum hysterectomy. Other procedures are used occasionally, including uterine devascularisation and internal iliac artery ligation. There is also a place for arterial embolisation using interventional radiology procedures.

Retained Products of Conception

Retained products of conception (RPOC), usually associated with infection, is a major cause of secondary PPH. Avoidance and realisation of retained placental tissue is key to the management of this problem. Following delivery, it is generally the midwife who checks the placenta and membranes and documents whether the placenta is complete or not and the membranes are complete or ragged. Active management of the third stage of labour significantly reduces the risk of PPH and reduces the likelihood of RPOC remaining. RPOC will lead to failure of adequate contractions of the uterus which may result in a primary PPH. If it is appreciated that placental or membranous tissue is absent, this is likely to lead to exploration of the uterus/manual evacuation of products of conception. Alternatively, the prostaglandin analogue misoprostol may be used.

In the post-natal period, retained products may present with vaginal bleeding to a varying extent. RPOC is often associated with infection of the decidua (endometrial lining), known as endometritis. This may present as local sepsis with an offensive vaginal discharge or systemic infection.

It may be difficult to distinguish bleeding secondary to RPOC from normal or physiologically heavy lochia. On clinical examination, an open cervix, as opposed to patulous cervix, is usually associated with clinically significant retained products of conception. Ultrasound examination of the post-partum uterus is known to be unreliable [16]. Products of conception may readily be confused with clot and blood. It is usually held that a cotyledon, i.e. segment of placenta measuring approximately 3 cm in diameter, should be recognised by the midwife checking the placenta and the failure to do so represents a breach of duty.

The options are firstly expectant management, usually combined with antibiotic therapy using a broad spectrum antibiotic such as co-amoxiclav or cephalosporin with metronidazole. Although expectant management is usually successful, a significant volume of likely RPOC requires active management. It may be appropriate to treat with misoprostol. The further in time from delivery, the less likely is misoprostol to be effective. Alternatively, surgical evacuation may be undertaken. This carries its own hazards, including an increased risk of perforation of the soft post-partum uterus and the development of uterine adhesions (Asherman's syndrome). The likelihood of this complication is greatest when evacuation of the uterus is performed three to four weeks post-partum. Although not standard practice, the use of ultrasound guidance may be considered for post-partum evacuation of the uterus. There is a strong argument for its use in repeat procedures. Persistent retained products may need to be treated several months later by hysteroscopic resection under direct vision, particularly where there is evidence of calcification of the RPOC.

Causes of Litigation

The NHSLA review of maternity claims 2000–2010 shows that 82 of 111 cases were in respect of retained products of conception, 25 in which haemorrhage was the primary issue and four others. However, 63% of the total £3 million value of these claims arose from the haemorrhage cases [4].

As indicated by the relatively high number of claims associated with RPOC, failure to adequately assess the placenta and membranes following delivery leads to litigation. Each claim must be considered on its merits depending on the extent of products identified.

Poor surgical technique at caesarean section may be evidenced by bleeding from a poorly sutured uterine angle or extension found at laparotomy for haemorrhage.

The feeling of vulnerability and imminent death from major haemorrhage may cause significant psychological consequences at a time when a woman feels particularly vulnerable following childbirth.

The need for hysterectomy and loss of reproductive function following massive PPH results in loss which may be recoverable in damages if due to negligence. It must be said that peripartum hysterectomy may often be life-saving.

Bleeding from perineal trauma may be associated with other morbidity such as scarring and dyspareunia (pain on sexual intercourse) leading to subsequent litigation.

Rare causes of litigation include damage to other organs associated with massive blood loss, for example, Sheehan's syndrome or post-partum hypopituitarism or renal failure.

Avoidance of Litigation

Adequate training of both midwifery and obstetric staff is crucial. This pertains to all aspects from assessment of placenta and membranes after delivery to good surgical technique at caesarean section.

Women should deliver in an appropriate setting. For example, the management of placenta accreta spectrum (PAS) is now being commissioned on a regional basis by NHS England. At a more straightforward level there should be appropriate discussion when necessary about home versus hospital delivery.

There is usually an antenatal discussion concerning active management of the third stage of labour between the midwife and pregnant woman. Active management should be positively encouraged.

The placenta and membranes should be checked adequately following delivery and any concerns voiced and documented.

Although many cases that come to litigation represent a failure of recognition of the extent of PPH, failure of anticipation often underlies this. Underestimation of blood loss leads to poor and tardy management with further complications which may give rise to claims.

There should be early recourse to hysterectomy in cases of massive PPH, before the patient becomes severely cardiovascularly unstable and clotting disturbances supervene (disseminated intravascular coagulation or DIC).

Clear and effective communication with the patient and her family may help reduce any psychological impact of PPH.

References

1. Knight, M, Bunch, K, Tuffnell, D et al., on behalf of MBRRACE-UK. Saving Lives, Improving Mothers' Care – Lessons learned to inform maternity care from the UK and Ireland Confidential Enquiries into Maternal Deaths and Morbidity 2015–2017. Oxford: National Perinatal Epidemiology Unit, University of Oxford; 2019.

2. Waterstone, M, Bewley, S, Wolfe, C. Incidence and predictors of severe obstetric morbidity: case-controlled study. *BMJ* 2001; 322: 1089–94.

3. Royal College of Obstetricians & Gynaecologists (RCOG). Antepartum Haemorrhage. Green-top Guideline No. 63. London: RCOG; 2011.

4. Royal College of Obstetricians & Gynaecologists (RCOG). Prevention and Management of Post-partum Haemorrhage. Green-top Guideline No. 52. London: RCOG; 2016.

5. https://resolution.nhs.uk/wp-content/uploads/2018/11/Ten-years-of-Maternity-Claims-Final-Report-final-2.pdf

6. Glantz, C, Purnell, L. Clinical utility of sonography in the diagnosis and treatment of placental abruption. *J Ultrasound Med* 2002; 21: 837–40.

7. Royal College of Obstetricians & Gynaecologists (RCOG). Placenta Praevia and Placenta Accreta: Diagnosis and Management. Green-top Guideline No. 27a. London: RCOG; 2018.

8. Royal College of Obstetricians & Gynaecologists (RCOG). Caesarean section for placenta praevia. Consent advice No. 12. London: RCOG; 2010.

9. Kamara, M, Henderson, JJ, Doherty, DA, Dickinson, JE, Pennell, CE. The risk of placenta accreta following primary elective caesarean delivery: a case-controlled study. *BJOG* 2013; 120: 879–86.

10. Rahaim, NS, Whitby, EH. The MRI features of placental adhesion disorder

and the diagnostics of significance: systematic review. *Clin Radiol* 2015; 70: 917–25.

11. National Institute for Health and Care Excellence (NICE). Intrapartum care for healthy women and babies. NICE Clinical Guideline 190. Manchester: NICE; 2014 (last updated February 2017).

12. Patel, A, Goudar, SS, Geller, SE, et al. Drape estimation vs visual assessment for estimating postpartum haemorrhage. *Int J Gynaecol Obstet* 2006; 93: 220–4.

13. Begley, CM, Gyte, GM, Devane, D, et al. Active versus expectant management for women in the third stage of labour.

Cochrane Database Syst Rev 2011; 11: CD007412.

14. Keriakos, R, Mukhopadhyay, A. The use of the Rusch balloon for management of severe post-partum haemorrhage. *J Obstet Gynaecol* 2006; 26: 335–8.

15. B-Lynch, C, Coker, A, Lawal, AH, et al. The B-Lynch surgical technique for the control of massive postpartum haemorrhage: an alternative to hysterectomy? Five cases reported. *Br J Obstet Gynaecol* 1997; 104: 372–5.

16. Edwards A, Elwood DA. Ultrasonographic evaluation of the postpartum uterus. *Obstet Gynecol* 2000; 16: 640–3.

Infection and Sepsis in Pregnancy

Adam S Gornall

CASE COMMENTARY
Swati Jha

Successful Claim

Colwill v Oxford Radcliffe Hospitals NHS Trust [2007] EWHC 2881 (QB)

The Claim

The claimant claimed damages for an infection she contracted during her admission to hospital. The infection was caused by the insertion of a cannula resulting in septicaemia which left her hemiplegic, almost blind and with severe cognitive impairment. It was claimed that all these injuries could have been avoided if the cannula had not been placed. It was claimed that placement of the cannula was not necessary, the crook of the arm should not have been used, the cannula should have been removed a day earlier and it was negligent to fail to recognise the infection and administer antibiotics earlier.

The Summary

Ms Colwill came to the United Kingdom from Nigeria. She suffered recurrent malaria and was admitted to hospital with rigors, headaches, malaise and a temperature. A cannula was sited in the crook of her arm to provide hydration, which was removed three days later. The cannula was used once for a saline drip on admission but was not used at all subsequent to this. There was no documentation of the presence of the cannula which resulted in a delay in its removal. It also meant it was not adequately monitored or removed. The cannula caused a staphylococcal septicaemia and pneumonia that left her with multiple disabilities. However, soon after removal she started to complain of pain in her arm at the site of the cannula and by the next day looked unwell. Antibiotics were not started till several days (two days) after the infection in the arm was recognised, as phlebitis is relatively common. She went on to develop septicaemia and severe respiratory distress syndrome and had to be transferred to the intensive care unit.

The Judgement

The placement of the cannula and its location in the crook of the arm were not deemed negligent as it was extremely widespread and commonly performed. However, the failure to remove the cannula in a well patient who did not require it as she was not dehydrated was unnecessary and was in breach of duty. Had the cannula been removed earlier, on a balance of probabilities, the infection is unlikely to have become so widespread. Commencement of antibiotics to treat the infection was also delayed, and the infection was more advanced and widespread as a result of this. This could have been started a day earlier, which would have contained the infection better and thereby prevented the extreme sequelae and admission to the ICU.

In the case of *Finnie v South Devon Healthcare NHS Foundation Trust*, the claimant underwent 23 separate operations due to a pelvic abscess and sepsis following surgery for a megarectum. The claim succeeded on the grounds that there had been a breach of duty in the performance of the surgery which was not absolutely necessary, hence the complications arising from its performance could have been avoided.

Unsuccessful Claim

Keh v Homerton University Hospitals NHS Foundation Trust [2019] EWHC 548 (QB)

The Claim

The claimant's wife developed an infection in the operation wound following a caesarean section (CS). This failed to respond to subsequent treatment leading eventually to her untimely demise. There was a high likelihood of the induction of labour failing in her given situation. It was claimed that the negligence of the defendant trust was in failing to perform an elective CS, failing to perform the CS earlier in labour and failing to perform a hysterectomy. All of these failures caused the infection to spread, resulting in her death.

The Summary

Mrs Keh was a Jehovah's witness. This was her first pregnancy and she was 40 years old when she was in this pregnancy. She had a two-year history of infertility. She suffered from hypertension and a plan was made for an induction of labour at 39 weeks but she was admitted a few weeks prior to the scheduled induction due to concerns with the baby. As she was a Jehovah's witness it was agreed that an attempt to avoid unnecessary surgery i.e. a CS was in her interests as this would increase the risk of bleeding.

During induction of labour there were concerns about the fetal heartbeat, so an emergency CS was performed. This was uneventful, with minimal blood loss, and her discharge was anticipated a few days later but she was found to have an MSSA infection. In view of this, she was isolated but was visited daily by her husband. She continued to show signs of infection so underwent a CT scan which showed evidence of endometritis. The purpose was to identify any collections or abscess that would benefit from drainage. Her blood cultures were reported as negative and blood results were improving, suggesting she was responding to the antibiotics. Over the next few days however, her condition deteriorated, and she went into respiratory failure and subsequently died. The post-mortem findings showed evidence of a continuing Gram-positive infection in the CS uterine wound site, and this was probably the source of the severe sepsis. However, there was no evidence to suggest carrying out a hysterectomy based on the investigations.

The Judgement

Given it would not be routine practice to offer women an elective CS purely on the grounds that an induction might fail, it was reasonable to attempt to deliver Mrs Keh vaginally.

The CS was performed adequately and performing the CS any sooner would not have changed the sequence of events. In the absence of abnormal investigations, there was also no indication to perform a hysterectomy. In view of these issues, the judgement was in favour of the defendant trust and, in spite of the tragic outcome, no liability attributed to them.

Legal Commentary

Eloise Power

Sepsis and Successive Causative Events

Most sepsis cases encountered in practice are multifactorial and will require the legal team and experts to consider the causative relevance of a series of events over the course of the development of the illness. The legal principles relating to causation in cases involving successive causative events were considered by the Judicial Committee of the Privy Council[1] in the influential case of *Williams v Bermuda Hospitals Board* [2016] UKPC 4.

Williams was itself a sepsis case, involving a patient who suffered a ruptured appendix with widespread pus throughout the pelvic region, leading to a myocardial ischaemic event and lung complications. It was common ground that there had been an avoidable delay in performing surgery. The issue before the Privy Council was whether the Court of Appeal in Bermuda had been entitled to hold that a "material contribution" (due to the delay) was sufficient to establish causation.

The Court approved the following formulation from the academic literature:[2]

> It is trite negligence law that, where possible, defendants should only be held liable for that part of the claimant's ultimate damage to which they can be causally linked... It is equally trite that, where a defendant has been found to have caused or contributed to an indivisible injury, she will be held fully liable for it, even though there may well have been other contributing causes.

Applying these principles to the facts, the Court rejected the defendant's argument that in the present case the sepsis attributable to the negligence had developed after sepsis had already begun to develop, and that the contributing causes of an indivisible injury had to be simultaneous, holding as follows [para 39, underlining added]:

> *The sequence of events may be highly relevant in considering as a matter of fact whether a later event has made a material contribution to the outcome... or conversely whether an earlier event has been so overtaken by later events as not to have made a material contribution to the outcome. But those are evidential considerations. As a matter of principle, successive events are capable of each making a material contribution to the subsequent outcome.*

On the facts of the case, the Court found that the development of sepsis, and its effect on the heart and lungs, was a *"single continuous process"* which had continued for at least two hours and 20 minutes longer than it should have done due to negligence.

---

[1] The Judicial Committee of the Privy Council is the court of final appeal for United Kingdom overseas territories, Crown dependencies and for certain independent Commonwealth countries that have retained a final right of appeal to the Crown or to the Judicial Committee. The members of the Committee are drawn from the justices of the United Kingdom's Supreme Court. See www.jcpc.uk.

[2] Professor Sarah Green, *Causation in Negligence*, Hart Publishing, 2015, Chapter 5, p97, cited at para 31 of the judgement in *Williams*.

Accordingly, the Court found that the negligence had materially contributed to the process of sepsis and hence to the claimant's injury.

The principles in *Williams* are relevant to all sepsis cases where causation is in dispute and are also applicable to other areas of clinical negligence involving successive events.

Colwill v Oxford Radcliffe Hospitals NHS Trust [2007] EWHC 2881 (QB)

Although *Colwill* was not a gynaecological/obstetrics case (it involved the development of sepsis consequent upon the presence of an in-dwelling intravenous cannula inserted due to malaria), the judgement is likely to be of interest to lawyers and to medical practitioners in all fields due to Dobbs J's detailed analysis of the witness evidence of a clinician who was found to have been negligent. On the facts, the key question for the Court was whether a particular doctor had failed to properly address his mind to the question of infection on a particular date. It was common ground that if antibiotics had been prescribed on that date, the complications suffered by the claimant would not have arisen.

In finding that the doctor in question was *"an unsatisfactory witness"*, the Court relied upon the following instructive points:[3]

(i) *He often gave answers before the full question had been asked, so much so that Counsel for the Claimant had to remind him to wait till the end of the question. He frequently did not listen properly to the question being asked in cross-examination, and gave an answer to a different question...*

(ii) *He was ready to defend the actions of Dr Ready without proper thought...*

(iii) *He contradicted himself in evidence...*

(iv) *He made previous inconsistent statements...*

(v) *His evidence is contradicted by other evidence...*

(vi) *He sought to justify his actions with little or no evidential foundation: (a) in evidence-in-chief, Dr Northfield indicated that the prescribing of antibiotics might have masked the "important" diagnoses which could have led to complications. In cross-examination, he conceded that antibiotics would not in fact have masked them; (b) in evidence-in-chief, part of his justification for not prescribing antibiotics on 25th September was that the white cell count did not support any relevant diagnosis. In cross-examination he conceded that he probably did not have the results of the white cell count at the time he conducted the examination of the patient as they would have come back later.*

(vii) *Given that he claims to write his notes chronologically, he had no credible explanation for (a) why the notes on 25th September were written in the margin; (b) why he found it necessary to underline the word "not" when he was not in the habit of emphasising negative findings; (c) why he made no note of redness and swelling/puffiness which he now says he found on 25th; and (d) why, if his diagnosis was that Miss Colwill was suffering from phlebitis and not an infection, this is not recorded in the notes.*

(viii) *He has been careless in his note-making and in his statement... He seemed unconcerned about the error, indicating that "it is very common for people to write down the wrong date in medical notes".*

(ix) *He was very defensive about criticism.*

---

[3] I have shortened the judge's criticisms for reasons of space; the complete account can be found at para 76 of the judgement.

The Court found that these and other examples gave *"the impression of a practitioner who is less than careful and attentive"*. Following a close review of the evidence, the Court rejected the doctor's evidence to the effect that he had given careful consideration to the issue of infection on the date in question and held that he had been negligent. The claimant's claim succeeded.

Keh v Homerton University Hospitals NHS Foundation Trust [2019] EWHC 548 (QB)

This case involved the tragic death of a mother who developed sepsis consequent upon an emergency caesarean section in her first pregnancy. The claimant, who was the deceased's widower and father of the baby, brought a claim on behalf of the dependents under the Fatal Accidents Act 1976 and on behalf of the estate under the Law Reform (Miscellaneous Provisions) Act 1934,[4] alleging (1) that the defendant should have been warned of the high risk that induction would be unsuccessful and should have been offered an elective caesarean section; (2) that when the emergency section was eventually performed, there was an unnecessary delay of an hour and the section took 18 minutes longer than it should have done; (3) that there was a negligent failure to perform a hysterectomy.

In relation to the first area, Stewart J found that the consultant was in breach of duty in failing to communicate to the deceased that she was at higher-than-average risk of requiring an emergency section. The Court also found that the deceased was not given the option of an elective section. Despite these identified failings, the first area of allegations failed on causation: the Court found that the deceased would probably not have chosen to have an elective section.

In relation to the second area, the Court found that the difference between the target time of 75 minutes and the actual time of 93 minutes was insufficient to prove a breach of duty; the Court accepted that a target was different from a mandatory requirement.

In relation to the third area, the Court conducted a detailed analysis of the evidence and found that it was not negligent to have failed to perform a hysterectomy. Although the defendant should have performed an MDT consultant review, this would not have led to a hysterectomy, as a radiologist would have said that there were no specific features on the CT scan which would have confirmed an infection of the uterus.

An area of interest arising from the judgement is the approach taken by the Court to the expert evidence of the obstetrician instructed by the claimant. The following criticisms made by Counsel for the defendant were approved by the Court and taken into account when assessing the reliability of the expert's evidence:[5]

(i) Professor X has not been in regular clinical practice (on call and on the labour ward) since August 2007...

(ii) Professor X gave his views without acquainting himself with the pleadings or witness statements. On the first day of his evidence he said he had not been supplied with these documents

---

[4] See the legal commentary at Chapter 26 (Gynaecological Malignancy) for further consideration of claims after death.

[5] Para 84 of the judgement; I have shortened the criticisms for reasons of space, and have also anonymised the expert in question.

by those instructing him. He was unable properly to explain why he took no steps to obtain them...

(iii) At the outset of the second day of his evidence, he said that, although he had checked and had in fact been supplied with some, but not all, of the witness statements and pleadings, he did not feel that they added anything factual or material to his view of the events.

(iv) The bulk of Professor X's professional career has been spent at the Chelsea & Westminster Hospital, which has a very high caesarean section rate... He did not seem to accept that this might affect his view as to the likelihood of Mrs Keh requiring a section following IOL...

(v) He appeared on a number of occasions to be unable to recognise a range of obstetric opinion extending beyond his own. This was illustrated by his criticism of not performing a vaginal examination before the plan to induce labour was agreed. The paper that he himself had cited demonstrated that even in 2015 there was a range of opinion, based on apparently reputable studies, as to the utility of the Bishop Score in decision-making in relation to IOL. Even having been taken to that paper, he seemed unwilling to acknowledge the existence/reasonableness of the alternative view...

(vi) In cross-examination he sought to advance, for the first time, criticisms of Miss Ray... These criticisms had not been put to Miss Ray, even though Professor X had been present throughout the trial. Despite them being obstetric matters, no satisfactory explanation as to why they had not been mentioned previously was forthcoming...

The duties of an expert are considered in more detail in Chapter 3. The instructive criticisms endorsed by Stewart J in the case of *Keh* emphasise the importance of good and thorough preparation: it is vital for experts to familiarise themselves with the crucial documents in the case, which will include the pleadings and the witness statements as well as the medical records, to give rational and objective consideration to alternative viewpoints and to consider any areas where their views may be affected by relevant biases.

Clinical Commentary
Adam S Gornall

Introduction

Infection during pregnancy, childbirth and in the postnatal period is relatively common and in many cases treated without problem. Some infections that occur in pregnancy primarily pose a risk to the mother whilst others can be transmitted to the fetus through the placenta or during birth. Pregnancy itself can make women more susceptible to certain infections and may also make such infections more severe. Even mild infections can occasionally lead to serious illness in pregnant women. In a few cases the infection may progress to sepsis and ultimately serious morbidity and mortality. Severe sepsis with acute organ dysfunction has a mortality rate of 20–40%. With the onset of septic shock, the mortality rate increases to 60%. The World Health Organization has described maternal sepsis as "a life-threatening condition defined as organ dysfunction resulting from infection during pregnancy, childbirth, post-abortion or postpartum period [1]." Sepsis involves an exacerbated systemic inflammatory response to the toxins produced by an infecting agent. Consequently, the defence cells in the body release large amounts of pro-inflammatory cytokines. In turn, the cytokines activate endothelial tissues, resulting in a wide range of systemic changes ultimately causing generalized tissue hypoperfusion, cell hypoxia, anaerobic metabolism, increased lactate, and acidemia. The process culminates in multiple organ dysfunction and death.

Unfortunately, despite being highly preventable, maternal sepsis continues to be a major cause of death and morbidity for pregnant or recently pregnant women and their babies.

In the last 10–15 years, sepsis in general has received increased attention due to the recognition that it poses a significant risk of serious morbidity and mortality. Studies have shown that survival rates following sepsis are related to early recognition and prompt, comprehensive management. Consequently, many organisations such as the UK Sepsis Trust and the Surviving Sepsis Campaign have produced guidance associated with publicity campaigns [2,3].

Changes in Maternal Immunity and Body Systems

Modulation of the immune system, in order to protect the mother and fetus from disease, will occur during pregnancy. Such changes also help to prevent the maternal immune system from attacking the fetus that is "foreign" to the mother. However, modulation can also make the mother prone to infections that do not normally cause illness.

In addition, there are significant changes to the maternal organs outside the uterus. Progesterone will lead to relaxation of the ureter and bladder muscles leading to an increased chance of urinary retention and urinary reflux into the kidneys. Coupled with the pressure caused by an expanding uterus, there is an increased risk of urinary tract infection in the bladder and kidneys. Increased fluid in the lungs may stimulate bacterial growth, raising the risk for lung infections such as pneumonia.

Risks for Mother

Infections in pregnancy, childbirth and the postnatal period will commonly involve the urogenital tract [4]. Other foci for infection may involve the lungs, surgical wounds and breasts. Many infections can be readily treated with antibiotics. However, failure to recognise and treat an infection may lead to deterioration and the onset of sepsis. Some women may have a higher risk for sepsis if they have an underlying condition such as diabetes, anaemia, obesity, congestive heart failure, liver disease, or lupus. Others may have undergone invasive procedures to help them get pregnant, or invasive tests, e.g. amniocentesis and procedures, e.g. cervical cerclage during pregnancy. Women of black or other minority ethnic group origins develop sepsis more frequently than their white counterparts.

In early pregnancy, intrauterine infection poses a risk after any miscarriage or induced abortion, particularly if there has been instrumentation of the uterine cavity. During pregnancy, infection of the uterine cavity may follow rupture of the membranes surrounding the amniotic cavity. At delivery, common surgical procedures such as episiotomy and caesarean section will provide a route for infection. If the surgery occurs after prolonged or obstructed labour or prolonged rupture of membranes, the chance of infection increases yet further. Once infection develops, it may in turn lead to necrotizing fasciitis and pelvic abscess. Group A streptococcal infection is more prevalent in the postnatal period and may be related to close contact with family members or small children carrying the organism.

Urinary tract infections are common in pregnancy and in the postnatal period. Without treatment, an infection of the urinary tract, commonly caused by the organism E. coli, may progress to urosepsis.

Risks for the Fetus and Neonate

Some maternal infections such as cytomegalovirus, toxoplasmosis, parvovirus, hepatitis, syphilis and HIV can all be transmitted and may have a direct impact on the fetus. Bacterial infections may present a risk to the fetus within the uterine cavity or may pose a risk in the neonatal period following infection in the uterine cavity or during childbirth.

Bacterial infection of the fetus during pregnancy is usually caused by infection ascending the genital tract from the vagina. Once infection establishes within the uterine cavity, the fetus and subsequently the neonate may be adversely affected. Outcomes may include perinatal death, asphyxia, early onset neonatal sepsis, septic shock, pneumonia, intraventricular haemorrhage (IVH), cerebral white matter damage, and long-term disability including cerebral palsy. The inflammatory process may sensitise the fetal brain to hypoxia and may have an impact upon the development of subsequent cerebral palsy.

Early onset neonatal sepsis is variably defined as infection occurring within 48–72 hours of birth. The risk of sepsis and mortality increases with decreasing gestational age and birth weight. The incidence is around 0.9 per 1000 live births in the United Kingdom. Group B streptococcus (GBS) and *Escherichia coli* are the most common causative organisms.

Good Practice Guidance
Ascending Infection and Chorioamnionitis

Acute chorioamnionitis is usually caused by ascending infection of the maternal genital tract. Whilst all pregnant women have microorganisms in the lower genital tract, most do not have intra-amniotic infection. The mucus plug within the cervix represents an anatomical and functional barrier to ascending infection during pregnancy. Microbial invasion of the amniotic cavity commonly occurs in women in spontaneous labour at term. It is usually of short duration and can occur after the initiation of labour. Bacteria can be introduced when the chorioamniotic membranes are exposed to the vaginal microorganisms during the course of digital examinations performed during labour to determine cervical dilatation. Such microbial invasion is typically low in amount and usually elicits only a mild intra-amniotic inflammatory response.

Risk factors for chorioamnionitis at term include prolonged labour, second stage of labour >2 hours, prolonged membrane rupture (typically >12 hours), multiple digital examinations, especially after membrane rupture, nulliparity, Group B streptococcus colonisation, bacterial vaginosis, alcohol and tobacco use, meconium-stained amniotic fluid, internal fetal heart rate monitoring and epidural anaesthesia.

Evidence of intra-amniotic infection or inflammation can be shown on microscopic examination of the placenta and membranes and is called histologic chorioamnionitis. Such a finding may be present in clinically unapparent (sub-clinical) chorioamnionitis as well as clinical chorioamnionitis. The latter is a clinical syndrome comprised of the combination of maternal pyrexia, maternal tachycardia (>100 bpm), fetal tachycardia (>160 bpm), uterine tenderness and foul-smelling amniotic fluid. Maternal fever is the most important clinical sign of chorioamnionitis.

Thus the definition of chorioamnionitis varies according to key diagnostic criteria, which can be clinical (presence of typical clinical findings), microbiologic (culture of microbes from appropriately collected amniotic fluid or chorioamnion) or histopathological (microscopic evidence of infection or inflammation on examination of the placenta or chorioamniotic specimens). Diagnosis of chorioamnionitis prior to birth will usually rely upon clinical symptoms and signs making diagnosis difficult at times. In the absence of overt clinical signs, particularly maternal, the fetus may be severely affected before the presence of chorioamnionitis has been recognised.

Usually prolonged membrane rupture, where microorganisms from the vagina have a direct route into the amniotic cavity, associated with other risk factors, is a typical scenario for the development of clinical chorioamnionitis. However, there is also experimental evidence that bacteria can cross intact membranes and therefore rupture of the membranes is not always necessary for bacteria to reach inside the amniotic cavity. Such infections can be subclinical in nature and again difficult to diagnose early.

Prelabour Rupture of Membranes

Prelabour rupture of membranes (PROM) after 37 weeks gestation occurs in 8% of cases [5]. Spontaneous onset of labour usually follows, with 79% of women labouring spontaneously within 12 hours, and 95% within 24 hours. Preterm prelabour rupture of membranes (PPROM) will occur in up to 3% of pregnancies and is associated with 30–40% of preterm births [6]. Over the years, guidance on the management of PROM at term has varied between immediate induction and expectant management whilst delivery timing for PPROM has also varied. A long interval between PROM and delivery increases the risk for fetal and neonatal infection. Early delivery following PPROM may lead to complications from prematurity but delayed delivery will increase the risk of complications related to chorioamnionitis.

In many women, PROM and PPROM can be diagnosed clinically with visualisation of clear fluid in the vagina. However, in other cases, additional tests are required such as a test for a specific biochemical marker found in the vagina using a commercial testing kit and assessment for reduced liquor volume using ultrasound. The clinician should bear in mind that none of the additional tests are completely diagnostic and follow-up is required if doubt remains.

Early identification of infection and subsequent delivery remains the cornerstone of expectant management. A combination of clinical assessment (pulse, blood pressure, temperature and symptoms), maternal blood tests including C-reactive protein (CRP) and white cell count, and fetal heart rate using cardiotocography, should be employed to diagnose clinical infection. In cases of PPROM, women may be observed as an outpatient for days or weeks prior to delivery following administration of corticosteroids to improve fetal lung maturity. They should be advised of the symptoms of chorioamnionitis, reviewed regularly one or two times each week for any signs of infection and be given open access if the woman has any concerns. It should be noted that the white cell count will rise 24 hours following administration of corticosteroids but then return to the baseline three days later. Although a raised CRP is the most informative maternal serum marker for predicting histological chorioamnionitis after PPROM, a systematic review and meta-analysis of 13 observational studies only found a sensitivity of 68.7% and specificity of 77.1%.

Maternal sepsis following PPROM may lead to serious morbidity and occasional mortality. In the MBBRACE report relating to maternal mortality in the UK 2016–2018, *Escherichia coli* (*E. coli*) was the causative organism leading to mortality from chorioamnionitis and sepsis in the mid-trimester [7]. Half of the women had experienced PPROM at less than 20 weeks of gestation and rapidly progressed to septic shock. In such a scenario, decision-making around active termination of pregnancy is difficult. There are challenging decisions around whether to continue a pregnancy with very early rupture of membranes. Counselling should involve a careful discussion about the risk of morbidity and mortality to the mother and to future pregnancies if sepsis should develop. If infection develops, the strong recommendation should be to terminate the pregnancy as quickly and safely as possible. A regular criticism within MBRRACE reports is the lack of senior involvement early in the decision-making process.

Prevention of Ascending Infection

Following PPROM, women should be offered antibiotics. A Cochrane review found that the use of antibiotics is associated with a reduction in chorioamnionitis, prolongation of pregnancy and a reduction in neonatal infection, use of surfactant, oxygen therapy and abnormal cerebral ultrasound prior to discharge from hospital [5]. However, there was no reduction in perinatal mortality or effect on the health of the children at seven years of age. The evidence for the use of a particular antibiotic is not present but co-amoxiclav should be avoided due to an increase in necrotizing enterocolitis in the neonate. It should also be noted that prophylactic antibiotics given to women with PPROM are not necessarily effective for the treatment of developing infection. Such infection requires additional immediate therapeutic treatment beyond prophylaxis.

Group B streptococcus (GBS) is present in the vagina or rectum in 20–40% of adults [8]. Colonisation with GBS can be transient, intermittent or chronic. Transmission from the mother to the fetus may occur during vaginal delivery. Infection in the early neonatal period can lead to serious and potentially life-threatening complications including sepsis, pneumonia, and meningitis in the newborn. Prevention of neonatal infection with GBS infection requires intrapartum antibiotic prophylaxis (IAP) to be most effective. Many countries adopt universal antenatal screening for GBS at 35–37 weeks gestation and IAP is then offered, at the onset of labour, to those women who are GBS-colonised. In the United Kingdom, the National Screening Committee has not recommended a universal maternal GBS screening programme. IAP is only recommended if a woman is found to be colonised with GBS when incidentally tested, or has had a previous baby with invasive GBS disease, or as part of broad-spectrum antibiotic therapy if she is febrile in labour, or has evidence of chorioamnionitis. She may be offered prophylactic antibiotics or a vaginal swab near term if she has had GBS detected in a previous pregnancy.

Identification and Management of Intrauterine Infection

Diagnosing sepsis in a pregnant woman or one who has recently given birth can be challenging. Pregnancy and childbirth are linked with a slightly faster heart rate and breathing, changes in blood pressure and an increased white cell count in the blood, all signs usually suggestive of infection. During childbirth, a mildly increased temperature and sweating are not uncommon. Pain is normal during labour but constant pain is not. Constant pain and tenderness, unrelieved by usual analgesia, may be caused by placental separation but may also be caused by intrauterine infection that can lead to sepsis. Women at risk of intrauterine infection, either following miscarriage or birth, may have signs and symptoms such as increasing pain, discoloured or malodorous vaginal discharge, abdominal tenderness, high temperature, fatigue and feeling unwell. Urinary frequency, often suggestive of a urinary tract infection, is normal in pregnancy but pain during urination is not. Other signs may include a rash, diarrhoea, vomiting or a productive cough. However, all such signs may be related to conditions other than sepsis.

A high index of suspicion for developing infection is therefore necessary, since disease progression to sepsis may be much more rapid than in the non-pregnant state. Within each of the recent MBRRACE reports, it is repeatedly stated that clinicians should consider the possibility of sepsis in order to achieve early recognition and treatment [7]. In the most recent MBRRACE mortality report, it is suggested that improved care may have changed the outcome for 68% of women.

Regular observations including pulse, blood pressure, respiratory rate, temperature and oxygen saturation will provide evidence that sepsis is developing. Each parameter can be scored, based upon deviation from the norm. A cumulative score, known as an early warning score, can then be derived from a complete set of observations. An increasing early warning score can alert the clinician to early deterioration. In pregnancy the scoring system is modified to take into account the changes in physiology during pregnancy. Failure to recognise deterioration may arise if observations are not performed frequently, are incomplete, or an increasing score does not prompt escalation. However, criticism has also been made when the clinician relies only on the early warning score and does not take into account other symptoms and signs.

Once sepsis has been considered as a diagnosis, prompt resuscitation with intravenous fluids and treatment with intravenous antibiotics is imperative. Senior clinician and intensive care team involvement is vital in continuing to manage a critically ill pregnant woman. The UK Sepsis Trust devised a resuscitation bundle known as the "Sepsis Six", consisting of six tasks to be ideally performed within the first hour of the diagnosis of sepsis [2]. The tasks include administration of broad-spectrum antibiotics, oxygen and intravenous fluids at the same time as obtaining blood cultures, measurement of the serum lactate, and checking the urine output.

Regular criticism in the recent MBRRACE reports are around the delay in administration of antibiotics and appropriate blood tests along with delay in senior involvement when sepsis was not considered in the first instance [7]. Although even when senior clinicians have been involved early in the case, they have not readily asked for advice from a colleague, either from the same specialty or a different specialty such as the critical care team. An increase in the serum lactate should alert the clinician to the development of septic shock and should prompt involvement of the critical care team. The expert advice of a consultant microbiologist or infectious disease physician should be sought urgently when serious sepsis is suspected. Another suggested area of improvement centres upon communication of the team members caring for the pregnant woman and the woman herself. A number of the women who died from sepsis were black or from other minority ethnic groups, particularly if English was not their first language. Failure to use an interpreter appeared to exacerbate the problem.

Postpartum Infection

Infection in the postnatal period or following miscarriage is relatively common [9]. Endometritis is an infection of the endometrial lining of the uterus, occurring up to six weeks after birth but most common between the second and tenth day after the delivery. It is caused by bacteria entering the uterus during birth and occurs in 1–3% of women who have delivered vaginally. For women who have delivered by caesarean section, the risk can be up to 20 times the risk of vaginal birth and therefore all women undergoing caesarean section are offered antibiotics as prophylaxis against endometritis. Other risk factors include prolonged labour, particularly if the membranes ruptured a long time before delivery, difficulty in removing the placenta, many internal examinations during labour and a history of pelvic infection including GBS. Clinically, endometritis causes pyrexia, pelvic pain, malodorous discharge and a relatively sudden increase in vaginal bleeding. Within the recent MBRRACE reports there are consistent failures regarding the postnatal assessment of women [7]. They include not recognising that a woman is unwell, not undertaking a full set of clinical observations, including respiratory rate, and not escalating concerns rapidly.

Postpartum endometritis needs treatment with antibiotics either orally or intravenously if the infection is more severe. Failure to institute appropriate, prompt treatment with antibiotics can lead to sepsis, particularly if the infection is caused by Group A streptococcus. In some cases, there may be retained tissue such as placenta or membranes within the uterus. Failure to recognise the presence of retained tissue and promptly remove the infected tissue can exacerbate the infection. In other cases, a pelvic abscess or peritonitis may develop, requiring more aggressive surgical treatment in the form of a laparotomy and occasionally hysterectomy.

Another cause of puerperal infection, typically streptococcal, is mastitis. Recognition of deterioration leading to sepsis, often despite treatment, has been a source of criticism.

Causes of Litigation

The reasons for litigation arising from infections and sepsis in pregnancy include the following failures in practice:

- Failing to follow RCOG guidance following rupture of membranes by omitting antibiotics and delay in delivery of the fetus
- Failing to follow NICE guidance on caesarean section by omitting prophylactic antibiotics
- Failing to consider prophylactic antibiotics in the presence of GBS
- Failing to adequately treat chorioamnionitis and then deliver the fetus in a timely fashion to prevent damage to the fetus
- Failing to promptly remove retained products of conception if present

Prevention of Litigation

- Prevention of infection by administering prophylactic antibiotics in the presence of GBS, following caesarean section or following PPROM
- Recognition when symptoms have become extraordinary and listening to the patient
- Recognition of the signs of developing sepsis by performing:

Regular observations

A complete set of observations

Using a modified early warning score for pregnant women

- Escalation if signs of sepsis and communicate with wider members of the multidisciplinary team
- Administration of intravenous fluids and intravenous antibiotics in a prompt fashion
- Using lactate as a means of assessing the development of septic shock
- Considering the presence of retained products of conception in cases of intrauterine infection and bleeding

References

1. The WHO Global Maternal Sepsis Study (GLOSS) Research Group. Frequency and management of maternal infection in health facilities in 52 countries (GLOSS): a 1-week inception cohort study. *Lancet* 2020: 8; e661–e671.

2. https://sepsistrust.org/professional-resources/clinical/

3. www.sccm.org/SurvivingSepsisCampaign/Guidelines

4. Royal College of Obstetricians and Gynaecologists (RCOG). Bacterial Sepsis in Pregnancy. Green–top Guideline No. 64a. London: RCOG; 2012.

5. Middleton, P, Shepherd, E, Flenady, V, McBain, RD, Crowther, CA. Planned early birth versus expectant management (waiting) for prelabour rupture of membranes at term (37 weeks or more). *Cochrane Database Syst Rev* 2017; Issue 1.

6. Thomson, AJ, on behalf of the Royal College of Obstetricians and Gynaecologists. Care of Women Presenting with Suspected Preterm Prelabour Rupture of Membranes from 24+0 Weeks of Gestation. *BJOG* 2019; 126: e152–166.

7. Knight, M, Bunch, K, Tuffnell, D, Shakespeare, J, Kotnis, R, Kenyon, S, Kurinczuk, JJ (eds.), on behalf of MBRRACE-UK. Saving Lives, Improving Mothers' Care – Lessons learned to inform maternity care from the UK and Ireland Confidential Enquiries into Maternal Deaths and Morbidity 2016–2018. Oxford: National Perinatal Epidemiology Unit, University of Oxford; 2020.

8. Hughes, RG, Brocklehurst, P, Steer, PJ, Heath, P, Stenson, BM on behalf of the Royal College of Obstetricians and Gynaecologists. Prevention of early-onset neonatal group B streptococcal disease. Green-top Guideline No. 36. *BJOG* 2017; 124: e280–e305.

9. Royal College of Obstetricians and Gynaecologists (RCOG). Bacterial Sepsis Following Pregnancy. Green–top Guideline No. 64. London: RCOG; 2012.

13 Caesarean Section Including Uterine Rupture and Full Dilatation Caesarean Deliveries

Emma Ferriman

CASE COMMENTARY
Swati Jha

Successful Claim

Yiqun Zhang (A Child Suing by his Mother and Litigation Friend, Shifang Liu) v Homerton University Hospitals NHS Foundation Trust

The Claim

During the claimant's delivery, labour was obstructed and a caesarean section (CS) performed by the registrar. The claimant's head was deeply impacted in the maternal pelvis and it was alleged that in the course of delivering and freeing the head, there was significant damage resulting in a depressed fracture of the skull and a subgaleal haemorrhage (bleeding between the scalp and the skull) as well as intracranial haemorrhage (bleeding into the cavern of the skull). These in turn caused permanent brain damage. It was claimed that this trauma was due to the use of undue force that was unnecessary for the purpose.

The Summary

The claimant's mother made good progress in labour initially but then failed to progress beyond 9 cm. Hence, after 2.5 hours of no progress, a decision was made to deliver by CS following discussion with the consultant on call.

The CS was performed by the Registrar and it took six minutes to deliver the head following the incision on the uterus. The head was in a deflexed right-occipito posterior (ROP) position and delivery proved very difficult.

The case centred around the method of breaking the "seal" between the head and soft tissues of the maternal pelvis when deeply impacted. This is usually achieved by insinuating the hand between the fetal head and symphysis at the front of the pelvis, but where this is not feasible, then the hand will need to be insinuated elsewhere around the circumference of the skull. The aim however is that the pressure exerted by the obstetrician's hand should predominantly be at the back of the hand which is in contact with maternal soft tissues rather than the palm of the hand which is in contact with the fetal skull, as the baby's head is relatively fragile. Where the head is deflexed, the aim is to flex the head along a longitudinal axis, to reduce the effective circumference of the head to allow disimpaction and delivery.

In this case it was not possible to break the seal by insinuating the hand between the pubic symphysis and fetal head, so the registrar insinuated the hand to the fetal right (left side of the pelvis) and felt a movement of the impacted head to the maternal right, managing to flex the head and deliver it.

The Judgement

It was conceded by the defendant that the trauma that ensued occurred during the manipulation of the head to disimpact it but this on its own would not equate to negligence. However, the claimant's expert made the point that there had been negligence during disimpaction on three counts: an attempt to rotate the head, deliberately moving the head laterally and the wedge effect of the hands causing undue pressure on the fetal skull. Usually once an impacted head had been disimpacted, rotation will occur spontaneously. It was alleged that any attempt at rotation or lateral movement of an impacted head was an inappropriate and dangerous manoeuvre. It was alleged that no reasonable doctor would perform rotation or lateral movement prior to disimpacting the head. Attempted rotation of an impacted head results in shearing forces to be applied in the plane between the scalp and skull which would cause subgaleal haemorrhage.

The registrar stated that the reference to rotation of the head in the records was meant to refer to rotation after disimpaction of the head, but the documentation of events in the records suggested that rotation was prior to disimpaction. This evidence together with the midwife accounts and the defence statement served to prove that rotation had been attempted prior to disimpaction.

The other issues of substandard care including lateral movement of the head and the wedge effect were described by the registrar when referring to the manoeuvres performed to insinuate the hand to flex the head. The other evidence provided by the claimant was that almost all cases of fractured skulls with difficult CS were after failed instrumental deliveries, hence a skull fracture of an impacted head in the absence of an attempted instrumental delivery must indicate the use of undue force.

On these bases the delivery was deemed substandard, with the defendant in breach of duty. The judgement found in favour of the claimant.

Another case of a successful claim with a deflexed head was of *Hollie Douse (a child suing by her father and litigation friend Chis Douse) v Western Sussex Hospitals NHS Foundation Trust*. In this case, a sub-optimal position for the head was noted (deflexed ROP) but in the absence of moulding and caput was not felt to be deeply impacted. The delivery of a head that is in a suboptimal position but not impacted should not be outside the experience of most obstetricians and should be achievable in five minutes from incision on the uterus to delivery of the head. A failure to do so resulted in a verdict of substandard care.

Unsuccessful Claim

CXB v North West Anglia NHS Foundation Trust

The Claim

A claimant and her twin brother were born at Hinchingbrooke hospital and the claimant suffered injuries during delivery. It was alleged by the claimant's mother that she had requested a caesarean delivery for both babies when seen at 36 weeks and 4 days in the antenatal clinic and had she been delivered by CS none of the complications suffered by the claimant would have occurred.

The Summary

When reviewed by the senior registrar at this appointment, the registrar made an entry in the records which stated: "Discussed mode of delivery at length. Patient keen for induction of labour (IOL)." The case was discussed with the consultant responsible for care and they agreed that the IOL should proceed. The registrar went on to record this in the hand-held records of the patient as well. This was in stark contrast to the patient's testimony of requesting a CS at this visit and gave a fundamentally different account of the sequence of events at this visit. The claimant's parents, in both their witness statements and their oral testimony, stated that they specifically requested a caesarean section and the registrar refused, and that they had not been offered a discussion on another day. When it was pointed out that the hand-held records contained a record of the discussions the defendant maintained that she was "completely stunned" and stated that this was "just wrong".

The claimant's mother stated in her witness statement that every time she saw a midwife or doctor she mentioned that she would really like a caesarean section. Following her initial diagnosis of twins, the consultant she saw actually recorded "I have discussed the risks and implications of twin pregnancy, and also mode of delivery depending on the gestation of twins." There were ample opportunities for the mother's delivery preference to be recorded, but there is no record in any of the notes of her expressing such a preference during the pregnancy. The defence admitted that if the claimant's mother had chosen at any stage delivery by way of elective caesarean section her choice would have been agreed and avoided the subsequent harm to the claimant, but this was never requested.

Following various contradictory statements from both her partner and herself, she conceded at cross-examination that she had not made up her mind on mode of delivery until the 36-week scan.

Following her ANC appointment at 36 weeks, the claimant's mother was visited by her midwife at home. The records from this visit do not reflect any concerns from the ANC appointment three days prior to this visit. The midwife also stated that had she been made aware of the patient's wishes to have a CS or found she was unhappy with the discussions in ANC she would document this in the notes and arrange a further appointment for her in the ANC. In addition, if the claimant's mother had stated during any of the midwifery appointments that she really wanted a caesarean section, it would be written in the notes and a second opinion sought if the claimant's mother had voiced her concerns. Midwives act as the woman's advocate and with a twin pregnancy it is unlikely that any doctor would refuse an elective caesarean section.

A few weeks after this appointment, the claimant's mother attended after her waters broke. Again, there was no note requesting a caesarean section. When she went into labour, under the heading "Birth Plan", the midwife wrote in the records: "Twins? epidural will decide at time", indicating that the plan had been discussed and there was no request for a caesarean section. When she was assessed by the specialist Registrar on admission to the labour ward, she was reviewed to check presentation and it was noted that the first twin was cephalic and the second was breach. The plan was to allow to labour with review in the second stage, and an epidural was discussed. Once again, there is no note that a caesarean section was requested. The absence of any contemporaneous records supporting the claimant's mother's version of events undermines the credibility and reliability of her assertion.

The Judgement

The defendant submitted that in a clinical negligence case the court should prefer the reliability and veracity of clinical notes over witness statements and oral testimony because of the unreliability of a witness's recollection of events. Judgement for the defendant was held.

Legal Commentary

Eloise Power

The judgements in *Zhang v Homerton University Hospitals NHS Foundation Trust* [2012] EWHC 1208 (QB) and *CXB v North West Anglia NHS Foundation Trust* [2019] EWHC 2053 (QB) turn on a key issue of legal principle: what approach should the Court take to credibility in cases where there is a conflict between contemporaneous records and witness evidence? As might be expected, the underlying legal principles are of wider application than the clinical negligence setting alone.

Perhaps the most authoritative statement of principle in relation to the importance of contemporaneous documentation in the assessment of witnesses' credibility derives from the judgement of Lord Pearce in *Onassis v Vergottis* [1968] 2 Lloyds Rep 403:

> "Credibility" involves wider problems than mere "demeanour" which is mostly concerned with whether the witness appears to be telling the truth as he now believes it to be. Credibility covers the following problems. First, is the witness a truthful or untruthful person? Secondly, is he, though a truthful person telling something less than the truth on this issue, or though an untruthful person, telling the truth on this issue? Thirdly, though he is a truthful person telling the truth as he sees it, did he register the intentions of the conversation correctly and, if so has his memory correctly retained them? Also, has his recollection been subsequently altered by unconscious bias or wishful thinking or by over much discussion of it with others?
>
> Witnesses, especially those who are emotional, who think that they are morally in the right, tend very easily and unconsciously to conjure up a legal right that did not exist. It is a truism, often used in accident cases, that with every day that passes the memory becomes fainter and the imagination becomes more active. For that reason a witness, however honest, rarely persuades a Judge that his present recollection is preferable to that which was taken down in writing immediately after the accident occurred. Therefore, contemporary documents are always of the utmost importance.
>
> And lastly, although the honest witness believes he heard or saw this or that, is it so improbable that it is on balance more likely that he was mistaken? On this point it is essential that the balance of probability is put correctly into the scales in weighing the credibility of a witness. And motive is one aspect of probability. All these problems compendiously are entailed when a Judge assesses the credibility of a witness; they are all part of one judicial process. And in the process contemporary documents and admitted or incontrovertible facts and probabilities must play their proper part (emphasis added).

Although *Onassis v Vergottis* was a contract case involving shipping, Lord Pearce's words are of general application and have been applied in the clinical negligence context. By way of an example, the famous statement of principle in *Onassis v Vergottis* was applied in *Speirs and another v St George's Healthcare NHS Trust* [2014] 12 WLUK 343. *Speirs and another* was a case involving alleged psychiatric injury of a mother consequent upon the birth injuries of her baby. The Court preferred the evidence contained in the mother's contemporaneous medical records over the later opinion of an expert psychiatrist instructed by the claimant.

In *Zhang*, Hickinbottom J (as he was) adopted a similar approach [para 48–53]. He reviewed the obstetrician's operation note and investigation statement very closely (the investigation statement was drafted relatively soon after the index events). He looked closely at the investigation statement of another witness, Midwife Harling. He also considered the stance taken by the defendant at earlier stages of the case; early correspondence and indeed the pleaded defence suggested that an attempt to rotate the impacted head had occurred. He concluded [para 51] that the doctor attempted to rotate the claimant's head while it was impacted.

It is evident from the judgement that Hickinbottom J gave considerable thought to the evidence as a whole: *"I have not found the issue of whether Dr Gupta attempted to rotate the Claimant's head whilst it was impacted an easy one"* [para 51]. He found that the doctor was a truthful witness: *"I have considered Dr Gupta's evidence very carefully. I have no doubt that, in giving it, she was attempting to assist and was genuinely attempting to recollect what happened."* However, he concluded that in the light of all of the evidence in the case: *"she does not have a true recollection of the events at the delivery of the Claimant."* In short, Zhang presented the Court with a situation of the kind envisaged in *Onassis v Vergottis*, involving a truthful witness with imperfect recollection in circumstances where the Court placed considerable weight upon the contemporaneous documentation.

The case of *CXB* raises a number of similar issues. The Court considered a number of first instance judgements, including a well-known Commercial Court judgement, *Gestamin SGPS SA v Credit Suisse (UK) Limited* [2013] EWHC 3560, where Leggatt J (as he was) observed that *"the best approach for a judge to adopt in the trial of a commercial case is, in my view, to place little if any reliance at all on witnesses' recollections of what was said in meetings and conversations, and to base factual findings on inferences drawn from the documentary evidence and known or probable facts."* Gore J reminded himself that the Commercial Court setting is very different from the clinical negligence setting and regarded the observations of Leggatt J as unhelpful. The Court's attention appears not to have been drawn to the authoritative House of Lords judgement of *Onassis v Vergottis* and other higher-court case law, and Gore J concluded that *"All that the decided cases to which I have made reference do is to remind judges that care has to be taken in making these assessments, and full and proper reasons have to be given for the conclusions reached, but beyond that I do not find anything in these judgments to be of assistance as a matter of principle in explaining how this task should be undertaken by judges."*

On the facts in *CXB*, the Court observed that the evidence of the claimant's witnesses, while not deliberately untruthful, was *"not internally, or externally, consistent and, in some cases, has changed over time"* as well as being inconsistent with the contemporaneous records. The witnesses changed their account in crucial respects. For example, the claimant's mother stated in her witness statement that she repeatedly mentioned to professionals that she would really like a caesarean section, whereas she stated in evidence that her actual and stated preference was always what was safest for the babies, and that she wanted a caesarean section if either baby were in anything other than a head down position. Under all of the circumstances, it is difficult to envisage a Court arriving at a different conclusion, regardless of the precise legal principles which were adopted.

It is important to remember that there can be circumstances where a clinical record is **not** preferred over later witness evidence. In *Synclair v East Lancashire Hospital NHS Trust* [2015] EWCA Civ 1283, the Court of Appeal upheld the judgement of a trial judge who had preferred the witness evidence of the claimant and his wife over an apparently contemporaneous clinical record of a ward round.

On the facts in *Synclair*, there were legitimate concerns in relation to the clinical record: the record appeared to have been written by a doctor who was not called to give evidence, there was a lack of evidence in relation to the precise circumstances in which the record was made, and inferences were drawn from other records that the record may not have been entirely accurate (the record stated *"patient well"*, whereas other records demonstrated that he had taken recent analgesia). Although the principles in *Onassis v Vergottis* and other authoritative cases were cited with approval and followed, the Court of Appeal found that on the facts, it was legitimate and appropriate for the trial judge to have preferred the witness evidence over the clinical record of the ward round. In the words of Tomlinson LJ, giving unanimous judgement for the Court of Appeal: *"However it is too obvious to need stating that simply because a document is apparently contemporary does not absolve the court of deciding whether it is a reliable record and what weight can be given to it"* [para 12].

Drawing the threads together, the following principles arise from the case law: (a) As set out in *Onassis v Vergottis*, contemporaneous documentation (such as medical records) are always of the utmost importance. A common thread running through all of the judgements discussed above is that each Court scrutinised the relevant records and other contemporaneous documents with considerable thought and care; (b) this does not, however, imply that medical records will always be preferred over other forms of evidence as an automatic principle. As the case of *Synclair* makes clear, the Court needs to assess the reliability and the weight to be given to the evidence even where this takes the form of a contemporaneous record; (c) as all of the cases discussed above establish, the Court will consider the evidence in the round and will assess the weight to be given to the contemporaneous records in conjunction with the other sources of evidence in the case.

Clinical Commentary

Emma Ferriman

Caesarean section (CS) is one of the commonest operations performed in the United Kingdom and rates continue to increase. According to Hospital Episode Statistics, the rates in 2018–2019 were approaching 30% [1]. The NHS litigation authority report, looking at 10 years of maternity claims, found that 13.24% were associated with CS and 1.67% with uterine rupture [2]. The medicolegal issues mainly relate to the complications of the procedure itself or the failure to deliver in a timely manner.

Caesarean section is commonly performed out of hours and by junior clinicians. It is therefore important to ensure that doctors are adequately trained and/or supervised as rates continue to rise and surgery becomes increasingly complicated. The NICE guidance states that one in four women will undergo a CS and because of this there should be appropriate evidence-based information given in the antenatal period. This should include the indications for operation including fetal distress, failure to progress, malposition or malpresentation, placenta praevia/accreta, previous CS, previous difficult delivery, previous obstetric anal sphincter injuries (OASIS) and maternal request. There should be a full explanation of the procedure, its associated risks and benefits and the implications for future pregnancies [3]. The consent process has been further complicated by the *Montgomery v Lanarkshire Health Board* ruling, where the patient must be informed of all the material risks associated of a procedure [4].

There are increasing numbers of women who request a CS without a clinical indication. NICE recommends that the reasons for this are explored and recorded. A clinician must discuss the overall risks and benefits of elective CS compared to vaginal birth. There should also be a discussion with other members of the multi-disciplinary team to include a midwife and anaesthetist. This will ensure that the reasons for the request are identified and explored and that the woman has accurate information. Where the request is based around anxiety surrounding childbirth, a referral should be made to a healthcare professional with experience in perinatal mental health. For women requesting CS after discussion and appropriate support in whom a vaginal birth is not an acceptable option, a planned CS should be arranged [3]. In 2018, Birthrights published a report on maternal request CS based upon the 2011 NICE guidance and the Montgomery ruling [4]. Of the 153 trusts providing maternity care, 148 provided a response (97%), only 26% offered a maternal request CS in line with NICE guidance [5]. The report found that the majority of Trusts in the United Kingdom made the process lengthy, difficult or inconsistent, creating further anxiety and distress. NICE also suggest that if an obstetrician does not feel able to support such a request, that the woman should be referred to an obstetrician who will carry out the procedure [3]. There have been a number of litigation cases based on the failure of an obstetrician to perform a CS for maternal request who subsequently develop complications of labour and delivery.

Although most CS will proceed without complication, it should be remembered that the procedure is a major open abdominal operation often performed as an emergency. The rate of a return to theatre post operation is between 0.12–1.04%, the commonest indications are intra-abdominal bleeding, intra-abdominal infection and abscess formation or bladder and bowel complications [6]. The complications of CS and suggested management strategies for avoidance are summarised in Table 13.1. When providing information regarding the potential complications of the operation, it is important to divide these into those occurring frequently (wound discomfort, risk of repeat operation, hospital readmission, postpartum haemorrhage and infection), and those that are less common but more serious (hysterectomy, requirement for further surgery, admission to intensive care unit, thromboembolic disease, bladder injury, ureteric injury and death). Women who are obese who have significant pathology, who have had previous surgery or with pre-existing medical complications must understand that the quoted risks for serious and frequent complications will be increased. The complication rates associated with elective surgery are on the whole lower than those undergoing emergency surgery (16 women per 100 compared to 24 women per 100). Complication rates are also higher at 9–10 cm dilatation when compared to 0–1 cm dilatation (33/100 compared to 17/100) [7].

Table 13.1. Complications occurring during or after caesarean section adapted from Field at al, "Complications of Caesarean Section", 2016 [4]

Complication	Incidence	Avoidance	Treatment
Postpartum haemorrhage	Approx. 5%	1. Antenatal diagnosis of abnormal placentation/ fibroids etc. 2. Meticulous surgical technique	1. Uterotonic agents 2. Prompt surgical repair 3. Balloon tamponade 4. Compression sutures 5. Uterine devascularisation 6. Interventional radiology 7. Hysterectomy
Sepsis	Wound 6.9–9.7% Endometritis: 3.9–18.4%	1. Antibiotics prior to skin incision 2. Vaginal decontamination 3. Meticulous haemostasis 4. Abdominal/wound drains where appropriate	1. Antibiotics 2. Radiological drainage 3. Wound exploration/ debridement 4. Re-laparotomy, debridement, washout
Bladder injury	Approx. 0.1%	1. Careful peritoneal entry 2. ?Avoid bladder flap creation 3. Avoid low uterine incision	1. Surgical repair 2. Consider ureteric damage 3. Bladder drainage 4. Cystogram 10–14 days

Ureter injury	Approx. 0.4%	1. Correct for dextro-rotation prior to uterine incision
		2. Caution when repairing extensions and operating near broad ligament
			1. Urology opinion
			2. Ureteric occlusion
			  i. Suture removal
			  ii. Ureteric stenting
			  iii. Nephrostomy
			3. Ureteric transection
			  i. Re-anastomosis
			  ii. Re-implantation

Bowel injury	Unknown	1. Careful peritoneal entry 2. General surgical assistance if extensive previous surgery 3. ?Exteriorisation when suturing near broad ligament	1. General surgical assistance 2. Primary repair 3. Resection and stoma formation
Postoperative ileus	Approx. 12%	1. Careful bowel handling 2. ?Chewing gum postoperatively	1. Exclusion of more serious pathology 2. IV fluids 3. Correction of electrolytes 4. Anti-emetics 5. Nasogastric tube

Table 13.1. (cont.)

Complication	Incidence	Avoidance	Treatment
Ogilvie syndrome	Unknown		1. As per postoperative ileus 2. Urgent surgical review 3. Consider neostigmine 4. Rectal flatus tube 5. Laparotomy

The incidence of CS performed at full dilatation is increasing. Approximately 5% of operations are performed at full dilatation in the United Kingdom and 50% occur without an attempt at operative vaginal delivery. This may be due to concerns of fetal compromise or safety concerns for difficult rotational deliveries. The reasons for the increasing rates are likely to be multifactorial with increased rates of failed operative vaginal delivery and reduced attempts at operative vaginal delivery. This may reflect reduced training times for junior clinicians or reduced exposure to more difficult deliveries. There is also the issue of whether there is adequate training in rotational delivery. In addition, there may be increasing concerns regarding the risk of operative vaginal delivery for both mother and baby. The risk of neonatal trauma and admission to the neonatal unit is increased when excess of three tractions are required for delivery or with the use of multiple instruments. Finally, there may also be concerns regarding the escalating levels of litigation within the maternity system which may contribute to increased numbers of full dilatation sections [9]. For the mother, CS in the second stage of labour is associated with double the risk of intraoperative trauma compared to operation in the first stage. These injuries include injury to bladder, bowel and uterine extensions. Haemorrhage of greater than 1000 ml occurs in between 5–10%. Currently there are no national guidelines for conducting CS at full dilatation. In the United Kingdom, the commonest skin incision for CS is low transverse, with NICE recommending the Joel-Cohen incision because of the reduced risks of postoperative febrile illness [3]. At full dilatation the uterine incision should be higher than usual as the lower segment is stretched obscuring the landmarks that differentiate between the vagina, cervix and uterine body. A standard lower segment incision may risk injury to the vagina or bladder and may be more prone to tearing and difficult repair.

Full dilatation CS also presents a risk to the fetus. The Early Notification Scheme interim report in 2018 reviewed all cases where term babies were diagnosed with either grade 111 hypoxic ischaemic encephalopathy, were actively cooled or had decreased central tone and coma and seizures. In this report 9 of the 96 cases reviewed (9%) had difficult delivery of the head at CS or a deeply impacted head. The reasons underpinning the difficult delivery were unclear. Theories proposed included changes in obstetric management, increasing rates of induction, prolonged labour, oxytocin use and full dilatation CS with a changing training or skill set for those obstetricians conducting the deliveries [9]. Impaction of the fetal head is usually not associated with cephalopelvic disproportion where the head fails to descend in the maternal pelvis. It has been proposed as a manifestation of an unduly long second stage of labour when the obstetrician has to decide on the mode of delivery, whether instrumental delivery or CS [10].

Techniques to aid head impaction include stopping oxytocin and using a uterine relaxant prior to delivery. The "push" technique relies on placing the woman in semi-lithotomy with a second assistant pushing the fetal head out of the pelvis at the same time as the surgeon attempts delivery of the head. There should be an equal spread of pressure across the fetal head during this procedure to avoid additional trauma and the head should be flexed to narrow the diameter and ease delivery. It is proposed that the "push" method may be associated with increased trauma to the lower uterine segment due to manipulation of the fetal head. There is also an increased risk of infection due to contamination from vaginal flora and a risk of scalp trauma to the baby. The reverse breech or "pull" technique involves delivering a cephalic baby as a breech by grasping one or both feet at the fundus of the uterus and applying steady downward traction. The buttocks are then delivered with flexion of the thoracolumbar spine allowing more space for delivery of the head. The "pull" technique may be associated with extension of the uterine incision and neonatal trauma due to traction on the limbs. In a randomised trial comparing the two techniques, reversed breech extraction was associated with a reduction in intraoperative blood loss, shorter operating time and reduced hospital stay. Maternal pyrexia was significantly increased in the "push" technique group (3.1% versus 19.8%). Neonatal outcomes were also better in the "pull" technique group, with fewer babies having an Apgar score less than 7 (8.3% compared to 21.9%) [11]. Patwardhan's method is also described to aid delivery of the impacted head, although less frequently. This involves delivery of both fetal shoulders through the incision followed by the trunk, breech and then the head [11,12]. A number of medical devices have been developed to aid delivery of the fetal head at CS. NICE issued preliminary guidance on the use of the fetal pillow in 2015 [12]. With the increasing rates of CS at full dilatation there is an impact on junior doctor training. The RCOG recommends that a consultant should be present for all full dilatation CSs, but this is not always practical or predictable. There is strong evidence that emergency simulation training improves outcomes and these training issues are addressed in the mandatory RCOG operative birth simulation training (ROBuST) course. The UK Obstetric surveillance system (UKOSS) MIDAS study has set out to investigate both the incidence and consequences of the impacted fetal head and its results are awaited [13].

A significant amount of the litigation surrounding CS occurs when there is a failure to deliver a potentially compromised baby in a timely manner. Lucas et al developed a classification system [14] which was further modified by the RCOG and Royal College of Anaesthetists (RCA) [15]. Category 1 is where there is an immediate threat to the life of mother or baby, category 2 is where there is maternal or fetal compromise which is not life-threatening , category 3 requires early delivery but with no maternal or fetal compromise and category 4 can be performed at a time suiting the woman and the maternity services [14,15]. NICE state that a category 1 CS should be performed as soon as possible (within 30 minutes) and category 2 within 30–75 minutes. The categorisation of CS raises two issues; firstly, that the clinician must accurately categorise the urgency for delivery and secondly, having chosen the category, must adhere to the recommended decision to delivery interval. Clinicians must ensure that these timings are accurately documented and communicated to the theatre team. Failure to assign the appropriate urgency to the delivery and to deliver within the recommended time is a common theme in litigation cases.

With increasing numbers of women undergoing CS, there are increasing women requiring management of a subsequent pregnancy by either vaginal birth after caesarean section (VBAC) or elective repeat caesarean section (ERCS). The RCOG recommend that women with a singleton cephalic presentation at 37 weeks with one previous CS with or without a previous vaginal delivery should be offered VBAC. Contraindications to VBAC include previous uterine rupture or classical uterine incision or women having absolute contraindications to VBAC irrespective of uterine scar (placenta praevia). An antenatal pathway is recommended to document informed consent and shared decision-making. The risk of uterine rupture occurs in approximately 1 in 200 cases where labour occurs spontaneously but is increased by a factor of 1.5 in induced or augmented labour. The decision for induction of labour should be made by a senior obstetrician [16]. When planning an ERCS this should be conducted at 39 weeks gestation.

Uterine rupture is a pregnancy complication associated with both maternal and fetal morbidity and mortality. In developed countries it is commonly associated with birth by previous CS. Current recommendations are to encourage women to attempt VBAC but worldwide VBAC seems to have reduced in numbers due to the perceived risks of rupture and its associated morbidities. Indeed, the commonest indication for CS currently is previous CS. In the UKOSS study of uterine rupture there were 159 cases, representing an estimated incidence of 1.9/10,000 pregnancies. Eighty-seven per cent of ruptures occurred in women with a previous CS. The most frequent clinical sign was an abnormal fetal heart rate followed by abdominal pain. In the NHSLA review of 10 years of maternity claims, there were 85 cases of uterine rupture and in 50% there was a delay in recognising rupture, with 55–87% showing an abnormal fetal heart rate pattern [2]. Risk factors for rupture were previous CS, trial of labour, number of previous CS, short interval between sections and induction of labour [17].

Good Practice Guidance

There should be detailed antenatal discussion regarding the risk of CS for all women. Women should sign a consent form (for category 1 procedures verbal consent is permissible). The WHO surgical safety checklist should be completed [19]. Regional anaesthesia is the preferred option for the procedure. For procedures where there is an increased risk of bleeding, blood and blood products should be available as well as intraoperative cell salvage. Where surgery is likely to be difficult, a senior obstetrician should be involved, including full dilatation CSs. An indwelling catheter should be sited, and prophylactic antibiotics given prior to the skin incision. There should be a venous thromboembolism (VTE) assessment prior to surgery. The skin incision will vary according to the indication for the procedure and the baby may be delivered manually or with the use of Wrigley's forceps. A neonatal team should be present for emergency deliveries and cord gases should be taken. The placenta should be delivered by either controlled cord traction or manual removal and the uterine cavity should be inspected to ensure it is empty. The uterus should be repaired in layers where possible with repair of the sheath and/or peritoneum. The skin should be repaired with either interrupted sutures or staples or a subcuticular absorbable material.

Reasons for Litigation

Common reasons for litigation include:

- – Inappropriate or incomplete antenatal counselling (VBAC)
- – Failure to document all the material risks
- – Delay in decision to delivery interval
- – Maternal complications of the procedure

– Fetal complications of the procedure
– Inappropriate use of oxytocin
– Failure to recognise uterine rupture in a timely fashion

Avoidance of Litigation

Women with a previous CS should have the risks and benefits for VBAC and ERCS clearly documented (Table 13.2) and undergo detailed counselling, ideally in a VBAC clinic. The risk of uterine rupture should be clearly documented following both spontaneous labour and induction of labour. Labour should be conducted in a consultant-led unit where there is immediate access to emergency CS with continuous fetal monitoring. The labour ward should have senior obstetric input, especially where consideration is made to induction or the use of oxytocin, and women should be aware that the risk of uterine rupture will increase two- to three-fold. Clinicians should be aware of the signs of impending uterine rupture and act on abnormal fetal heart rate patterns in labour and abdominal or scar pain unrelated to uterine contractions.

Table 13.2. Taken from the Royal College of Obstertricians and Gynaecologists Green-top Guideline No. 45, "Birth after Caesarean Section"

	Planned VBAC	ERCS from 39 weeks
Maternal outcomes	72–75% of successful VBAC with shorter hospital stay and recovery	Ability to plan a known delivery date in most patients. Individual circumstances may change according to antenatal factors in mother or fetus
	Approximately 0.5% risk of uterine rupture associated with maternal and fetal morbidity/mortality	Virtually avoids the risk of uterine rupture (less than 0.02%)
		Longer recovery
		Reduced risk of pelvic organ prolapse and urinary incontinence in comparison to vaginal birth
		Option for sterilisation if family complete. Regret rate is higher than failure rate of procedure. Ideally consent should be obtained two weeks before procedure
	Increases likelihood of future vaginal birth	Future pregnancies likely to require caesarean delivery, increased risk of placenta praevia and accreta and adhesions with successive operations
	Risk of OASI is 5% and birthweight is the strongest predictor. Rate of instrumental delivery is approximately 39%	
	Risk of maternal death with planned VBAC of 4/100,000	Risk of maternal death with ERCS of 13/100,000

Table 13.2. (cont.)

	Planned VBAC	ERCS from 39 weeks
Infant outcomes	Risk of transient respiratory morbidity of 2–3%	Risk of transient respiratory morbidity of 4–5% (6% if delivery performed at 38 weeks). Risk reduced with antenatal steroids but there are concerns about potential long-term adverse effects
	10 per 100,000 (0.1%) prospective risk of antepartum stillbirth beyond 39 weeks while awaiting spontaneous labour similar to nulliparous women	
	8 per 100,000 (0.03%) risk of hypoxic ischaemic encephalopathy (HIE)	<1 per 100,000 (0.01%) risk of delivery-related perinatal death or HIE
	4 per 10,000 (0.04%) risk of delivery-related perinatal death comparable to nulliparous in labour	

References

1. NHS maternity statistics 2018–2019. Published 31st October 2019.

2. NHS Litigation Authority. Ten years of maternity claims. An analysis of NHS Litigation Authority Data. 2012.

3. National Institute for Health and Care Excellence (NICE). Caesarean section (CG132). Clinical guideline. Published 23 November 2011.

4. Montgomery v Lanarkshire Health Board 2015.

5. Birthrights. Maternal request caesarean section. August 2018.

6. Field, A, Haloob, R. Complications of caesarean section. *Obstet Gynaecol* 2016; 18: 265–72. https://doi.org/10.1111/to g .12280

7. Royal college of Obstetricians and Gynaecologists (RCOG). Consent advice No.7. Caesarean section. October 2009.

8. Vousden, N, Cargill, Z, Briley, A, Tydeman, G, Shennan, AH. Caesarean section at full dilatation: incidence, impact and current management. *Obstet Gynaecol* 2014; 16: 199–205.

9. NHS Resolution. The early notification scheme progress report: collaboration and improved experience for families. An overview of the scheme to date together with thematic analysis of a cohort of cases from year 1 of the scheme 2017–2018. Published September 2019.

10. Chopra, S. Disengagement of the deeply engaged fetal head during caesarean section – Conventional method versus reverse breech extraction: review of literature [Electronic resource]. *Clin Mother Child Health* 2016; 13(2).

11. Nooh, AM, Abdeldayem, HM, Ben-Affan, O. Reverse breech extraction versus the standard approach of pushing the impacted fetal head up through the vagina in caesarean section for obstructed labour: a randomised controlled trial. *J Obstet Gynaecol* 2017; 37(4): 459–63.

12. National Institute for Health and Care Excellence (NICE). Insertion of a balloon device to disimpact an engaged fetal head before an emergency caesarean section. Interventional procedures guidance. Published 27 March 2015.

13. UK Obstetric Surveillance System (UKOSS). MIDAS study of the impacted

fetal head at caesarean section. Available at: www.npeu.ox.ac.uk/ukoss/completed-surveillance/ifh

14. Lucas, DN, Yentis, SM, Kinsella, SM, Holdcroft, A, May, AE, Wee, M, Robinson, PN. Urgency of caesarean section: a new classification. *J R Soc Med* 2000; 93(7): 346–50.

15. Royal College of Obstetricians and Gynaecologists (RCOG) and Royal College of Anaesthetists (RCA). Classification of urgency of caesarean section: a continuum of risk. Good practice No. 11. April 2010.

16. Royal College of Obstetricians and Gynaecologists (RCOG). Green-top Guideline No. 45. Birth after caesarean section. October 2015.

17. Fitzpatrick, KE, Kurinczuk, JJ, Alfirevic, Z, Spark, P, Brocklehurst, P, et al. Uterine rupture by intended mode of delivery in the UK: a national case-control study. *PLoS Med* 2012; 9(3): e1001184. https://doi.org/10.1371/journal.pmed.1001184

Assisted Vaginal Birth

Emily J Hotton, Joanna F Crofts

CASE COMMENTARY

Swati Jha

Successful Claim

JRM (By his Father and Litigation Friend TRM) v King's College Hospital Foundation Trust Case Number HQ15C01040

The Claim

JRM was one of twins, delivered by forceps at 29 weeks and suffered serious injury to his spinal cord around the time of his birth. The forceps caused traumatic injury and tearing of the lining of the spinal artery (arterial dissection), and subsequent clot formation within the vessel resulting in vascular injury to the spinal cord due to occlusion of a branch of the anterior spinal artery. It was alleged that this was due to the negligent use of forceps with the claimant in the occipito-lateral (OL) position at birth.

The Summary

The claimant's mother presented in preterm labour and JRM (twin 1) was noted to be cephalic with twin 2 in a breech presentation. They were dichorionic twins and health problems had been identified on scans in the second twin. A Neville Barnes forceps was used and when applied properly on an occipito-anterior or occipito-posterior head should sit over the lateral aspect of the head with no part lying over the scalp, centre forehead, chin or nose of the child. If incorrectly applied in an OL position, there would be consequent bruising of the central part of the face including the tip of the nose and the right side of the eye.

The Judgement

The extent and severity of bruising on the face was indicative of excessive force and traction from instrumental delivery being used during the delivery. This suggested that the forceps was applied on a head that was mispresenting in an OL position and this was a breach of duty. This in turn was responsible for the injury to the spinal cord and therefore the judgement was in the claimant's favour.

In the case of *FE v St George's University Hospitals NHS Trust* [2016] EWHC 553 (QB), 2016 WL 01032317, there was a delay in delivery and following a failed ventouse and forceps a caesarean section (CS) was performed with the baby delivered 46 minutes after the decision to delivery was made. Judgement was in favour of the claimant.

In the case of *P (a child) v Royal Berkshire NHS Foundation Trust* [2013] 5 WLUK 724, damages were approved for an inadvertent laceration to P's neck which required surgery under general anaesthetic the day after birth. P was born in otherwise good condition.

Unsuccessful Claim

Reeve v Heart of England NHS Trust [2011] EWHC 3901 (QB), 2011 WL 6329549

The Claim

A claim was made following delays in delivering a child leading to cerebral palsy occurring due to acute cord compression. It was claimed that if the consultant obstetrician had been called earlier and been present on site, the delivery could have been completed earlier in the hypoxic event and therefore have prevented the injury to the baby.

The Summary

Following an uneventful pregnancy, the claimant was induced at term for raised blood pressure. There was no evidence of fetal compromise. During labour, the liquor was initially clear but later stale meconium was noted, and the CTG remained normal. During the labour, she had a syntocinon infusion and an epidural for pain relief. For reasons that were unclear, the syntocinon infusion was stopped at 9 cm dilatation by the registrar in charge of the labour ward although slow progress was identified. A plan to review in two hours was made with a view to proceeding to a CS if there was no progress. Immediately after this examination, the registrar had to go to theatres for an emergency CS, and they spoke to the consultant on call at the time to discuss the management plan of both the claimant and the impending emergency CS. There was no indication at this point for the consultant to be called into hospital.

There was a fetal bradycardia while the registrar was still busy with the emergency CS. The consultant was called but by the time they arrived the registrar had delivered the baby by forceps (failed ventouse).

The Judgement

Following review of the CTG, it was felt that there was no indication for the registrar to call the consultant on site prior to proceeding with the emergency CS on another patient. The first point at which the consultant should have been called into hospital was acted upon and this would not have shortened the period of hypoxia to which the baby was exposed thus leading to the HIE. The ruling was therefore in favour of the defendant.

Legal Commentary

Eloise Power

JRM (By His Father and Litigation Friend TRM) v King's College Hospital NHS Foundation Trust [2017] EWHC 1913 (QB)

This case involved an acute spinal injury to a new-born baby causing four-limb paralysis, the requirement for a tracheotomy and ventilator dependency. Prior to trial, the parties managed to narrow the issues significantly, reaching agreement upon the following issues:

a) The parties agreed that JRM had suffered an acute spinal injury at around the time of birth, which consisted of a vascular injury to the spinal cord due to occlusion of a branch of the anterior spinal artery.

b) There were two potential mechanisms of injury: (i) a traumatic injury causing arterial dissection and subsequent clot formation within the vessel or (ii) occlusion due to a blood clot or placental emboli lodging in the arterial lumen. The second mechanism was agreed to be exceedingly rare.

c) The parties agreed that *if* the Court accepted that there had been excessive force and traction from instrumental delivery (via Neville Barnes forceps), then the arterial dissection was the most likely mechanism of injury. If there was no significant trauma, an embolic cause was more likely.

d) The parties also agreed that JRM could only have sustained a traumatic injury if he had been in the occipito-lateral (OL) position when the forceps were used. The injury could not have been caused if JRM had been in the occipito-anterior (OA) position.

The judgement of Gilbart J consequently focused upon the crucial issues of JRM's position at the time when the Neville Barnes forceps were used and upon the factual evidence relating to his condition following delivery. In addition to the witness evidence of the obstetrician who delivered JRM, there were three further sources of evidence: the witness evidence of JRM's father, the subsequent clinical records relating to the condition of JRM, and the photographs taken by the parents which demonstrated the bruising on JRM's face.

The obstetrician who delivered JRM claimed that he had checked that JRM was in the OA position and that he gave two gentle pulls to achieve a forceps delivery; nothing occurred during delivery which would cause significant bruising.

The father's evidence accorded with the subsequent clinical records: he stated that the nurses in NICU told him that they had never seen a baby with such bad bruising to the face and chest. Importantly, the clinical records described extensive bruising *on arrival* at NICU, i.e. before JRM had undergone any further procedures which could potentially have caused bruising. The Court placed significant weight upon the consistency between the father's evidence and the NICU records, finding that it was *"impossible to reconcile the account given in that substantial body of evidence of a difficult forceps delivery, which caused extensive bruising"*, with the witness statements of the obstetrician and his assistant [para 77].

The Court also placed significant weight upon the photographs, recognising that the location and degree of the bruising was relevant in determining whether JRM was in the OL or OA position. Having heard expert evidence, the Court found as follows:

> I turn now to the location of the bruising. This is an important matter, as it can indicate whether the forceps were properly applied. I regard it as most significant that there was bruising to the nose and to other parts of the central facial area. There was also some bruising to the scalp, although the extent is unknown. In my judgement, while the location of the bruising is consistent with the forceps being applied to the baby in an OL position, it is not consistent with the baby being in an OA position [para 76].

These comments serve as a salient reminder of the importance of ensuring that enquiries are made at the earliest possible point about any photographs which may have been taken by injured patients or their relatives. Photographs can often be of crucial relevance, even where (as here) they are not professional or medical photographs or part of the clinical records.

Finally, the Court took into account that no other witnesses who were present during the delivery (such as midwives and nurses) had been called to give evidence, nor had any of the clinicians who treated JRM in the NICU. For further discussion of the inferences which can be drawn from the absence of a witness, please see the legal commentary at Chapter 10, which includes a discussion of the principles in *Wisniewski v Central Manchester Health Authority* [1998] Lloyds Reports Med 223.

The Court concluded that:

> had Dr Mahfouz examined the mother properly, he would have found that the baby was in the OL position. His subsequent application of the forceps to the Claimant in the OL position resulted in increased force being required. I find that JRM was delivered with excessive force, with the forceps being placed in the wrong position, and then pulled vigorously [para 82].

Accordingly, the obstetrician fell below a reasonable standard of care, and there was judgement for the claimant.

Going beyond this, the Court questioned whether the defendant should have fought the case at all [para 83]:

> in the light of the terms of the NICU records, notes and reports, and the other documents to which I have referred, I am very critical of whoever it was in the Defendant Trust or in the NHSLA who considered that this claim should be resisted on the basis (among others) that the delivery was a straightforward and unremarkable forceps delivery. It must have been known for a long time that Dr Mahfouz' evidence about the delivery was, to say the least, difficult to reconcile with the internal notes and records, where the obvious injuries to the baby had excited so much concern and comment by those treating him. It was an obvious lacuna in the Defendant's case that, in a claim where so much turned on the evidence that this child was injured at round the time of his birth, no midwife or nurse present at the birth was called, nor, perhaps more concerningly, none of the clinicians or nursing staff who dealt with the consequences of the labour when C was admitted to NICU.

These comments illustrate the importance of (a) good case selection for trial from the viewpoint of defendants; (b) proper evaluation of witness evidence against other contemporaneous and objective sources of evidence; (c) ensuring that all relevant witnesses of fact are contacted and, where appropriate, called to give evidence – particularly eyewitnesses who were present during disputed and crucial points of the history.

Reeve v Heart of England NHS Trust [2011] EWHC 3901 (QB)

This case concerned a baby who suffered brain damage consequent upon acute cord occlusion and hypoxia. At the point in time when the obstetric emergency became obvious, the registrar on duty was engaged in performing an emergency CS upon another patient. The only other doctor on duty, a SHO, was not trained to perform an instrumental or surgical delivery. The key question for the Court was whether the on-call consultant should have been called to attend at an earlier point in the chronology. The defendant accepted that if the on-call consultant had been present, the baby would have been delivered uninjured.

In addressing this issue, the Court looked closely at the CTG trace and considered the expert evidence relating to the interpretation of the trace. The parties agreed that the

CTG trace showed variable decelerations at five points in time. The claimant argued that the trace was suspicious of hypoxia. The defendant argued that the decelerations were intermittent and did not form a pattern which made the trace suspicious of hypoxia. The Court acknowledged that the CTG trace needed to be seen in the context of the clinical picture, and also that it should be viewed holistically. Having considered the expert evidence, the Court concluded that the midwife and registrar had been entitled to consider the trace as satisfactory, and the claimant's case accordingly failed. Further consideration of CTG interpretation can be found at Chapter 9.

In finding for the defendant, HHJ Clark observed as follows [para 23]:

> *I would add that I have been shown no written guidance as to the circumstances in which a consultant on call should be summoned to the hospital. Pausing there, I note that no criticism is made of the staffing levels that night, a registrar and SHO on duty at the hospital with the consultant on call. Plainly in the emergency which arose after 6.37 a.m. Sister Ajayi was right to call Mr Churchill, having established Dr Hady's lack of availability. However, it is not suggested that Mr Churchill ought to have been called simply because Dr Hady was engaged elsewhere. First, there must be signs that a risk of acute cord occlusion existed in this case. For the reasons I have given, I am not satisfied that those signs were present such as to cause a reasonably competent registrar or midwife to consider it necessary to call in Mr Churchill. That it would, with hindsight, have prevented the injury to Jack, is nothing to the point when applying the proper legal test in this case.*

These comments illustrate the importance (for both claimants and defendants) of identifying all relevant written hospital policies and protocols, particularly where issues relating to systems or resources may be raised. On the facts in the case of *Reeve*, there was no wider criticism raised in relation to the staffing levels on the ward; the claimant's case turned upon the narrower question of whether the baby's condition mandated an earlier call to the consultant. The Court's comments also contain a helpful warning against judging negligence from a position of hindsight.

Clinical Commentary

Emily J Hotton and Joanna F Crofts

Background

An assisted (or operative) vaginal birth (AVB) is a birth in which an accoucheur (a medical practitioner or a midwife who has undergone specialist training) uses a medical device to guide the baby through the birth canal in the second stage of labour. The devices in the United Kingdom are metal forceps or ventouse (which may also be referred to as vacuum extractor, vacuum or suction device). The purpose of an AVB is to enable a vaginal birth whilst minimising maternal and neonatal morbidity [1], the alternatives being a CS at full cervical dilatation or awaiting a spontaneous vaginal birth. Situations in which AVB is indicated are often time critical, stressful and can be challenging for both parents and clinicians. In the United Kingdom, AVB is the mode of birth in 10–15% of all births [2].

Indication for Assisted Vaginal Birth

Indications to perform an AVB include presumed fetal compromise, maternal fatigue and inadequate progress in the second stage of labour. Less commonly, an AVB may be performed to shorten the second stage for women with pre-existing medical conditions that may be affected by a pushing in the second stage [2].

Assisted vaginal birth, when performed by a skilled operator in an appropriate setting, is associated with better maternal and neonatal outcomes than CS at full dilatation [3]. Specifically, women having an AVB have reduced rate of postpartum haemorrhage and reduced length of stay, whilst their babies are less likely to be admitted to the neonatal intensive care unit (NICU) [3].

A CS may be performed in the second stage of labour when AVB is deemed inappropriate or unsafe, or is attempted but fails to complete the birth. However, a CS at full dilatation is a difficult procedure and is associated with an increased risk of complications including major obstetric haemorrhage, damage to internal structures (e.g. bladder, ureters) and neonatal skull fractures secondary to the disimpaction required to free a deeply engaged fetal head. CS in the second stage of labour is also associated with prolonged hospital stay and neonatal hospital admission when compared to completed AVB [3]. Furthermore, a CS increases maternal and neonatal risks in future pregnancies including the risk of scar rupture, abnormal placentation, increased risk of late miscarriage and preterm birth and a 1.5 times increased risk of unexplained stillbirth [4–7]. Moreover, AVB can be expedited more quickly and women are much more likely (>80%) to have a spontaneous vaginal birth in their next pregnancy [8]. Therefore, AVB is often the best option for the mother and baby in the second stage of labour if assistance is required.

Pre-requisites for an Assisted Vaginal Birth

Current United Kingdom guidance [2] provides clear pre-requisites for performing an AVB. The presentation should be the fetal vertex, with full cervical dilatation, the fetal head must be less than a fifth palpable per abdomen and the membranes must have ruptured. A full assessment of caput and moulding must be achieved as well as the exact position and station of the fetal head. In the United Kingdom, an AVB can be performed at any station at the level of, or below, the ischial spines.

Clear informed consent must be obtained; adequate analgesia must be in place and the maternal bladder emptied pre-procedure.

Location of Assisted Vaginal Birth

An AVB can be conducted in a birth room or in an operating theatre. The decision on where the birth should take place should be based on the probability of failure, with a consideration for the speed in which the birth needs to be expedited, together with analgesic requirements.

"Lift out" and non-rotational low-pelvic AVBs in which the vertex is 2 cm below the ischial spines have a low probability of failure. Most procedures can be conducted safely in a birth room.

Assisted vaginal births that have a higher risk of failure should be attempted in an operating theatre where immediate recourse to CS can be undertaken. This is often referred to as a "trial of assisted vaginal birth" and women will be consented along the lines of *"trial of forceps delivery +/–proceed to Caesarean section"*. The biggest predictor of a failed AVB is the station of the vertex; the higher the vertex the more difficult the AVB and the more likely the attempt is to fail, especially if any of the fetal head is palpable on abdominal examination. A fetal malposition (e.g. ccciput posterior (OP) or occiput transverse (OT)) also significantly increases the chance of failure, as rotation of the fetal head is required during the AVB. This rotation can be performed manually before the application of an instrument or with the assistance of an instrument (e.g. Keilland's forceps, posterior metal cup or single-use ventouse). In the OP position a non-rotational birth may be attempted using forceps (known as a direct OP delivery), however this is associated with a higher risk of failure and complications due to the larger presenting diameter of the vertex in the OP position.

Additional risk factors for a failed AVB include maternal BMI greater than 30, short maternal stature, neonatal birth weight greater than 4 kg, and neonatal head circumference above the 95th percentile [2]. It should, however, be noted that the neonatal birth weight and head circumference are not known until after the AVB. Antenatal growth scans or abdominal palpation may be used to predict neonatal size at birth, but have a large margin of error [9].

The "decision to birth time" is longer if the woman is transferred to theatre for an AVB [2]. Therefore, the risks of unsuccessful AVB in the birth room need to be balanced with the risks associated with the transfer time for an AVB in an operating theatre.

Choice of Device to Assist Birth

The devices used to perform assisted vaginal births can be broadly divided into "metal forceps" or "ventouse" and "rotational" or "non-rotational" devices (Table 14.1).

In England, the rate of use of forceps and ventouse is similar (7.3% of births in 2019/2020 were assisted with forceps and 5.0% with ventouse) [10].

Forceps (see Figure 14.1) and ventouse (see Figure 14.2) are associated with different benefits and risks. Forceps are the better instrument in terms of achieving a "successful" birth (i.e. the baby is delivered vaginally with the assistance of forceps). However, forceps are associated with higher rates of complications for the mother including perineal trauma, tears, requirements for pain relief and incontinence [11]. Comparisons between different types of ventouse demonstrate that the metal cup is better at achieving successful delivery than the soft cup, but with more risk of injury to the baby. A Cochrane review found no significant differences between the handheld (e.g. Kiwi and Mityvac) and the standard ventouse (e.g. silastic) in terms of effectiveness or rate of injury [11].

Table 14.2 (adapted from the Royal College of Obstetricians and Gynaecologists (RCOG) AVB Guideline) summarises the differences in outcomes in vacuum extraction as compared with forceps assisted birth [2].

Decisions as to which device should be used depend upon individual situations, where the urgency with which the baby needs to be delivered is balanced against potential risks to the mother and baby. The current RCOG AVB guideline [2] states "the operator should choose the instrument most appropriate to the clinical circumstances and their level of skill". There is little evidence of increased maternal or neonatal morbidity following failed AVB compared to immediate caesarean birth where immediate recourse to caesarean birth is available [2].

User Technique, When to Discontinue and Sequential Use of Instruments

One of the key skills of performing an AVB is knowing when to discontinue the procedure.

Table 14.1. Detail of the devices for assisted vaginal birth

Type of device		Name of device	Key features	Use
Forceps	Non-rotational	Rhodes, Neville-Barnes, Anderson	"Standard" double blade design	OA positions at any station
		Wrigley's	Short handle	At CS if head difficult to deliver For a "lift out" vaginal birth
	Rotational	Keilland's	Shallow pelvic curve to enable rotation Sliding lock used to correct asynclitism	To rotate the fetal head from OP or OT to an OA position within the maternal pelvis To assist the birth of a slow after-coming head in a vaginal breech birth (no rotation used)
Ventouse	Non-rotational	Silastic	Reusable Vacuum from a connected electrical pump	OA position only
		Kiwi, Mityvac	Single use Vacuum via integral hand-pump	Any fetal position (OP, OT, OA)
	Rotational	Kiwi, Mityvac	Single use Vacuum via integral hand-pump	Any fetal position (OP, OT, OA)
		Posterior metal cup	Reusable Vacuum from a connected electrical pump	Generally used in OP position

The RCOG guidance states that "vacuum birth should be completed within three to four contractions" [2]. The use of forceps following failed ventouse-assisted birth may be judicious in avoiding a difficult caesarean birth but must be balanced with the increased risk of neonatal trauma associated with sequential instrument use [2].

Ventouse devices are known to suddenly disconnect ("pop off") the baby's head during AVB. This usually causes no additional harm to the baby but can be alarming for the woman and her birth partner. The RCOG guidance states to "discontinue vacuum-assisted birth if there have been two 'pop-offs' of the instrument. Less experienced operators should seek senior support after one 'pop-off' to ensure the woman has the best chance of a successful assisted vaginal birth" [2], as incorrect placement of the

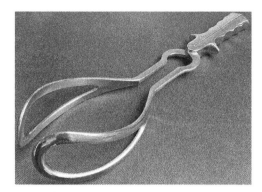

Figure 14.1 Example of forceps device (Neville-Barnes Forceps).

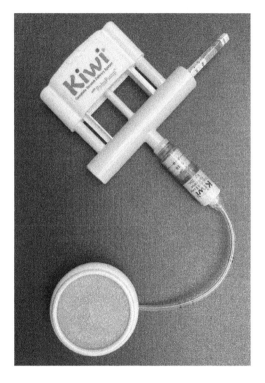

Figure 14.2 Example of ventouse device (Kiwi Ventouse).

ventouse is associated with a higher chance of failure. The ventouse device "popping-off" can be viewed as a "safety feature" as it stops continued and sustained traction being applied to the fetal head when an AVB is not progressing; this contrasts with the forceps which do not "pop-off". Therefore, any decision to stop using forceps must be consciously instigated by the operator and the forceps manually removed.

If forceps cannot be applied easily, or the forceps handles do not approximate ("lock") easily, the attempted forceps birth should be stopped. Once the forceps are applied, if there is a lack of progressive descent with moderate traction, the operator should consider whether the application of the forceps is suboptimal, the position of the fetal head has been incorrectly diagnosed, or there is cephalopelvic disproportion (i.e. the

Table 14.2. Outcomes following ventouse-assisted birth compared with forceps-assisted birth [2]

Outcome	Odds ratio (95% confidence interval)
More likely to fail at achieving vaginal birth	1.7 (1.3–2.2)
More likely to be associated with cephalohaematoma	2.4 (1.7–3.4)
More likely to be associated with retinal haemorrhage	2.0 (1.3–3.0)
More likely to be associated with maternal worries about baby	2.2 (1.2–3.9)
Less likely to be associated with significant maternal perineal and vaginal trauma	0.4 (0.3–0.5)
No more likely to be associated with birth by caesarean birth	0.6 (0.3–1.0)
No more likely to be associated with low 5 min Apgar scores	1.7 (1.0–2.8)
No more likely to be associated with the need for phototherapy	1.1 (0.7–1.8)

fetal head is too big to fit through the maternal pelvis). Accurate instrument placement influences the probability of success and the risk of maternal and neonatal trauma. Suboptimal instrument placement is associated with a four-fold increased risk of neonatal trauma, use of sequential instruments and caesarean birth for failed AVB [2].

If there is a lack of progressive descent with moderate traction, or birth is not imminent following three pulls of a correctly applied instrument by an experienced operator, the attempted vaginal birth should be stopped. When rotational forceps are used, if rotation is not easily achieved with gentle pressure, this should also signal discontinuing the procedure [2].

The sequential use of ventouse and forceps compared with forceps alone is associated with an increased risk of intracranial haemorrhage, retinal haemorrhage, requirement for neonatal ventilation, and feeding difficulty [2].

Complications of Assisted Vaginal Birth

Systematic reviews comparing forceps- and ventouse-assisted births have repeatedly reported increased vaginal and anal sphincter trauma with the use of forceps. Forceps use is commonly associated with an episiotomy (~90% of attempts) and perineal tears (~20%). Obstetric anal sphincter injury (OASI) is reported in around 10% of AVBs [2].

Forceps have also been associated with greater rates of lasting complications such as faecal and flatus incontinence [11]. Interestingly, studies have begun to suggest that ventouse-assisted births could be protective against late development of pelvic floor complications [12]. Evidence surrounding mid-cavity rotational deliveries suggests that both maternal and neonatal outcomes are comparable, regardless of the method used for rotation (i.e. manual or forceps) [13]. Comparative studies demonstrate that maternal and neonatal morbidity is greater in rotational ventouse births than direct ventouse births; this is thought to be reflected by the increase in sequential instrument use with such rotational assisted births [13–15]. Any AVB has a risk of failure; it has associated risks of consecutive instrument use on the pelvic floor but also risk of caesarean birth if an AVB cannot be achieved, despite the use of a second instrument [15].

The existing Cochrane Systematic Review on assisted vaginal birth summarised that, when comparing births assisted by forceps or ventouse, there was no difference in umbilical cord pH, neonatal admission to NICU, length of stay or risk of low Apgar score [11]. The risk of facial injury was significantly increased with forceps as compared with ventouse [11,16]. Known complications of a birth assisted by forceps include soft tissue injury (bruise, laceration and graze), facial nerve injury and skull fracture [17,18]. Visual effects of ventouse-assisted births on the neonate include a chignon and cup discolouration, with softer cups known to have fewer aesthetic effects than ridged cups [11]. The incidence of cephalohaematoma is increased in ventouse births as compared to forceps [11]. Interestingly, for all neonatal outcomes examined in the review, all results were clinically non-significant. This is compounded by a wealth of observational studies implying that subgaleal haemorrhage is more common in births assisted by ventouse [19].

Information for Women

The RCOG has clear guidance on what information should be provided to women during the process of receiving informed consent for AVB [20]. The risk-based information can be summarised into key maternal and perinatal outcomes.

Maternal Outcomes

Episiotomy is very commonly used with forceps (>90%) and with ventouse (50–60%). Significant vulvo-vaginal tears are twice as common with forceps (20%) than ventouse (10%), with obstetric anal sphincter injuries being found in 8–12% of forceps births and 1–4% of ventouse births. The risk of postpartum haemorrhage is found in 10–40% of AVBs and urinary or bowel incontinence is stated as common at six weeks, but it said to improve over time.

Perinatal Outcomes

Cephalohaematoma is predominantly associated with ventouse births (1–12%) whilst facial and scalp lacerations are seen in 10% of ventouse and forceps births. Neonatal jaundice or hyperbilirubinaemia is present in 5–15% of AVB. Retinal haemorrhage and subgaleal haemorrhage are complications more associated with ventouse births and reported rates are variable between 17–38%, and 0.3–0.6%, respectively. More serious complications such as intracranial haemorrhage, cervical spine injury (mainly seen following Kielland's rotational forceps), skull fracture, facial nerve palsy and fetal death are rare.

Governance

The use of a standard proforma to document AVB is recommended by the RCOG [2]. This ensures for precise and concise contemporaneous notes. Key details to document should include but are not limited to: decision-making, conduct of the procedure, any adverse outcomes or complications and plan for postnatal care. Obstetricians should document that women meet the inclusion criteria and pre-requisites for a safe AVB. Key timings and procedure aspects should be documented, such as the number of tractions and the number of "pop-offs", if applicable.

It is recommended that for all cases of *"trial of forceps delivery +/–proceed to Caesarean section"* in the operating theatre, there should be documented written consent [2]. This ensures that the woman has been fully consented for both potential procedures, AVB and CS. For all cases of AVB in a birth room there should be documentation of written or verbal consent. Verbal consent is appropriate, especially in assisted births where there is presumed fetal compromise and an expedited birth is of paramount importance.

Obstetric trainees should have appropriate training that is both gained from simulation and clinical training under direct supervision.

Reasons for Litigation

Common reasons for litigation include:
- Failure to obtain fully informed consent
- Failure to document all the material risks
- Delay in decision to birth interval
- Failure to categorise urgency
- Inappropriate use of force
- Incorrect positioning of the device
- Inappropriate use of instrument (forceps or ventouse)
- Strategies employed to minimize maternal perineal trauma
- Fetal complications of the AVB
- Maternal complications of the AVB
- Inappropriate or incomplete counselling

Avoidance of Litigation

- Information regarding AVB provided to women and partners in the antenatal period
- Obstetrician has undergone training in AVB
- Senior supervision of inexperienced operators
- Clear reasoning behind choice of location for the birth
- Single instrument use
- Appropriate Neonatal team present at the birth
- Clear documentation

Summary

Assisted vaginal birth is a complex intervention that requires a diverse range of technical and non-technical skills by both the obstetrician and the team supporting the birth. When utilised correctly and appropriately it is associated with positive outcomes for both the woman and her baby. Obstetricians must be thorough and clear in their assessment, communication and documentation of why an AVB was indicated, how it was attempted and the clinical outcomes associated with the birth.

References

1. Keriakos, R, Sugumar, S, Hilal, N. Instrumental vaginal delivery – back to basics. *J Obstet Gynaecol* 2013; 33(8): 781–6.

2. Murphy, D, Strachan, B, Bahl, R, on behalf of the Royal College of Obstetricians and Gynaecologists. Assisted Vaginal Birth. *BJOG* 2020; 127 (9): e70–112.

3. Murphy, DJ, Liebling, RE, Verity, L, Swingler, R, Patel R. Early maternal and neonatal morbidity associated with operative delivery in second stage of

labour: a cohort study. *Lancet* 2001; 358 (9289): 1203–7.

4. Royal College of Obstetricians and Gynaecologists (RCOG). Birth after Previous Caesarean Birth: Green–top Guideline No. 45 [Internet]. 2015. Available from: www.rcog.org.uk/ globalassets/documents/guidelines/gtg_ 45.pdf

5. Norman, JE, Stock, SJ. Birth options after a caesarean section. *Br Med J* (Clinical research ed) 2018; 360: j5737.

6. Clark, EAS, Silver, RM. Long-term maternal morbidity associated with repeat cesarean delivery. *Am J Obstet Gynecol* 2011; 205(6 Suppl): S2–10.

7. Moraitis, AA, Oliver-Williams, C, Wood, AM, Fleming, M, Pell, JP, Smith, G. Previous caesarean delivery and the risk of unexplained stillbirth: retrospective cohort study and meta-analysis. *BJOG* 2015; 122(11): 1467–74.

8. Bahl, R, Strachan, B, Murphy, DJ. Outcome of subsequent pregnancy three years after previous operative delivery in the second stage of labour: cohort study. *Br Med J* (Clinical research ed) 2004; 328 (7435): 311.

9. Gupta, M, Hockley, C, Quigley, MA, Yeh, P, Impey, L. Antenatal and intrapartum prediction of shoulder dystocia. *Eur J Obstet Gyn R B* 2010; 151(2): 134–9.

10. NHS Digital. NHS Maternity Statistics, England 2019-2020 [Online]. Available from: https://digital.nhs.uk/data-and-information/publications/statistical/nhs-maternity-statistics/2019-20

11. O'Mahony, F, Hofmeyr, GJ, Menon, V. Choice of instruments for assisted vaginal delivery. *Cochrane Database Syst Rev* 2010; 16(11): 201–7.

12. Handa, VL, Blomquist, JL, McDermott, KC, Friedman, S, Muñoz, A. Pelvic floor disorders after vaginal birth: effect of episiotomy, perineal laceration, and operative birth. *Obstet Gynecol* 2012; 119 (2 Pt 1): 233–9.

13. Bahl, R, Venne, MV de, Macleod, M, Strachan, B, Murphy, DJ. Maternal and neonatal morbidity in relation to the instrument used for mid-cavity rotational operative vaginal delivery: a prospective cohort study. *BJOG* 2013; 120(12): 1526–33.

14. Macleod, M, Strachan, B, Bahl, R, Howarth, L, Goyder, K, Venne, MV de, et al. A prospective cohort study of maternal and neonatal morbidity in relation to use of episiotomy at operative vaginal delivery. *BJOG* 2008; 115(13): 1688–94.

15. Murphy, DJ, Macleod, M, Bahl, R, Strachan, B. A cohort study of maternal and neonatal morbidity in relation to use of sequential instruments at operative vaginal delivery. *Eur J Obstet Gyn R B* 2011; 156(1): 41–5.

16. Black, M, Murphy, DJ. Forceps delivery for non-rotational and rotational operative vaginal delivery. *Best Pract Res Cl Ob* 2019; 56: 55–68.

17. Demissie, K, Rhoads, GG, Smulian, JC, Balasubramanian, BA, Gandhi, K, Joseph, KS, et al. Operative vaginal delivery and neonatal and infant adverse outcomes: population-based retrospective analysis. *Br Med J* 2004; 329(7456): 24.

18. Caughey, AB, Sandberg, PL, Zlatnik, MG, Thiet, M-P, Parer, JT, Laros, RK. Forceps compared with vacuum: rates of neonatal and maternal morbidity. *Obstetrics Gynecol* 2005; 106(5, Part 1): 908–12.

19. Uchil, D, Arulkumaran, S. Neonatal subgaleal hemorrhage and its relationship to delivery by vacuum extraction. *Obstet Gynecol Surv* 2003; 58(10): 687–93.

20. Royal College of Obstetricians and Gynaecologists (RCOG). Operative Vaginal Delivery. Consent Advice No. 11. [Internet]. 2010. Available from: www .rcog.org.uk/globalassets/documents/ guidelines/ca11-15072010.pdf

Breech Presentation and Delivery

Myles JO Taylor

CASE COMMENTARY

Swati Jha

Successful Claim

TW (A Child) v Royal Bolton Hospital NHS Foundation Trust [2017] EWHC 3139 (QB)

The Claim

The claimant was born vaginally presenting as a breech baby. Earlier in the course of labour the claimant's mother called hospital but was advised not to come into hospital at that point in time. This resulted in a delay and by the time the patient attended hospital it was too late to perform a caesarean section (CS), resulting in the circulatory collapse and consequent brain injury arising from a vaginal breech delivery.

The Summary

The claimant was not known to be a breech presentation prior to the start of labour and the mother had a very rapid labour. When the mother's waters broke, she was in pain and the contractions were at five-minute intervals lasting 30 seconds and she wanted to come into hospital. Instead, she was advised to stay at home, put on a pad, walk around and call back in half an hour. A second call was made 40 minutes later, and in spite of the advice to stay home, the claimant's mother was brought into hospital. On arrival in the hospital, she was found to be fully dilated and a scan confirmed a breech presentation at the level of ischial spines. Options for delivery including a vaginal breech and CS were discussed, but due to quick progress and descent of the breech so it was visible at the vaginal opening, it was too late to perform a CS. As a result, a plan was made to proceed with a vaginal delivery. Following on from this there was a circulatory collapse and consequent brain injury.

The defendant trust initially denied that this call was made but at the time of the incident it was not routine practice to log such calls. Subsequent assessment of phone records found this to be the case, but they were unable to identify the midwife who took the call.

The Judgement

On a balance of probabilities, if, following the initial call after the mother's waters broke, she had been given permission to attend hospital (as opposed to being told not to attend), it would have been identified that the baby was breech earlier. The options of delivery would have been discussed and she would have opted for CS. This would have prevented the subsequent problems with delivery and the injury to the claimant would therefore have been avoided. The claimant's case therefore succeeded on liability.

Unsuccessful Claim

Smithers v Taunton and Somerset NHS Trust [2004] EWHC 1179 (QB)

The Claim

During the assisted vaginal breech delivery of the claimant there was a period of profound hypoxia resulting in brain injury. A vaginal breech delivery is a high-risk labour and it was claimed that the defendant failed to adequately plan for an entirely foreseeable event, namely fetal distress requiring further obstetric intervention. They also claimed that an obstetrician should have attended labour sooner to facilitate a breech extraction delivery and if immediate delivery of the breech was not feasible, an emergency CS should have been performed. The claims made changed during the course of the trial.

The Summary

The claimant was the second child of Mrs Smithers, whose first delivery had been an uncomplicated vaginal delivery of a baby in the normal cephalic presentation. During the antenatal period the baby was noted to be breech and this was maintained at subsequent antenatal visits. The baby was in a frank breech position with hips flexed and legs extended up towards the head. The options of delivery were discussed, and she wished a vaginal delivery. Mrs Smithers was induced and had an uneventful labour and reassuring fetal heart throughout. When she was in the second stage and breech found to be descending in the birth canal, fetal heart decelerations were noted and the registrar called. As they were dealing with another emergency in theatres at the time, they could not attend immediately. On arrival, the registrar performed an assisted breech delivery as opposed to a breech extraction as this was obsolete in obstetric practice due to its inherent risks. Whereas an assisted breech delivery involves delivery by a combination of uterine contractions and maternal pushing, with assistance to ensure the positioning of the baby is correct during the delivery to ensure a slow and controlled delivery of the head, a breech extraction would require actively pulling the baby out using traction. The assisted breech delivery was performed competently and could not have been achieved any sooner. The claimant weighed 4.192 kgs at birth.

The Judgement

The options and discussions regarding mode of delivery in the antenatal period were in keeping with the practice of the time as this delivery predated the Term Breech Trial, which has since affected breech deliveries significantly. The obstetric registrar was dealing with another obstetric emergency at the time of the onset of the fetal bradycardia and could not have attended any sooner. The assisted breech delivery was performed competently. Even if an emergency CS had been performed, a delivery would not have been achieved any sooner than it was by an assisted breech delivery.

The claim was therefore dismissed.

Legal Commentary

Eloise Power

TW (A Child) v Royal Bolton Hospital NHS Foundation Trust [2017] EWHC 3139 (QB)

This case ultimately turned upon the advice which the claimant's mother was given in a telephone call with an unnamed midwife at the hospital at 4 am on 26 March 2008. The defendant had initially denied that the telephone call was made. By the time the case came to trial, telephone records were available, and the defendant conceded that the telephone call had taken place. At the material time, the defendant had no system for taking records of telephone calls, and there was no available evidence from the midwife who had taken the call. The evidence from the claimant's mother was that she informed the midwife that her waters had broken and that she was in a lot of pain, with contractions at five-minute intervals. The midwife seemed uninterested and advised her to stay at home. The mother said *"but my waters have broken"*. The midwife advised her to put a pad on and walk around for about 30 minutes. By the time the mother eventually reached the hospital (following a further telephone call), it was too late to perform a CS as the descending breech was below the ischial spines. The claimant suffered brain injury at birth.

At trial, the defendant made two crucial concessions: first, that the mother's account of the telephone call at 4 am should be accepted, and second, that if she had been admitted to hospital sooner, she would have elected a delivery by way of a CS. The question which the Court had to consider was whether the advice given by the midwife at 4 am was acceptable. The Court found that, as a minimum, the mother should have been invited to attend hospital (although there was no need to express this advice in urgent terms). On the facts, she was actively discouraged from attending hospital. This amounted to a breach of duty. The Court accepted that if the mother had been invited to attend hospital, she would have attended within 30 minutes.

The Keefe Principle

The case of *TW* raises the important issue of the approach which the Courts should take to cases where defendants have not kept relevant records, made relevant observations or taken relevant measurements. Perhaps unsurprisingly, this is an issue which has been the subject of various judgements, and which comes up regularly in practice.

In *TW*, the Court did not make a clear finding as to whether the defendant's failure to have a proper system in place for keeping records of telephone calls amounted to a breach of duty in itself. However, the following observations were made:

> the fact is no records were kept and the lack of evidence as to what was said (other than that of the family), and the lack of evidence from the material midwives who took the calls, has to be laid at the door of the Defendant.

The Court relied upon a well-known principle from the case of *Keefe v Isle of Man Steam Packet Co Ltd* [2010] EWCA Civ 683. Keefe was a case involving noise-induced hearing loss. Longmore LJ found as follows [para 19]:

If it is a defendant's duty to measure noise levels in places where his employees work and he does not do so, it hardly lies in his mouth to assert that the noise levels were not, in fact, excessive. In such circumstances the court should judge a claimant's evidence benevolently and the defendant's evidence critically (underlining added).

The *Keefe* principle should not be seen as an automatic route to victory for claimants in cases involving deficiencies of measurements or record-keeping. It does not amount to a reversal of the burden of proof. It has been considered in various clinical negligence cases, with differing degrees of success for claimants. Several examples are listed below.

In *Executors of the Estate of John Raggett (Deceased) v King's College Hospital NHS Foundation Trust and others* [2016] EWHC 1604, Sir Alistair MacDuff applied the *Keefe* principle in favour of a claimant in a multi-defendant case involving various deficiencies of measurements and record-keeping. One of the defendants, an orthopaedic surgeon, had failed to make records of tests which he had allegedly carried out to the pedal pulses of the deceased's feet. On the facts, the Court found that the tests had not been carried out, and that if the tests had been carried out, the pedal pulses would have been absent, leading to vascular referral and prevention of amputation.

By contrast, in *H (a child, by her mother and litigation friend) v Southend Hospital NHS Trust*, May J declined to apply the *Keefe* principle in a case involving a partial rather than a total absence of records. The case involved a home birth. The midwives had recorded regular observations of the fetal heart rate. However, their records stopped during a 20-minute period. The claimant alleged that if the midwives had observed the fetal heart rate during this period, they would have detected bradycardia and the baby would have been delivered earlier, avoiding brain damage consequent upon a hypoxic ischaemic event. The Court found that neither a positive nor a negative inference could be drawn from the fact that the record of observations had stopped during the critical period. The midwives were regarded as candid and honest witnesses, and the Court declined to make a finding that they had failed to observe the fetal heart rate (as distinct from failing to make a record of their observations).

In *ZZZ v Yeovil District Hospital NHS Foundation Trust* [2019] EWHC 1642, Garnham J declined to apply the *Keefe* principle in relation to causation. Counsel for the claimant submitted that as a consequence of the defendant's breach of duty, no proper neurological examination was carried out upon the claimant, and the Court should therefore draw an inference that the claimant's deterioration in limb function would not have occurred. This submission was robustly rejected given that, *"in sharp contra-distinction from Keefe"* there was clear expert evidence dealing with the issue of deterioration in limb function (para 142).

By contrast, in *Younas v Dr Okeahialam* [2019] EWHC 2502, the Court was prepared to apply the *Keefe* principle at the causation stage in considering what would have happened if a GP had made a referral to the cardiology department of his local hospital. The Court observed that *"Applying proper 'claimant benevolence' without reversing the burden of proof requires care"* (para 38), but nevertheless took into account that *"it is the fault of the defendant that we are having to undertake this exercise at all"* (para 46). The claimant's claim succeeded.

In the light of the different approaches taken in *ZZZ* and in *Younas v Dr Okeahialam*, it is to be hoped that the higher courts will give further consideration to the applicability or otherwise of the *Keefe* principle at the causation stage of clinical negligence matters.

On the facts in *TW*, it is unsurprising that the Court was prepared to invoke *Keefe* in the claimant's favour, given that there was a total absence of evidence from the defendant and a credible and comprehensive account of the telephone call from the claimant witnesses.

For a discussion of the related issue of the approach which the Court should take to cases where a party has not called a witness who might be expected to have relevant evidence to provide on a particular issue, please see the legal commentary at Chapter 10. On the facts in *TW*, it seems unlikely that the defendant would have had any way of knowing which midwife took the telephone call at 4 am, given the absence of any record-keeping system. The case illustrates the importance of maintaining solid record-keeping systems, not just as a matter of good medico-legal practice but also to promote account-ability and high standards.

Smithers v Taunton and Somerset NHS Trust [2004] EWHC 1179 (QB)

As an initial observation, this case may well have been approached differently if the underlying events had happened after the publication of the Term Breech Trial (pub-lished in October 2000).[1] Although the judgement in *Smithers* postdates the Term Breech Trial, the underlying events took place in March 2000 and therefore predated the publication of the Term Breech Trial. As discussed at Chapter 6, the standard of care is assessed at the time of the underlying events rather than by reference to later standards which might exist by the date of trial.

The case of *Smithers* raises the interesting issue of how the courts approach compet-ing emergencies and resource considerations. On the night in question, there was another labouring mother who required delivery by emergency CS. The consultant on call was aware that the registrar on duty was in theatre with this patient, and that if there were any *"competing emergencies or potential emergencies"* he would have to come in. On the facts, the Court accepted that the registrar and the on-call consultant reasonably believed that there was no need for the on-call consultant to attend: viewed prospectively, they reasonably believed that the other patient's condition would be controlled locally within 10–15 minutes, and that the registrar would then have been able to attend to the claimant's mother. The Court rejected the submission that an *off*-call consultant should have been summoned as a precautionary measure, observing that *"this would mean that the hospital's consultants were in reality permanently on-call"*.

Essentially, the Court in *Smithers* approached the issue of the competing emergency by way of a close examination of the facts rather than by reference to any wider points of principle (except when considering the submission relating to the off-call consultant). One can contrast the approach taken in the case of *Mulholland v Medway NHS Foundation Trust* [2015] EWHC 268, where the Court held that the standard of care of an Accident and Emergency doctor working in a pressurised environment *"must be calibrated in a manner reflecting reality"*. The implications of *Mulholland* are considered in more detail at Chapter 10.

It remains to be seen how the immense resource pressures placed on the NHS system as a whole due to the Covid-19 crisis will be taken into account by the court system. In the case of *University College London Hospitals NHS Foundation Trust v MB* [2020]

---

[1] *Lancet* 2000; 356(9239).

EWHC 882, Chamberlain J was prepared to grant an interim injunction to require a patient to vacate a neuropsychiatric bed which was urgently required for the use of other patients due to the Covid-19 crisis. The Court observed:

> Decisions taken by a health authority on the basis of finite funds are, in my judgment, no different in principle from those taken by a hospital on the basis of finite resources of other kinds. In each case a choice has to be made and, in making it, it is necessary to consider the needs of more than one person.

This was a Human Rights Act/public law/possession matter rather than a clinical negligence case. Clinical negligence cases, by their nature, are slower to reach trial. However, it seems likely that in the clinical negligence context, the courts will look closely at the reasonableness or otherwise of decisions made on the ground, bearing in mind the reality that resources are finite. NHS Resolution has established a Clinical Negligence Scheme for Coronavirus to meet liabilities arising from the special healthcare arrangements which were put in place in response to the Covid-19 situation.

Clinical Commentary

Myles JO Taylor

Background Information

Breech presentation occurs in around 3% of fetuses at term [1] and refers to the presenting part, or lowermost aspect, of the fetus being the buttocks or feet.

The main types of breech presentation are:

- Extended or frank breech (50–70%), the commonest form, where both hips are flexed and both knees are extended
- Flexed or complete breech, where both hips and both knees are flexed (5–10%)
- Footling or incomplete breech, where one of both hips are not completely flexed (10–40%).

Significance

The key problem with breech vaginal delivery is that the most important part of the baby to be born, the head, is by definition, delivered last. With the baby's body dangling outside the mother, particularly if this process has been relatively easy with a footling breech, the head can become entrapped, and, with the cord at risk of being compressed, the risks of hypoxia and birth-related trauma are increased.

Perhaps the most vivid example of what can go wrong occurred well before CS became available, with the birth of Kaiser Wilhelm II in 1859 [2] .

Kaiser "Bill", as he affectionately became known by the British soldiers, was born with a withered arm, and somewhat erratic behaviour which, according to some, may have contributed to the outbreak of World War I and, indirectly, to World War II.

The delivery was difficult because, with only his buttocks delivered, there was a "weakening of the pulse in the umbilical cord" and "the Prince appeared quite lifeless". Analysis of the delivery suggests that the obstetrician, in dealing with this situation, was forced to manoeuvre the hapless Prince, and in so doing probably injured his left arm and, due to the interval between delivery of body and head, possibly also sustained a hypoxic brain injury. Whether or not Kaiser Wilhelm's birth injuries were at least to some extent responsible for the start of World War I is open to question, but his delivery was certainly traumatic for him, and highlights what can be at stake when things go wrong.

More than a century later, breech presentation and delivery continues to be a potential cause of harm and major source of litigation. Only recently, for example, a delay in arranging an emergency CS because the fetus was in the breech position, which led to serious hypoxic brain injury, resulted in one of the biggest out-of-Court settlements in medical negligence claims in NHS history, at over £37 million [3].

Modern Evidence

Two trials transformed modern obstetric practice. The first, in 1992, compared the outcome of 3,447 women who presented and delivered at term with breech presentation. The incidence of intrapartum and neonatal death associated with vaginal birth was 8/961 (0.83%) compared with only 1/2486 (0.03%) in babies born by CS – a staggering 20-fold increase in risk of demise. The authors concluded that: "The good neonatal outcome associate with elective caesarean delivery . . . may influence the decision of women and their obstetricians about mode of delivery". The results were devasting for devotees of vaginal delivery, but attracted considerable criticism, principally focused on the hazards of drawing too many conclusions from retrospective analysis of a computerised database. At the very least, however, as a result of this trial, vaginal delivery was put on notice.

The second, and to my mind the "nail in the coffin" for planned vaginal delivery, came in 2000 with "Term Breech Trial" (TBT) [4], a multi-centre randomised controlled trial in which 2,088 women with a frank or complete breech were randomised to planned CS or planned vaginal birth. These results were not quite so dramatic, but nevertheless showed that perinatal mortality, neonatal mortality, or serious neonatal morbidity was significantly lower for planned CS (17/1039 [1.6%]) than for the planned vaginal delivery (52/1039 [5.0%]) – a two-thirds reduction in the risk of serious perinatal complications. Criticism of the TBT have been made, but in short, this, along with other randomised controlled trials has meant that very few mothers currently opt for planned vaginal delivery in the UK. This itself has inevitably resulted in a reduction in experience in delivering breech babies vaginally by obstetricians. Inevitably, because of inexperience, the belief that vaginal delivery will all but disappear, has become a self-fulfilling prophecy. Thus, even if vaginal delivery were safe, the lack of experienced hands has rendered it potentially the opposite.

Vaginal Birth: Putting the Risks into Perspective

Whilst dramatic, the plight of Prince Wilhelm needs to be put in context, as does the evidence from the scientific literature. In 2015, the Montgomery [5] ruling prompted a need to understand what constitutes a material risk to the mother in modern obstetric practice. Thus, as can often occur, if the relative risk of an adverse outcome is reviewed in isolation, when the actual, or absolute risk remains very low, the mother may be misinformed or become unnecessarily alarmed. On the other hand, even if the absolute risk is low, but the outcome in question extreme, this issue should be addressed.

To help in this regard, the risk of dying on the day of birth has been compared with other hazardous activities [6]. When expressed in "micromorts", or the number of one in a million chances of dying, the overall risk of dying on the day of birth in the United Kingdom for a term baby who was alive at the onset of labour is 430 micromorts (0.43 per 1000). Thus, the risk of dying on the day of birth exceeded that of any other day of an individual's life until the ninety-second year. For comparison, unsurprisingly, the risk of coronary artery bypass graft is much higher, at 3800 micromorts. However, and to many somewhat surprisingly, the risk of dying from vaginal breech delivery is higher still at 5870 micromorts [7]. This figure is put further into perspective when calculating the risk of dying per day when climbing Mount Everest [8], where the risks are much lower at 820 micromorts (0.82/1000).

Finally, in any discussions, it is worth mentioning who is mainly at risk in this situation. The fetus is clearly at increased risk of demise with vaginal delivery, whilst the mother has some increased risk of morbidity – but not so much of dying – particularly in future pregnancies, with CS.

Therefore, in my experience, when things go wrong, most mothers, when asked in retrospect what they would have chosen had they been properly counselled, invariably reply that they would not have chosen any option that put their baby at any undue risk and would instead have accepted the increased risk of maternal morbidity and opted for CS.

Antenatal Counselling

Thus, when a mother presents with a breech presentation in the third trimester, the obstetrician has a duty of care to inform the mother of the risks of planned vaginal delivery versus planned CS, provided the baby does not spontaneously turn to cephalic presentation, which occurs in only 8% of primigravid women after 36 weeks' gestation.

A third option, which requires consideration, is external cephalic version (ECV), where, through external manipulation of the maternal abdomen after 36–37 weeks' gestation, the fetus is turned to cephalic presentation.

The RCOG [9] recommends informing mothers that the success rate of ECV is approximately 50% and has a very low complication rate. Its use is therefore supported, but only when performed by an appropriately trained practitioner. After a successful ECV, there is an approximately two-fold increase in risk of requiring an emergency CS (21% versus 11%) and modest increase in the risk of requiring an instrumental delivery (14% versus 12.6%) compared to spontaneous cephalic presentation.

The decision process needs to be thorough and complete, taking advantage of widely available patient decision aids produced locally or nationally. It is also important that a record is kept in the medical notes of such counselling and a note made of any decision that the mother has reached.

National Guidance

In 2017, the RCOG published updated guidance [10] on the management of breech presentation, including a detailed description of the information that mothers should be given to help them reach an informed choice on mode of delivery. It is recommended that breech delivery take place in a hospital in an obstetric-led unit, where immediate facilities for emergency CS are available, not least because around 40% of mothers planning a vaginal delivery will require an emergency CS. During labour, anaesthetic support should be immediately available, and a paediatrician present at the birth.

Essential to minimising the risks of breech vaginal delivery is the presence of a skilled birth attendant. How to acquire the necessary skills and experience is a moot point, given the diminishing number of vaginal deliveries. To address this, many units provide simulation training where manikins are used to help obstetricians and midwives improve and maintain their delivery skills.

Intrapartum Management

The specific management of a vaginal breech delivery is beyond the scope of this chapter. Nevertheless, a few points are worth highlighting.

First Stage of Labour

The management of the first stage is essentially no different to that of a cephalic presentation, except that continuous electronic fetal monitoring is recommended.

Second Stage of Labour

A passive second stage (i.e. without the mother pushing) is recommended to allow descent of the breech. If the breech is not visible within two hours of the second stage, CS should be recommended.

The active second stage of labour is when specific obstetric skills may be called for. Once the buttocks are beyond the perineum, a hands-off technique is usually recommended until the umbilicus appears. Traction may be required, however, if poor progress occurs. The RCOG has recommended: "intervention to expedite breech birth is required if there is evidence of poor fetal condition or if there is a delay of more than five minutes from delivery of the buttocks to the head, or of more than three minutes form the umbilicus to the head".

Various manoeuvres, such as Lovset's to secure delivery of the arms, or Mauriceau-Smellie-Viet to deliver the head, may be required. All obstetricians and midwives should be familiar with these and other techniques which should be practised in the simulation setting.

Special Situations

Undiagnosed Breech in Labour

The discovery of the undiagnosed breech in labour is a midwife's or obstetrician's heart-sink moment. Unless the baby has unexpectedly turned on its own since the last examination, it usually means that breech was missed antenatally – an uncomfortable, but recurring event in many maternity units. Management is challenging. The mother needs concise but nevertheless careful counselling on the options available. Counselling about the risks of vaginal delivery on the basis of evidence from the TBT is common, but not strictly justified, since women were entered into this trial prior to the onset of labour. Nevertheless, the option of emergency CS should be given as early as possible because delay may result in either a vaginal delivery occurring, if labour progresses rapidly, or result in an increasingly difficult emergency CS if labour reaches the second stage.

Furthermore, any undue delay may reach the point of no-return, where baby is hanging outside the mother's body, with the difficult part – the head – yet to come, with CS well-nigh impossible.

The undiagnosed breech is particularly challenging in the non-hospital birth settings, at home or in stand-alone midwifery birthing units. These are birth-settings chosen for low-risk mothers who, by definition, have often not required antenatal fetal ultrasound scans, and thus presentation has only been assessed clinically by midwives. It is for this reason that in late pregnancy, particularly when delivery is planned in such low-risk settings, if there is any doubt about fetal presentation, an ultrasound to confirm fetal presentation should be requested. In early labour, again, if there is any doubt, the ready availability of portable ultrasound scans can be of assistance.

If breech presentation is found to be present, the decision to request immediate transfer to the nearest maternity unit will depend on the balance of risks of remaining in that particular setting, as opposed to the hazards of delivering in the back of an ambulance whilst trying to reach a place of safety.

Multiple Pregnancy – Twins

In twins, CS is usually recommended if the presenting twin, Twin 1, is breech. For Twin 2, even if cephalic during labour, there should be realisation that following the birth of Twin 1 that its co-twin can turn spontaneously into any presentation. Hence, once Twin 1 is delivered, careful examination, usually assisted by ultrasound, is recommended. Management of vaginal breech delivery for Twin 2 is essentially the same as for a singleton. However, at this point, the advantages of having sited an epidural earlier in labour become apparent, particularly if internal version of Twin 2 to breech is required.

Preterm Labour

Unfortunately, the evidence on what is the optimal mode of delivery for preterm breech fetus is lacking. An attempt at a randomised controlled trial was abandoned after only 13 mothers were recruited in 27 months [11]. Therefore, clinicians, even if clear in their own minds what the best mode of delivery is, should nevertheless counsel mothers about the paucity of data on this issue, and base any decision on an individualised basis, including, as the RCOG [10] recommends, an assessment of the "stage of labour, type of breech presentation, fetal wellbeing and availability of an operator skilled in vaginal breech delivery."

Causes/Avoidance of Litigation

The reason litigation arises with breech presentation is almost invariably because injury occurs to the baby during planned or unplanned vaginal delivery. Thus, at each point in the pregnancy where labour itself, or least delivery by the breech, might have been prevented, allegations of negligence may arise.

Diagnosis of Breech Presentation

In most pregnancies, particularly those deemed to be at low risk, fetal presentation is determined clinically. As one might expect, and even in the best of hands, this assessment is not 100% accurate. That said, if, in the antenatal notes there is any hint of uncertainty over fetal presentation, any failure to confirm or refute the clinical findings by requesting a presentation scan makes those responsible open to allegations of negligence. Therefore, to avoid litigation, clinicians should have low threshold for requesting a presentation scan as it is readily available, often by means of a portable/in-roomer scanner. If this approach is observed, it follows that any incriminating documentation expressing uncertainty of fetal presentation will be avoided. Also, in this regard, many units currently advocate routinely scanning all mothers late in pregnancy planning to deliver in a low-risk setting, to reassure the mother that baby is cephalic and avoid the hazards of the undiagnosed breech.

Counselling

Planned Vaginal Delivery: Failure to Provide Proper Counselling

When injury to the baby occurs during vaginal breech delivery, attention will inevitably be focused on the quality of antenatal counselling, with any failure to give the mother sufficient information to allow her to make an informed decision on the risks and benefits of planning for a vaginal delivery attracting criticism. To avoid litigation, therefore, clinicians should not only counsel mothers properly, but document that this has occurred, and also support this by recording that the mother has been provided with patient choice information sheets, such as those provided by the RCOG.

Undiagnosed Breech in Labour: Failure to Provide Proper Counselling

The same issues apply for the undiagnosed breech as for when breech is diagnosed before labour. However, in labour, time is short, and the mother stressed – all the more so for having been diagnosed with breech presentation. Thus, providing sufficient and digestible information to ensure that the mother is fully informed is challenging. Therefore, to avoid litigation, proper counselling, probably by an experienced obstetrician and midwife, is required, and a full record kept of the discussion in the maternity notes.

Delivery

Mismanagement in Labour: Failure to Demonstrate Appropriate Delivery Skills

When injury occurs, close scrutiny will be focused on labour management – particularly of the second stage. To avoid litigation, obstetricians and midwives should ensure that they have learnt and maintained the necessary skills not only in their training, but also by means of regular skills drills, often with the benefit of manikins in simulated breech deliveries. A record should be kept of attendance at such training sessions. The Trust should ensure that it can provide an experienced obstetrician and midwife at all times to deal with vaginal breech delivery.

Conclusions

Planned vaginal breech delivery is fast becoming vanishingly rare, but still remains potentially hazardous for the baby. Midwives and obstetricians need to be aware of this important issue in order to provide proper counselling for when breech presentation is diagnosed before and during labour. Any lack of direct clinical experience in managing vaginal breech delivery should be mitigated by appropriate simulation training. Every effort should be taken antenatally to avoid the undiagnosed breech in labour.

References

1. Hofmeyr, GJ. Overview of breech presentation. In *UpToDate* [Online]. Published in the United States by Wolters Kluwer; 2019.

2. Ober, WB. Obstetrical events that shaped Western European history. *Yale J Biol Med* 1992; 65: 201–10.

3. 1 Crown Office Row. £37 million awarded to young boy left brain damaged at birth. 2021. Available from: www.1cor.com/london/2020/07/21/37-million-awarded-to-young-boy-left-brain-damaged-at-birth/

4. Hannah, ME, Hannah, WJ, Hewson, SA, Hodnett, ED, Saigal, S, Willan, AR. Planned caesarean section versus planned vaginal birth for breech presentation at term: a randomised multicentre trial. Term Breech Trial Collaborative Group. *Lancet* 2000; 356(9239): 1375–83.

5. Montgomery (Appellant) v Lanarkshire Health Board (Respondent), 2015. UKSC 11

6. Walker, KF, Cohen, AL, Walker, SH, Allen, KM, Baines, DL, Thornton, JG. The dangers of the day of birth. *BJOG* 2014; 121(6): 714–18.

7. Hickson, C, Hoskins, F, Ogollah, R, Walker, KF, Thornton, JG. The risks of a range of maternal pregnancy choices, expressed as "baby micromorts" (risk of death per million births). *Eur J Obstet Gynecol Reprod Biol* 2020; 251: 194–8.

8. Thornton, JG. Birth Risks. 2014. Available from: https://ripe-tomato.org/2014/04/24/birth-risks/

9. Impey, LWM, Murphy, DJ, Griffiths, M, Penna, LK. External cephalic version and reducing the incidence of term breech presentation. Green-top Guideline No. 20a. *BJOG* 2017; 124(7): e178–e92.

10. Royal College of Obstetricians and Gynaecologists. Management of Breech Presentation. Green-top Guideline No. 20b. *BJOG* 2017; 124(7): e151–e77.

11. Penn, ZJ, Steer, PJ, Grant, A. A multicentre randomised controlled trial comparing elective and selective caesarean section for the delivery of the preterm breech infant. *Br J Obstet Gynaecol* 1996; 103(7): 684–9.

Chapter 16

Multiple Pregnancy

Mark D Kilby

CASE COMMENTARY

Swati Jha

Successful Claim

SXX (By Litigation Friend NXX) v Liverpool Women's NHS Foundation Trust [2015] EWHC 4072 (QB)

The Claim

The claimant was the first twin and born by forceps delivery. At the time of the delivery, he suffered an intracerebral bleed, hydrocephalous and permanent neurological disability. It was claimed that the parents had informed the midwife they wished an elective caesarean section (CS) and there was a breach of duty in communicating this to the consultant in charge of her care. Had they been referred to the consultant, they would have asked for an elective CS which would have prevented the subsequent injury.

The Summary

The claimant was conceived through IVF and the father of the claimant had a brother and sister-in-law who had lost a twin during a vaginal delivery a few years before the claimant was due to be born. The parents of the claimant therefore had concerns about a vaginal delivery. The consultant also made clear that in view of this family bereavement, had a request been made for an elective CS, this would have been agreed, even though a vaginal delivery was still deemed to be safe in this scenario. The parents made it known to the midwife they saw at their initial Twin Clinic that they wished for an elective CS at their initial booking appointment but were told this was a discussion to be had later in the pregnancy. The claimant's mother saw a consultant during a threatened miscarriage in early pregnancy and again expressed a wish for an elective CS. The pros and cons were discussed at length and it was noted that they should have a CS if that was their wish.

Closer to the EDD, the midwifery review resulted in an induction of labour being booked. It was claimed that their request for an elective CS was dismissed. The parents felt they were coerced into agreeing to vaginal delivery even though they had previously indicated they wanted a CS on the basis that they were assured no risks would be taken. Labour started a few days before the scheduled induction and the claimant's mother felt that she was coerced again into agreeing to vaginal delivery by the attending midwifery team. The claimant was delivered by forceps and his sister was born by CS shortly after.

The Judgement

The parents had set out all along that they wanted a CS for delivery but felt obliged to agree to a natural birth as this was the clear advice being given by the midwife. They were not aware they had a right to have the matter referred to a consultant for a further discussion about the method of delivery. Based on discussions following the threatened miscarriage with the consultant obstetrician, the parents claimed they had asked for a CS repeatedly but were coerced into a vaginal delivery and that there was a failure to refer to see a consultant to discuss mode of delivery, The ruling was in favour of the claimant and but for the attempted vaginal delivery the claimant would not have suffered the harm they came to.

Unsuccessful Claim

Sarah Louise Cox v The Secretary of State for Health [2016] EWHC 924 (QB)

The Claim

The claimant mother Mrs Cox was pregnant with twins. Following a vaginal delivery of the first twin, the umbilical cord of the second twin prolapsed and an emergency CS was performed for delivery but resulted in oxygen deprivation and a serious brain injury. It was claimed that the negligence of the hospital staff, which the Secretary of State for Health is now responsible for, was responsible for this injury. The defendant hospital failed to deliver the baby sooner due to the absence of facilities for a general anaesthetic to carry out an emergency CS and a failure to perform a vaginal breech extraction, as this would have been quicker. These factors made the environment for delivery unsafe.

The Summary

Mrs Cox went into spontaneous labour and was transferred to the labour ward. She progressed to full dilatation and the first twin was delivered uneventfully vaginally. Following delivery, it was noted that the presenting part of the second twin was not palpable and this was followed soon after by a cord prolapse. A decision was made for an emergency CS, as the presenting part of twin 2 was a breech but very high in the birth canal. For a breech extraction, this would have required the baby to be pulled out feet first. To keep the presenting part off the cord, the obstetrician kept their hand in the vagina up until the CS could be performed. The fetal heartbeat before the CS was 40 bpm. At the time of delivery there was no requirement to deliver twins in theatres, hence there was a 20-minute interval from delivery of the first twin to delivery of the second, with the claim made that the delay was because of the operating theatres being on a separate floor of the hospital. It was claimed that there should have been facilities to perform the CS in the delivery room. The defendant argued that this was a reasonable interval in which to perform an urgent CS.

The alternative claim was centred around a failure to perform a vaginal breech delivery. It was accepted that this may have been quicker than an emergency CS, however given that the second twin was still very high in the birth canal this was deemed to be too risky.

The Judgement

There was no requirement to be able to perform a CS in the delivery room hence the only way of achieving delivery was to transfer the patient to the operating theatres. Once the cord prolapse was detected it was appropriately managed and this was acted on promptly with the subsequent transfer to theatres and delivery being in a timely manner. The claim regarding a vaginal breech delivery was rejected on the grounds it would have been too dangerous, hence there was no breach of duty in this regard either. Given the case failed on both accounts of breach, it was dismissed.

Legal Commentary

Eloise Power

SXX (By Litigation Friend NXX) v Liverpool Women's NHS Foundation Trust [2015] EWHC 4072 (QB)

The cases considered in this chapter illustrate the additional risks of pregnancy and birth in multiple pregnancies. In the case of *SXX*, Recorder Elleray QC considered the case of one of two twins who suffered an intracerebral haemorrhage and hydrocephalus consequent upon an instrumental delivery. The twins' parents were well aware of the risks of vaginal delivery of twins: the father's brother and sister-in-law had previously suffered the loss of one of their twins in the course of a vaginal birth. The judge found that the father's family had always had concerns about the prospect of vaginal delivery where twins were to be born.

The key issue which fell for consideration by the Court was whether, on the facts, the mother had made a request to her treating midwife for delivery by elective CS. It was common ground between the parties that if such a request had been made, this should have led to a referral to a senior obstetrician. The defendant acknowledged that if the parents had seen the relevant consultant and had made a request for a CS, the consultant would have agreed to this request.

In addressing the question of whether the mother had made a request for delivery by elective CS, the Court had regard to the clinical records as well as to the witness evidence of the parents and the midwife. Importantly, at an earlier stage in the pregnancy, the mother had experienced bleeding and was admitted to hospital overnight for monitoring. She was reviewed by a consultant obstetrician, who made a clear record that there had been a lengthy discussion about possible mode of delivery and had noted *"For elective section if wishes"*. The Court found that although no formal decision had been made at this stage, the mother had been reassured that she would be able to elect a CS. Although the subsequent midwifery records seem not to have recorded further requests for a CS, it is notable that around a month after the delivery a doctor recorded *"They feel they were coerced into agreeing to vaginal delivery when they previously indicated they wanted a C/S"*.

On the facts, the Court found that the parents had wanted an elective CS all along, but that they felt obliged to agree to a vaginal delivery because of advice they had received from their treating midwife. The parents were unaware that they had a right to have the matter referred to the treating consultant. Under all the circumstances, the Court found that the treating midwife was in breach of duty in failing to refer discussion of the mode of delivery to a consultant obstetrician, and that if the mother had seen the consultant, she would have requested a CS. The defendant had already acknowledged that this would have led to an elective CS.

Interestingly, the Court did not regard the Supreme Court's decision in *Montgomery* as particularly relevant to the issues under consideration (at the relevant time, *Montgomery* was a recent development in the law). This may have been because of the extensive concessions which had already been made by the defendant. In contextualising the judgement in *SXX*, it is suggested that the principles in *Montgomery* are relevant. As Baroness Hale found [para 115]:

> A patient is entitled to take into account her own values, her own assessment of the comparative merits of giving birth in the 'natural' and traditional way and of giving birth by caesarean section, whatever medical opinion may say, alongside the medical evaluation of the risks to herself and her baby. She may place great value on giving birth in the natural way and be prepared to take the risks to herself and her baby which this entails. The medical profession must respect her choice, unless she lacks the legal capacity to decide... There is no good reason why the same should not apply in reverse, if she is prepared to forgo the joys of natural childbirth in order to avoid some not insignificant risks to herself or her baby.

Applying these principles to the situation in SXX, it is evident that the family history of bereavement during twin delivery formed an important part of the mother's values and fed into her own assessment of the comparative merits of giving birth by CS rather than by vaginal delivery. As the Court found, the treating midwife had failed to respect that choice.

Sarah Louise Cox v The Secretary of State for Health [2016] EWHC 924 (QB)

This case reached trial before Garnham J in April 2016, but it concerned underlying events which occurred almost 30 years previously, in May 1986. The claimant had at all times lacked capacity to conduct legal proceedings, with the result that the normal statutory limitation period[1] did not apply.[2] The historic nature of the underlying events caused some practical difficulties for the Court. In particular, the complete delivery records for the claimant were no longer available, having been destroyed in a flood. There was also a significant dispute about whether or not a labour-ward handbook had been in existence in 1986 rather than later in the 1980s. The memories of witnesses of fact had understandably faded over the intervening decades.

The claimant was one of a pair of mono-chorionic, mono-amniotic and mono-zygotic twins; in practical terms, this meant that the twins shared the same amniotic sac. The claimant suffered a serious brain injury consequent upon cord occlusion, the two cords having become entangled and wrapped around her body. On the facts, 20 minutes elapsed between the detection of the cord prolapse and the claimant's delivery by CS.

---

[1] Under section 11 and section 14 of the Limitation Act 1980.

[2] Section 28 of the Limitation Act 1980 provides for the extension of the limitation period for persons under a disability at the point in time when a right of action accrued to three years after the date when the person ceased to be under a disability or died (in personal injury cases; other time limits apply to other types of claim).

The key issue which fell to be determined was whether the defendant had failed to ensure that the claimant's delivery was conducted in an environment where there could be immediate resource to an anaesthetist and to a CS if an emergency occurred. This amounted to an allegation that the CS should have been performed on the labour ward rather than in theatre.

In essence, the claimant team had set themselves the significant evidential challenge of proving that there was a duty to ensure that a delivery room on a labour ward should have been equipped to the same standards as an operating theatre applying the standards of 1986. In the course of analysing the issue, the Court had regard to historic handbooks from the 1980s, as well as factual evidence relating to the hospital in question and expert evidence about reasonable practice in 1986. The evidence in support of the claimant's case was tenuous; at best, it amounted to evidence that some hospitals in the 1980s had facilities for conducting operative deliveries on the labour ward, rather than evidence to the effect that there was a duty to have such facilities in place.

The Court found as follows:

> In my judgment, however, the Claimant has not established that provision of equipment on this scale, and the establishment of a system for using it in circumstances such as this, was part of what a reasonably competent obstetric unit would have provided in 1986. In truth, there was no evidence to support such an assertion [para 131].

As a secondary case, the claimant also argued that the delivery should have been performed by means of a vaginal breech extraction which would have been markedly quicker. The treating obstetrician explained that the baby was lying obliquely, the liquor had already drained, and that there was a risk of damage to the organs of the baby. The expert obstetrician instructed by the claimant acknowledged that the treating obstetrician was in an unenviable position. The Court held that that there were *"no possible grounds for finding her in breach of duty... her professional decision was beyond criticism."* [para 154–155]. The claimant's case accordingly failed.

In many ways, it is surprising that the defendant chose to take the case of *SXX* to trial, and that the claimant chose to take the case of *Cox* to trial. In both cases (in the opinion of the present author), the losing party faced almost insurmountable evidential hurdles. The potential value of both cases was high, which may have affected the willingness to take the cases to trial notwithstanding the considerable difficulties.

Conjoined Twins: Re A (Children) (Conjoined Twins: Medical Treatment) (No. 1) [2001] Fam 147; [2001] 2 WLR 480

Consideration of the legal principles relating to twins would not be complete without a brief look at the judgement in *Re A*, the case relating to the six-week-old conjoined twins Jodie and Mary. The Court of Appeal was faced with the agonising question of whether it was lawful for doctors to perform a separation procedure in circumstances where separation would inevitably lead to the death of the weaker twin, Mary, but where both twins would die within around three to six months if the separation procedure were not performed. The parents, who were devout Roman Catholics, opposed the procedure.

As a starting-point, Ward LJ held that each child was alive and each child was separate for the purposes of the civil and criminal law. On the evidence, the Court held firmly that the separation procedure was in the best interests of Jodie, the stronger twin:

if the separation procedure were performed, she could expect a normal expectancy of life with limited disability. The Court found that the analysis of the best interests of Mary, the weaker twin, was more difficult. In the course of the extensive analysis, Ward LJ held that it was *"impermissible to deny that every life has an equal inherent value"* [para 7.5] and that the proposed separation procedure could not be in Mary's best interests: *"It will bring her life to an end before it has run its natural span. It denies her inherent right to life. There is no countervailing advantage for her at all"* [para 7.9].

Having made these findings, the Court was thereafter faced with the difficulty of what course of action to take in circumstances where the best interests of the two children involved pointed so sharply in different directions. The Court's findings included the following:

> *Given the conflict of duty, I can see no other way of dealing with it than by choosing the lesser of the two evils and so finding the least detrimental alternative. A balance has to be struck somehow and I cannot flinch from undertaking that evaluation, horrendously difficult though it is* [para 8].

> *The universality of the right to life demands that the right to life be treated as equal. The intrinsic value of their human life is equal. So the right of each goes into the scales and the scales remain in balance. The question which the court has to answer is whether or not the proposed treatment, the operation to separate, is in the best interests of the twins. That enables me to consider and place in the scales of each twin the worthwhileness of the treatment. That is a quite different exercise from the proscribed (because it offends the sanctity of life principle) consideration of the worth of one life compared with the other. When considering the worthwhileness of the treatment, it is legitimate to have regard to the actual condition of each twin and hence the actual balance sheet of advantage and disadvantage which flows from the performance or the non-performance of the proposed treatment"* [para 10 (ii)].

The conclusion was that it was lawful for the separation procedure to take place: balancing the interests of the twins against one another, the Court was "wholly satisfied" that it was lawful for the operation to be performed. The distinction which Ward LJ made between the inherent value of life on the one hand and the worthwhileness of treatment on the other hand remains relevant and important today.

Clinical Commentary

Mark D Kilby

Good Practice Guidance

Initial Designated Risk in Twin Pregnancies

Multiple pregnancy rates are increasing globally with the more liberal use of assisted reproductive techniques, deferment by women of their first pregnancy to a more advanced age and with free movement of peoples globally increasing ethnic diversity. The most common form of multiple pregnancy is twins, making up 97% of the total.

Overall, multiple pregnancy is associated with an increased risk of maternal and perinatal morbidity and mortality [1]. This may predispose such pregnancies to potential litigation [2]. Within the United Kingdom, the challenge to deliver effective care to women with a multiple pregnancy led to the publication of recommendations by two Scientific Study Groups of the Royal College of Obstetricians and Gynaecologists (RCOG) and, in 2011, the publication of first national antenatal guidance (CG129) from the National Institute for Health and Care Excellence (NICE) [3] and updated in 2019 to include intrapartum care [4]. Subsequently, to emphasise the specific risks of mono-chorionicity, the RCOG published a "Green-top" guideline for the management of monochorionic twins (2008 and updated in 2016) [5,6]. These Guidelines have devised evidence-based management that is predicated upon twin chorionicity. One of the main principles of modern antenatal care in twins (since the early 1990s and in the United Kingdom, since the publication of the NICE Guidelines on the management of twin and triplet pregnancy in 2011) is designation of a twin pregnancy by chorionicity and amnionicity. This is allocated with a high degree of certainty at an 11–14 weeks ultrasound scan (with ~99% sensitivity).

Approximately 80% of twins are dichorionic diamniotic, where there are two fetuses in two separate amniotic sacs and with two placentae. The majority of these twins are dizygotic but 20% are monozygotic (but have separate placentae). In effect, these are two singleton pregnancies within the uterus but confer generic increased maternal risk of pre-eclampsia, thromboembolic disease and in-utero infection and the fetal risks princi-pally of preterm birth. Monochorionicity (single "shared placenta") complicates approxi-mately 20% of all twin pregnancies, with 99% of these being diamniotic (two amniotic sacs). A single amniotic sac (monoamnionicity) in monochorionic twins confers very high risk associated with high rates of miscarriage, preterm birth and congenital malformations.

Monochorionicity has a negative influence on gestational age-specific fetal mortality, compared with dichorionic twins, as a consequence of the complications arising from the conjoining of fetal circulations by placental anastomoses within a single shared placenta. These complications of twin-to-twin transfusion syndrome (TTTS), selective growth restriction (sGR), and twin anaemia polycythaemia sequence (TAPS) are associated with high risks of single or double fetal demise [4,6]. Although the death of any fetus is a tragedy, a single twin death in a monochorionic pregnancy is a particularly adverse event, as the presence of placental vascular anastomoses are not only responsible for the underlying aetiology and pathogenesis of TTTS, but their presence also leads to a substantial risk (up to 15%) of co-twin demise (if one baby dies) but may lead to acute fetal anaemia and hypoperfusion with ischaemic brain injury in at least 24% of surviving twins [7,8]. Monochorionicity is further associated with adverse neonatal outcomes, with an increased incidence of preterm birth, low birthweight, and more complicated mor-bidity, often resulting in a prolonged stay in the neonatal intensive care unit [1]. Recent MBRRACE-UK data published in the Perinatal Surveillance report noted that the stillbirth rate for twins nearly halved between 2014–2016; whereas the stillbirth rate for singletons remained unchanged [9]. Further analysis indicated that the "lion share" of stillbirths and neonatal deaths in twins were as a consequence of monochorionicity [10].

The first NICE Guidelines on the management of twin and triplet pregnancy were published in 2011 [3] and the Royal College of Obstetricians and Gynaecologists had published a Green-top Guideline (GTG) in 2008 outlining risks and good clinical practice for the management of twins based upon chorionicity [5]. Both these guidelines have been subsequently updated but were in the public domain and being utilised for guidance in 2015 [4,6].

The NICE and RCOG Guidelines recognised the increased prenatal risks of mono-chorionic twin pregnancies and indicated that all twin pregnancies (but specifically monochorionic twins) should be managed in a designated twin clinic. This recognises the increased risks of maternal morbidity and the global increased risk of late miscarriage and preterm birth complicating all twin pregnancies. This clinic should be comprised of a multidisciplinary team, with clinical expertise including an obstetrician, midwife and ultrasonographers with expertise in performing ultrasound of twin pregnancies. This allows the global risks of twin pregnancies to be discussed with parents, as well as specific chorionicity-based risks, allowing individualised care in each twin pregnancy. Often the lead clinician responsible for this Twin Clinic and leading the multidisciplinary team should have undergone advanced training in one of the following:

- Advanced Training Skill Module in Fetal Medicine
- Advanced Training Skill Module in High-risk Pregnancy
- Subspecialty Training in Maternal and Fetal Medicine

Management of Twin Pregnancies

Both the published NICE and RCOG Guidelines recognise and recommend (as good clinical practice) the use of obstetric ultrasound to screen twin pregnancies for morbid complications. Specifically, this guidance recommends obstetric ultrasound scans of the babies at two-weekly intervals from 16 weeks gestation in monochorionic twins and monthly in dichorionic twins. As well as a measurement of the twins (fetal) biometry, an assessment of amniotic fluid volume and umbilical artery Doppler assessment should be made [3,4,5,6] (see Figure 16.1). Fetal ultrasound is the "cornerstone of the antenatal management of twins to detect congenital malformations, abnormal fetal growth in all twins, as well as the specific risks of monochorionicity outlined above.

Preterm birth complicates nearly 60% of all twin pregnancies and is a significant contributor to perinatal mortality and morbidity. The screening of asymptomatic twin pregnancies with transvaginal-ultrasound-measured cervical length at 20 weeks has benefits in allocation of risk of preterm birth but sadly no evidence-based treatments have been demonstrated to significantly reduce the rate of preterm birth or long-term outcome in childhood. Again, monochorionicity increases risks of preterm birth, with high rates of iatrogenic prematurity associated with treatments of pathologic morbidities. In uncomplicated twin pregnancies, the length of gestation is arbitrarily curtailed to minimise risks of late gestation mortality. It is recommended that dichorionic twins are delivered at the end of 37th week of gestation and monochorionic diamniotic twins by the 36th week (Figure 16.1). Monoamniotic twins (in the rare event they are uncomplicated) are usually delivered by CS between 32–34 weeks gestation.

It is important that parental choices and healthcare professional opinions on timing and attempted mode of delivery are discussed, so care may be individualised. There is also a need to discuss the use of epidural analgesia during labour, continuous electronic fetal monitoring of birth twins and potential obstetric manoeuvres required to deliver the second twin. When vaginal delivery is planned, and delivery occurs at ≥32 weeks of gestation with the first twin in cephalic presentation, uncomplicated monochorionic diamniotic twin pregnancy is not associated with a higher rate of composite intrapartum mortality and neonatal morbidity and mortality compared with dichorionic twin pregnancy.

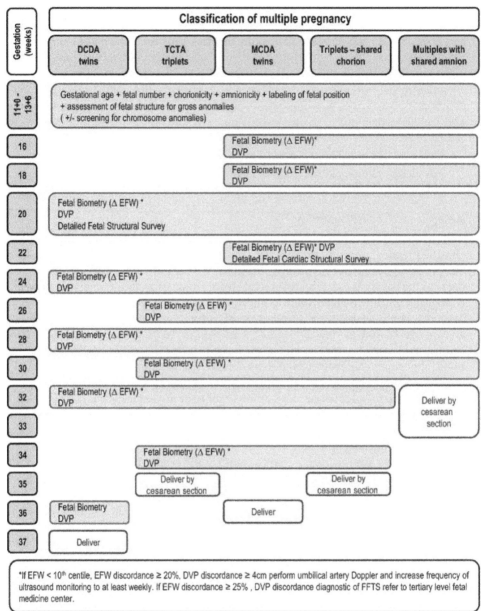

Figure 16.1 Individualised management of twin pregnancy [10].

In cases of extreme preterm birth, discussions around individualised twin pregnancy risks, place, mode of delivery and potential maternal therapies to reduce neonatal morbidity (i.e. maternal betamethasone and magnesium sulphate) are paramount, and if not managed optimally may lead to miscommunication, misunderstanding and potential risks for complaint and litigation.

Once the babies are delivered, then active management of the third stage is advised.

Concluding Discussion

In many instances of twin medicolegal litigation, there is associated medical clinically substandard care that may substantially contribute to injuries sustained by the unborn or newborn child [15]. This risk is significantly increased in monochorionic twins that are at significant risk of complex morbidities. This may be because of failure of obstetric surveillance to identify or healthcare professionals not recognising the abnormality/ complication and acting in a timely manner. Obstetricians, midwives and other health-care professionals providing care for pregnant women are held to a high standard of care when it comes to the health and safety of the mother and fetus. In twin and multiple pregnancy, this can be aided by recognising that such pregnancies are potentially complex and may develop complications. Institutional organisation of professional, multidisciplinary specialist clinics may aid both protocols for obstetric surveillance and enhance patient and professional communication. In addition, with reference to twin pregnancies, there are a number of national guidelines, in the United Kingdom, that are evidence based and designed to enhance the surveillance and delivery of care to the pregnant woman and her unborn babies. Such guidance should enhance communication and patient expectations, as well as explaining when and why such obstetric care is instituted.

The timely recognition of morbid twin complications and then discussion with the patent (and her family), as well as referral for specialist assessment and treatment is mandatory. Failure to adhere to safety protocols, clinical practice guidelines, best prac-tice recommendations, and to properly produce documentation reflecting such adher-ence, will most likely result in courts ruling against healthcare providers and professionals. Therefore, it is important that national/international institutions devise (and regularly update) evidence-based, standardised guidelines that set out best practice, both for the sake of patients and healthcare professionals.

Causes of Litigation

The potential causes of litigation in the management of twin pregnancies with a cumulative risk of adverse or morbid outcome are:

- Failure to diagnose and allocate chorionicity of twin pregnancy by the end of the first trimester.
- Failure to discuss with the patient (pregnant woman) and her family, the potential prospective risks of monochorionicity and the need for close and careful screening and surveillance.
- Failure to follow and adhere to national guidance issues by NICE and/or the RCOG. This gives recommended institutional and organisational guidance, as well as recommended intervals of obstetric ultrasound screening/surveillance. Failure to adhere to these recommendations is a common cause of litigation.
- Failure in communication. This is true both of professional communication between midwives, paediatricians and obstetricians; between obstetricians in a district general maternity hospital and a tertiary centre; and most importantly between healthcare professionals and the patient.
- Failure to diagnose a morbid complication of monochorionic twin pregnancy (such as TTTS) or a delay in referral for specialised care.

- Incomplete counselling and written consent taken before further complex and specialised treatment of morbid complications of monochorionic twin pregnancies (such as TTTS). Such a discussion always includes the potential adverse effects and complications of fetal therapy and indeed the effects of pathogenesis of the original pathology (consistent with the spirit of *Montgomery v Lanarkshire Health Board*).
- Failure to provide informed and expert follow-up after complex fetal therapy (most likely in monochorionic twins). This should involve obstetric ultrasound and additional investigations (such as in-utero magnetic resonance imaging) to detect ischaemic brain injury or haemorrhage and twin anaemic polycythaemia sequence [11,12,13]. This should also include a discussion and communication relating to timing and mode of delivery, as well as recommendations relating to intrapartum care.

Furthermore, MBRRACE-UK performed a perinatal confidential enquiry into stillbirths and neonatal deaths in twin pregnancies [14]. This audited all causes of twin stillbirth and neonatal death in 2018. It highlighted that *"In just over half of pregnancies, improvements in care were identified which may have made a difference to the outcome for the twins"*. Specifically relevant to the claimant's case was that *"For two fifths of women (20 of 50) care was not provided by a specialised multidisciplinary team as recommended by national guidance. For only 5 of the 50 women was care documented as including a specialist midwife and specialist sonographer involvement. In addition, discussions concerning the risks of twin pregnancy before 24 weeks were documented for only half of women"*.

Of specific concern was that *"emergency assessment in maternity triage was particularly problematic in TTTS which went unrecognised in women presenting with maternal concerns of classical 'red flag' signs and symptoms"*.

From this recent United Kingdom national audit, it is clear that clinical substandard care is not uncommon in complex twin pregnancy, with a significant delay in diagnosis and management of morbid clinical situations. This is particularly the case in monochorionic twins, when pregnancies should be managed by healthcare teams aware of specific complications and having a low clinical threshold for investigation and, if necessary, referral in a timely manner.

Avoidance of Litigation

- Offer a clear and prospective management plan for all twin pregnancies based upon evidence from current NICE and RCOG Guidelines (this is especially important in monochorionic twins).
- Communicate in a timely manner to patients and their families about the potential risks of twin pregnancies and the prospective antenatal surveillance and screening in place and managed within a specialist multidisciplinary obstetric team. Where possible shared decision-making is optimal.
- Communicate both verbally and in writing with the patient and other healthcare professions (often in other institutions) when the pregnancy develops (potential) complications.
- If complications develop, then timely explanation and referral to specialist centres should be facilitated. Authoritative counselling of the benefits and risks of fetal

surgery (including theoretical maternal and fetal risks) with shared decision-making tools and aids should be used.

- Patients should be given time to consider the potential options for management.
- Patient written information should be given to families to add their decision-making.
- Informed written consent should be obtained and ideally signed by both mother and father.
- Clear follow-up of the woman and her twin pregnancy post-specialist treatment should be arranged and delivered in a centre (and by healthcare professionals) with experience and expertise to monitor these complex pregnancies.
- If morbid fetal complications occur, then these should be investigated and discussed with the couple and appropriate options discussed (redress to potential selective or total termination of the twin pregnancy).
- To have a post-pregnancy consultation and debrief (especially if morbid complications have occurred).

References

1. Kilby, MD, Oepkes, D. Multiple pregnancy. In: Dewhurst's Textbook of Obstetrics and Gynaecology, edited by Keith Edmonds, Christoph Lees, and Tom Bourne. Oxford: John Wiley & Sons Ltd; 2018, p268–81. https://doi.org/10.1002/9781119211457

2. Hodgekiss, A. Mother Pregnant with Twins Lost both Her Babies after a Midwife Misdiagnosed Agonising Pains as a "Pulled Muscle". London: Associated New Papers Ltd. 9 November 2015.

3. National Institute for Health and Care Excellence (NICE). Multiple Pregnancy: Antenatal Care for Twin and Triplet Pregnancies. NICE Clinical Guideline [CG129]. Published September 2011. Available at: www.nice.org.uk/guidance/cg129/history

4. National Institute for Health and Care Excellence (NICE). Twin and Triplet Pregnancy. NICE Guideline [NG137]. Published 4 September 2019. Available at: www.nice.org.uk/guidance/ng137

5. Royal College of Obstetricians and Gynaecologists (RCOG). Monochorionic Twin Pregnancy, Management. Green-top Guideline No. 51. Guideline developers Professors J Neilson and MD Kilby. 2008.

6. Royal College of Obstetricians and Gynaecologists (RCOG). Monochorionic Twin Pregnancy, Management. Green-top Guideline No. 51. Published 16 November 2016. Available at: https://www.rcog.org.uk/en/guidelines-researchservices/guidelines/gtg51/

7. Mackie, FL, Rigby, A, Morris, RK, Kilby, MD. Prognosis of the co-twin following spontaneous single intrauterine fetal death in twin pregnancies: a systematic review and meta-analysis. BJOG 2019; 126 (5): 569–78.

8. Morris, RK, Mackie, F, Garces, AT, Knight, M, Kilby, MD. The incidence, maternal, fetal and neonatal consequences of single intrauterine fetal death in monochorionic twins: a prospective observational UKOSS study. PLoS One 2020; 15(9): e0239477.

9. MBRRACE-UK. Perinatal Mortality Surveillance Report 2018. Available at: www.hqip.org.uk/resource/mbrrace-uk-perinatal-mortality-surveillance-report-2018/

10. Kilby, MD, Gibson, JL, Ville, Y. Falling perinatal mortality in twins in the UK: organisational success or chance? BJOG 2019; 126(3): 341–7.

11. Morris, RK, Selman, TJ, Harbidge, A, Martin, WI, Kilby, MD. Fetoscopic laser coagulation for severe twin-to-twin transfusion syndrome: factors influencing perinatal outcome, learning curve of the procedure and lessons for new centres. BJOG 2010; 117(11): 1350–7.

12. Slaghekke, F, Lopriore, E, Lewi, L, Middeldorp, JM, van Zwet, EW, Weingertner, AS, Klumper, FJ, DeKoninck, P, Devlieger, R, Kilby, MD, Rustico, MA, Deprest, J, Favre, R, Oepkes, D. Fetoscopic laser coagulation of the vascular equator versus selective coagulation for twin-to-twin transfusion syndrome: an open-label randomised controlled trial. *Lancet* 2014; 383(9935): 2144–51.

13. Stirnemann, J, Chalouhi, G, Essaoui, M, Bahi-Buisson, N, Sonigo, P, Millischer, AE, Lapillonne, A, Guigue, V, Salomon, LJ, Ville, Y. Fetal brain imaging following laser surgery in twin-to-twin surgery. *BJOG* 2018; 125(9): 1186–91.

14. Draper, ES, Gallimore, ID, Kurinczuk, JJ, Kenyon, S (eds.) on behalf of MBRRACE-UK. MBRRACE-UK 2019 Perinatal Confidential Enquiry: Stillbirths and neonatal deaths in twin pregnancies. The Infant Mortality and Morbidity Studies, Department of Health Sciences, University of Leicester: Leicester, 2021. Available at: www.npeu.ox.ac.uk/assets/downloads/mbrrace-uk/reports/perinatal-report-2020-twins/MBRRACE-UK_Twin_Pregnancies_Confidential_Enquiry.pdf

15. Zaami, S, Masselli, G, Brunelli, R, Taschini, G, Caprasecca, S, Marinelli, E. Twin-to-twin transfusion syndrome: diagnostic imaging and its role in staving off malpractice charges and litigation. *Diagnostics (Basel)* 2021; 11(3): 445.

The Cervix: The Nemesis of Obstetrics and Gynaecology

Janesh K Gupta

CASE COMMENTARY

Swati Jha

Successful Claim

Lynn Scaddon v Phillip Morgan [2017] EWHC 1481 (QB)

The Claim

Ms Scaddon was reviewed by the consultant gynaecologist on the independent sector for heavy bleeding. She claimed that owing to his failure to detect a fibroid protruding through the cervix at the time of the primary consultation, there was an unnecessary delay in further investigations and treatment. It was also claimed that she should have been referred for a hysteroscopy urgently, which would have culminated in the performance of her hysterectomy seven months earlier than when it was finally performed. This unnecessary delay caused her to suffer continuing physical symptoms and develop a generalised anxiety disorder.

The Summary

The claimant was approximately 50 when she came to see the defendant. She had four children all delivered vaginally. She had a Mirena coil in situ, but when she started to suffer heavy menstrual bleeding and pain, a referral was made to gynaecology. Due to delays in the review appointment on the NHS and ongoing problems, she went to see the defendant privately. It was noted that she was difficult to examine and whereas an abdominal and speculum exam were performed, a bimanual was not performed to avoid discomfort. The threads of the coil were not seen, however it was not made clear whether the cervix was visualised or not. Both parties agreed that it would be negligent to fail to identify a fibroid protruding through the cervix. However, whereas the claimant's case was that it had already protruded through the cervix and should have been identified at the speculum exam, the defendant's case was that the fibroid had not yet protruded through the cervix hence could not be identified. The patient was then referred for an NHS scan, which identified the coil in situ but no fibroid. There were further delays in her subsequent review and hysteroscopy which could not be performed under local anaesthesia due to the presence of the pedunculate fibroid, so had to be performed under general anaesthetic. This also failed so she eventually underwent a hysterectomy.

The Judgement

In making a judgement, the main issue was whether the fibroid had already prolapsed through the cervix at the time of the primary consultation. The defendant made the case that an inability to visualise the threads implied that the cervix had been seen. However, the claimant's recollection of the consultation was that it was rushed, and the consultant made the comment that he had been unable to complete the examination. Based on the size of the fibroid at the time of removal and its rate of likely growth, which was significantly disputed, on a balance of probabilities it was likely that the fibroid had already prolapsed at the time of the primary consultation. The claimant therefore succeeded in her primary claim of breach of duty in failing to identify the prolapsed fibroid at the time of the initial exam nine months prior to the hysterectomy. The defendant made the case that the treatment would not have changed and she would still have required a hysterectomy even if the prolapsed fibroid had been identified, however the claimant's secondary case of an unnecessary delay resulting in prolonged physical pain and development of an anxiety disorder therefore also succeeded on the basis of the breach in the primary case.

Unsuccessful Claim

C v North Cumbria University Hospitals NHS Trust [2014] EWHC 61 (QB)

The Claim

The claim was made on behalf of the deceased patient's (M) partner. The patient suffered a uterine rupture during induction, and it was claimed that it was below a reasonable standard of care to give a second dose of Prostin which caused the uterine rupture, resulting in hypoxic ischaemic injury to the baby and demise of the patient.

The Summary

She was admitted for induction of labour in her second pregnancy. Both pregnancies were IVF pregnancies and in this pregnancy a plan was made for induction at term. The first pregnancy was delivered vaginally.

Following admission, the CTG was reassuring. The first dose of Prostin to ripen the cervix was given, and as there were no contraindications to the insertion of the second dose, this was given 7.5 hours later. Five hours following the second dose, M started to experience substantial discomfort and the cervix progressed from 2 cm to 9 cm in a short time span. At this time her waters broke (meconium stained), and she commenced pushing. She was transferred to theatres where a forceps delivery was performed and the baby delivered in a poor state and was affected by hypoxic ischaemic encephalopathy. She was then transferred to another room and when she collapsed and arrested it was identified that she was bleeding internally and she would need a hysterectomy to stop the bleeding. Following the hysterectomy, she was on ITU but deteriorated and she passed away a few days later. The defendant trust admitted liability for M's death based on substandard care but denied liability in the administration of the second dose of Prostin. There had been a failure to identify that M had suffered excessive amounts of blood and was allowed to leave theatres in this hypovolemic state due to a failure to appreciate the gravity of the situation.

Regarding the second dose of Prostin, the existing guidelines at the time recommended that a second dose be administered six to eight hours after the first if labour was not established and in the absence of contraindications. M had no contraindications and was not established in labour when her second dose of Prostin was given.

The Judgement

The risk of uterine rupture following on from the administration of Prostin is exceedingly rare and the second Prostin was inserted in keeping with existing guidelines with no contraindications. The pain and discomfort at the time of insertion of the second tablet were at a level to be expected with Prostin induction, hence the midwife who inserted the second dose was prima facie not acting negligently. The claim was therefore dismissed.

Legal Commentary

Eloise Power

Scaddon v Morgan [2017] EWHC 1481 (QB)

The key issue in the case of *Scaddon v Morgan* was whether the defendant, a consultant gynaecologist, had failed to see that a uterine fibroid had prolapsed through her cervix. As HHJ Worster (sitting as a Judge of the High Court) observed, *"The issue on this primary case reduces to a question of fact. Had the fibroid prolapsed through the cervix by 23 July 2010?"* [para 3]. It was common ground that if the fibroid had prolapsed through the cervix, it would have been negligent not to see it.

The approach taken by the Court to the evidence in the case is of interest. Essentially, the Court took a holistic approach, considering the claimant's witness evidence, the defendant's records, the defendant's witness evidence (albeit that he had no recall of the appointment and was relying on his usual practice), the findings on other examinations, the claimant's symptoms and (crucially) the expert evidence about the usual growth rate of such a fibroid.

On the facts, the Court acknowledged that the evidence was *"certainly not all one way"*. Counsel for the defendant invited the Court to draw an inference that it was unlikely that an experienced consultant would have missed a prolapse. The defendant's records indicated that the threads of the claimant's Mirena coil had been seen, and the Court was invited to infer that the fact that the threads were seen made it likely that the cervix had also been visualised. The Court placed considerable weight upon the expert evidence as to the growth of a uterine fibroid:

> The problem for the Defendant is the evidence about the growth of a fibroid such as this one. The one fact that I can be sure of is that in February 2011, there was a large prolapsed fibroid. There is factual evidence as to its size in April 2011, and findings which inform the experts' evidence of its rate of growth between February and April 2011.

The Court preferred the claimant's expert evidence as to the normal growth of the fibroid, and found that the fibroid had prolapsed by the date of the consultation with the defendant. The claimant's case accordingly succeeded.

Although the principles in *Penney and others v East Kent Health Authority* [2000] Lloyd's Rep Med 41 and subsequent cases were not referenced in the judgement in *Scaddon v Morgan*, the approach taken is clearly analogous to the approach recommended in *Penney*. The Court addressed the question of whether the prolapsed fibroid was present on the date of the consultation as a pure question of fact, to be resolved by reference to the expert and factual evidence. The question of whether it was negligent to have failed to see the prolapsed fibroid, if it was present, was a separate issue. The defendant had already conceded this issue, and the Court did not seek to go behind the defendant's concession. However, the possibility was floated in passing that the speculum examination had been so difficult to perform that the defendant had been unable to complete it at all, or to complete it to the required standard [para 60]. The Court did not develop this, as it had not been part of the defendant's case. For further discussion of the approach in *Penney*, please see the legal commentary at Chapter 25.

C v North Cumbria University Hospitals NHS Trust [2014] EWHC 61 (QB)

In this High Court case, Green J considered the question of whether a midwife had been negligent in administering a second dose of Prostin to induce labour. The underlying facts of the case are particularly tragic: the mother suffered a ruptured uterus and died from a cardiac arrest, and the claimant (the baby) suffered a hypoxic cerebral injury typical of a period of acute profound asphyxia commencing immediately prior to birth, leading to microcephaly and dystonic athetoid cerebral palsy. It was common ground between the parties that the second dose of Prostin was causative of the claimant's catastrophic injuries. The defendant also accepted that the mother's death had been caused by negligent post-natal care.[1]

In analysing the question of whether the midwife had been negligent in administering the second dose of Prostin, the Court described its task in the following terms:

> This involves examining, closely, the precise events preceding and to some degree following the administration of that second dose and placing them in context of such matters as: the guidelines produced for the use of the drug by the manufacturer and other relevant guidelines; the existence of any contra indications at the time militating against the administration of the second dose; the level of risk involved which includes a consideration of whether the midwife in question should have sought the advice and assistance of the consultant Registrar and, if so, what that "hypothetical" advice might have been; and the extent to which the midwife addressed herself to all the relevant considerations [para 8].

It can readily be seen that even the narrowest questions which fall for resolution by the Courts often require a very detailed and thorough analysis of evidence from multiple sources.

The Court's comprehensive judgement in this matter is well worth reading in full, as it covers a number of points of general interest and applicability, including (a) the role of expert witnesses; (b) the approach which the Court should take to the hypothetical advice which would have been given if the treating clinician (here, a midwife) had sought such advice; (c) the approach which the Court should take to the clinical records; (d) the approach which the Court should take to relevant clinical guidance.

Role of Expert Witnesses

The Court gave detailed consideration to the role of expert witnesses in clinical negligence cases [para 25]. The following points are of particular interest:

---

[1] The claim arising out of the mother's death was not considered in the judgement and was presumably dealt with separately.

(a) On good faith: *"A sine qua non for treating an expert's opinion as valid and relevant is that it is tendered in good faith. However, the mere fact that one or more expert opinions are tendered in good faith is not per se sufficient for a conclusion that a defendant's conduct, endorsed by expert opinion tendered in good faith, necessarily accords with sound medical practice."*

(b) On the meaning of the words competent, responsible and respectable (which are sometimes used interchangeably): *"'Competence' is a matter which flows from qualifications and experience. In the context of allegations of clinical negligence in an NHS setting particular weight may be accorded to an expert with a lengthy experience in the NHS. Such a person expressing an opinion about normal clinical conditions will be doing so with first-hand knowledge of the environment that medical professionals work under within the NHS and with a broad range of experience of the issue in dispute. This does not mean to say that an expert with a lesser level of NHS experience necessarily lacks the same degree of competence; but I do accept that lengthy experience within the NHS is a matter of significance. By the same token an expert who retired 10 years ago and whose retirement is spent expressing expert opinions may turn out to be far removed from the fray and much more likely to form an opinion divorced from current practical reality. 'Respectability' is also a matter to be taken into account. Its absence might be a rare occurrence, but many judges and litigators have come across so-called experts who can 'talk the talk' but who veer towards the eccentric or unacceptable end of the spectrum. Regrettably there are, in many fields of law, individuals who profess expertise but who, on true analysis, must be categorised as 'fringe'. A 'responsible' expert is one who does not adapt an extreme position, who will make the necessary concessions and who adheres to the spirit as well as the words of his professional declaration (see CPR35 and the PD and Protocol)."*

(c) On logic, the Court observed that the responsibility, competence and respectability of the expert may not be determinative of the question of whether their opinion is logical. The logic of the expert opinion tendered is *"far and away the most important consideration. . . A Judge should not simply accept an expert opinion; it should be tested both against the other evidence tendered during the course of a trial, and, against its internal consistency. For example, a judge will consider whether the expert opinion accords with the inferences properly to be drawn from the Clinical Notes or the CTG."*

Further consideration is given to the duties of clinical experts in Chapter 3.

The Court's Approach to Hypothetical Advice

The Court considered the issue of what advice an obstetric registrar would have given in relation to the second dose of Prostin if the midwife had sought such advice. On the relevant principles at play, the Court found as follows:

> In my view it would at least in principle to have been open to the Claimant to contend that the hypothetical advice was negligent and that the only advice that would or could have been reasonable was the very precautionary approach which is at the heart of their case. This dictum[2] and the general tenor of the Bolitho judgment indicates, in my view, that *the test is not what Dr*

---

[2] "A defendant cannot escape liability by saying that the damage would have occurred in any event because he would have committed some other breach of duty thereafter": *Bolitho v City and Hackney Health Authority* [1997]. UKHL 46; [1998] AC 232.

Bukhari would in fact have said or done but what a reasonable consultant should or would have said [para 70, italics added].

When the Court applied these principles to the facts, it was held that it would not have been negligent for a third-party obstetrician to have administered the second dose of Prostin [para 87].

The Court's Approach to the Clinical Records

The Court's comments upon the clinical records are of general interest and applicability:

First, considerable care must be exercised in analysing the Clinical Notes. They are not to be construed as if they were a literary or scientific text. The Notes reflect the views of a number of successive midwives who were on duty at the relevant times. They are prepared as a form of shorthand intended to be understood by other midwives and medical professionals. They reflect the impressions and conclusions of the various midwives as to the state of wellbeing of M over time [para 41].

The Court observed that there was a "degree of subjectivity" in the Notes (giving the example of descriptions of pain) and made the point that

a further reason for caution is that the recollection of the midwives who gave evidence was essentially based upon their interpretation as at the trial of the Clinical Notes. None of them had sufficiently clear recollection of the actual events to be able to say with confidence what they meant by a specific entry when they recorded it on the Clinical Notes [para 42].

Notwithstanding these caveats, the Court gave detailed consideration to the evidence contained in the records.

The Court's Approach to Clinical Guidance

In relation to the use of relevant clinical guidance (in this case, British National Formulary guidance together with a Data Sheet on Prostin), the Court observed that: *"in this case there was consensus that the guidelines were not complete or comprehensive"* [para 84]. The experts for both sides took a more cautious approach than the approach set out in the relevant guidance: the Court fairly observed that:

There may well be a serious point of criticism to be made about the guidelines in these respects; not least because, as I have already observed, all of those who gave evidence accepted that it was not automatically proper to administer a second dose before labour was established [para 84].

The Court held as follows:

In conclusion my view is that prima facie a midwife who acts in accordance with the guidelines should be safe from a charge of negligence. However, in the present case since it is common ground that in some regards the guidelines are not satisfactory I do not decide this case upon the basis that adhering to guidelines is sufficient. I consider the fact that Midwife Bragg acted in accordance with the guidelines is a factor militating against negligence but I also assess Midwife Bragg's conduct against the benchmark of the other surrounding facts and circumstances [para 84].

For further discussion of the approach taken by Courts to clinical guidance, see the legal commentary to Chapter 9, which contains a discussion of the case of *Sanderson v Guy's and St Thomas' NHS Foundation Trust* [2020] EWHC 20 (QB). In *Sanderson*, Lambert J held that *"the Guidelines are a practical tool to be used in conjunction with clinical judgment"*. Although she did not hold that adherence with guidance amounted to a prima facie defence to an allegation of negligence, the effect of her judgement is arguably similar to the effect of Green J's judgement in *C*.

Having considered all of the evidence, the Court's conclusion, applying *Bolam/ Bolitho* principles, was as follows:

> I therefore conclude that Midwife Bragg acted within the bounds of reasonable judgment. I of course accept that she might, equally reasonably, have adopted a very cautious approach and had she done so this tragedy would not have occurred. But this reflects the fact that there are a range of possible reasonable actions that might have been taken in this case and Midwife Bragg's decision was within that range.

The claimant's claim accordingly failed.

Clinical Commentary
Janesh K Gupta

Good Practice Guidance
The Cervix
The cervix is a tubular structure which is found between the vagina and the uterine body and is an opening into the uterine cavity. It is primarily made up of collagen fibres [1]. In order to access or exit from the uterine cavity, the cervix is the organ that needs to be dilated or opened. Therefore, the cervix is a crucial gynaecological organ that can create various challenges for the operating surgeon. There are many ways to manipulate the cervix to reduce risk of complications (see Table 17.1) in obstetrics and gynaecology. To illustrate this, three examples are presented below.

Management of Abnormal Uterine Bleeding
In the non-pregnant uterus, the cervix is a firm elongated tubular structure which becomes shorter during the reproductive years. Usually, the cervix is the most prominent organ of the uterus during the pre-pubertal and menopause years, i.e. cervix representing two thirds and the uterus just one third . During reproductive life, the cervix shortens relative to the uterus, i.e. cervix representing one third and the uterus two thirds. Therefore, the elongated cervix poses extra challenges, particularly in the menopause. Women with post-menopausal bleeding (PMB) represent extra risk.

Ultrasound diagnosis is now the main stay of initial assessment of the endometrial thickness in women with PMB. If the endometrial thickness is >4 mm then an endo-metrial biopsy should be performed in an outpatient setting to exclude an endometrial carcinoma. Failing to achieve a biopsy by failing to insert the endometrial catheter through the cervix beyond 5 cm distance would normally mean that the cervix is stenosed and is an obstruction. This means that a hysteroscopy is required, ideally in the outpatient setting as it is a safer procedure, reducing the risks of cervical/uterine perforation. Most gynaecological units should now be offering this service but should advise women to take oral analgesia before the procedure. The use of miniaturised hysteroscopes <5 mm is now recommended. Therefore, a see and treat hysteroscopy in a single setting should be feasible. If a woman declines the use of outpatient hystero-scopy, then general or regional anaesthesia should be offered [2].

Table 17.1. Complications

False passage created with blind cervical dilatation

Cervical trauma and perforation

Uterine perforation

Hysterectomy when there is uncontrolled life-threatening bleeding

The use of dilation and curettage should not be performed in the management of abnormal uterine bleeding (AUB). The use of blind dilators is associated with an increased risk of cervical and uterine perforations, particularly with a tight or stenosed cervix found in postmenopausal women. Blind cervical dilatation was traditional practice used under general anaesthesia. The use of outpatient hysteroscopy (or under general anaesthesia) should be a prerequisite before attempting to dilate the cervix so that the access and angle of the cervix and uterus (anteverted or retroverted) can be identified to reduce the risks of perforation.

Induction of Labour

The cervix has a mechanical role in ensuring that a pregnancy can progress to term, i.e. beyond 37 weeks gestation. However, pregnancy must be interrupted before 42 gestational weeks as there is an increased risk of stillbirth. Therefore, induction of labour in low-risk pregnancies should be performed between term + 10–14 days [3]. The cervix prior to term must remain closed and has to resist the weight of the growing pregnancy but at the time of delivery, the cervix needs to soften and dilate (up to 10 cm) to allow the pregnancy to pass through the cervix. Women will usually undergo spontaneous labour any time between 37 to 42 weeks gestation, but in certain circumstances, e.g. fetal growth restriction and prevention of prolonged pregnancy beyond 42 weeks gestation, induction of labour is recommended.

It is known that the cervix undergoes a natural modelling of softening and dilatation during spontaneous labour processes, and this is achieved by endogenous prostaglandins. Also, as a result of periodic uterine contractions, forceful cervical dilatation occurs. This is optimally achieved by having moderate to strong uterine contraction rates between three to five contractions in every 10 minutes. This results in progressive cervical dilatation, but it is known that the progress of labour is quicker if the baseline cervix is soft prior to uterine contractions starting.

The favourability of the cervix, i.e. being soft and ripened, is a main factor for better outcomes and this is assessed by using the Bishop score. The Bishop score is a measurement of five parameters i.e. station, dilatation, effacement (or length), position and consistency of the cervix. Generally, a score of six or more is indicative of a ripe or favourable cervix, with a high chance of spontaneous labour or response to interventions subsequent to induction of labour, i.e. amniotomy ± use of oxytocin.

There are many methods by which the cervix can be prepared for induction of labour [3]:

1. In nulliparous women it is recommended that membranes sweeping should be offered between 40–41 gestational weeks. This is known to induce endogenous prostaglandin stimulation by the method of separating the chorionic membranes

from the decidua through the process of a digital examination. If the cervix is closed, then massaging around the cervix in the vaginal fornices can achieve a similar effect.

2. Surgical methods such as amniotomy (ARM), i.e. rupturing the fetal membranes, is associated with a natural release of prostaglandins which increases uterine activity rate and allows labour to progress. It is known that uterine activity rate usually starts within two hours of ARM. If this does not occur, then the use of oxytocin is used to start the labour process by increasing the uterine activity rate. It is also now recognised that when amniotomy is performed and the cervix is not soft, then the labour processes can be prolonged.

3. There are several pharmacological agents that are now recommended for induction of labour in the United Kingdom. The principal mode of action is cervical softening but also to start uterine activity. They are primarily prostaglandins (PGE2), which are given either as a pessary, tablet or gel followed by subsequent doses six hours later if labour is not established (maximum of two doses). A controlled release pessary over 24 hours can be used and, in some instances, up to 36 hours. The use of prostaglandins is known to cause hyperstimulation, i.e. uterine contraction rates more than five in 10 minutes. Misoprostol (PGE1) can also be used and is recommended by WHO as it is a relatively cheaper option but in much smaller doses [4]. It is not currently recommended for use in the United Kingdom as it is associated with a higher risk of uterine hyperstimulation and uterine rupture in women with previous caesarean compared to PGE2 prostaglandins. Therefore, the safety profile of the two types limits the use of the PGE1 in the United Kingdom.

4. Insertion of mechanical devices into or through the cervix can soften or ripen the cervix. These include balloon catheters or osmotic dilators. Currently these are not recommended for use in the United Kingdom but there is increasing evidence that maternity hospitals are using these methods as they are associated with no risk of hyperstimulation. Compared to prostaglandins this is particularly useful for women who have had previous caesarean section. Mechanical methods are generally known to be effective within a 24-hour time period whereas multiple doses of prostaglandins may be required.

Termination of Pregnancy

Up to and including 13+6 Weeks' Gestation –– Termination of pregnancy is when a pregnancy needs to be interrupted before 23+6 weeks gestation, as per the legal requirements in the United Kingdom. To access the uterine cavity, the cervix needs to be dilated before surgical abortion can be performed. Before dilatation can be achieved safely, the cervix needs to be softened. Forceful cervical dilatation in an unprepared 'hard' cervix is associated with increased risks of complications, such as cervical tears, perforation or uterine perforation. The commonly used cervical ripening methods are prostaglandin E1 (PGE1 misoprostol) either in sublingual 400 mcg dose one hour before abortion or 400 mcg of vaginal misoprostol given three hours before abortion. If misoprostol cannot be used, then 200 mg oral mifepristone (anti-progesterone) can be given 24–48 hours before abortion. The risks of giving misoprostol are causing pain and/or bleeding before the procedure. The latter methods are commonly used to achieve medical abortion by way of expelling the pregnancy, ideally through a softer opened cervix.

After 14 weeks to 23+6 Weeks' Gestation -- Osmotic dilators can be used with or without the use of mifepristone 24–48 hours prior. In pregnancies beyond 18 weeks, the use of osmotic dilators are effective if placed at least 24 hours before surgery. The mechanism of action of osmotic dilators is that they dehydrate the cervix by osmosis of fluids from the cervix into the dilator and by a mechanical effect. Usually, this process softens the cervix enough that the cervix does not require formal cervical dilatation during surgery [5].

Causes of Litigation

The reasons for litigation include the following:

- Failure to adhere to national or local guidance. In general, a reasoned justification for not following such guidelines would be required to avoid litigation.
- Preoperative counselling/choices provided
- Consent and discussion of complications
- Failing to use cervical softening methods which are associated with reducing risks of cervical trauma and cervical/uterine perforation.
- Failing to adhere to the optimum time of use for cervical softening agents, e.g. uterine perforation occurring during surgical abortion when a short period of time was used for cervical softening
- Failure to recognise complications either immediately or promptly when recovery is outside the normal expected standards

Avoidance of Litigation

- Offer conservative or no treatment options
- Ensure medical treatments are considered where appropriate
- All risks and complications of the various options should be discussed
- Adhere to optimum type, doses and times for the cervical ripening agent

References

1. Yao, W, Gan, Y, Myers, KM, Vink, JY, Wapner, RJ, Hendon, CP. Collagen fiber orientation and dispersion in the upper cervix of non-pregnant and pregnant women. *PLoS One* 2016; 11(11): e0166709.

2. Royal College of Obstetricians and Gynaecologists (RCOG). Best Practice in Outpatient Hysteroscopy. Green-top Guideline No. 59. 2011. Available at: www.rcog.org.uk/en/guidelines-research-services/guidelines/gtg59/

3. National Institute for Health and Care Excellence. Inducing Labour. Clinical Guideline [CG70]. 2008. Available from: www.nice.org.uk/guidance/cg70

4. World Health Organization. Induction of Labour Guideline. 2011. Available from: www.who.int/reproductivehealth/publications/maternal_perinatal_health/9789241501156/en/

5. National Institute for Health and Care Excellence. Abortion Care. NICE Guideline [NG140]. 2019. Available from: www.nice.org.uk/guidance/ng140/chapter/Recommendations#cervical-priming-before-surgical-abortion

18

Hysterectomy for Heavy Menstrual Bleeding

Janesh K Gupta

CASE COMMENTARY

Swati Jha

Successful Claim

EG v Kettering General Hospital NHS Foundation Trust (2018)

The Claim

The claimant underwent a hysterectomy at the defendant trust. Five years following surgery she was found to have a chronic left hydronephrosis and hydroureter with only 9% of renal function on the affected side. It was claimed that the hysterectomy had been performed negligently resulting in injury to the left ureter with a loss of kidney function.

The Summary

The claimant underwent a hysterectomy five years prior to the recognition of the injury. She suffered chronic left-sided loin pain and underwent a CT scan which confirmed a hydronephrosis and hydroureter with significant reduction in renal function. She was advised a nephroureterectomy and suffered significant psychological symptoms following the diagnosis, including depressed mood and severe panic attacks. This resulted in a loss of income and a premature end to her career.

The Judgement

This resulted in an out-of-court settlement for £500,000. This was for the total duration of injury (11 years since the injury) and on the grounds that there would be a resolution of symptoms following further surgery but she was likely to require further treatment in future.

In the case of JD V Shrewsbury and Telford Hospital NHS Trust (2017), the trust admitted that there was a failure to recognise the damage at the time of surgery and in Hendy v Milton Keynes Health Authority (No 2) [1992] 3 Med LR 119, the cause of ureteric injury was because the bladder was not pushed down enough during the operation and this amounted to negligence.

Unsuccessful Claim

Gail Marie Duce v Worcestershire Acute Hospitals NHS Trust, Case No: B3/2016/0826, Court of Appeal (Civil Division) [2018] EWCA Civ 1307, 2018 WL 02724487

The Claim

The claimant underwent a total abdominal hysterectomy and bilateral salpingo-oophorectomy (TAH and BSO) for heavy and painful periods. She developed neuropathic pain post-operatively and claimed that the defendant had been negligent in failing to warn her of the risks of developing chronic post-surgical pain (CPSP).

The Summary

The claimant suffered from menorrhagia which worsened over time and was associated with low back pain. When reviewed by the gynaecologist, she was offered several less invasive options. She was informed that a hysterectomy was very major surgery and the recommendation would be to try less invasive options in the first instance. The claimant made clear she would not consider other options and "she wanted it all taken away", despite known serious risks. She was informed that the operation may not alleviate her existing pain, though there would be no reason to discuss CPSP following surgery. She was informed of other major risks associated with surgery and was willing to go ahead despite this. The operation was performed non-negligently. Post-surgery she developed pain in her abdominal wall due to nerve damage which was different to the pain she had before surgery and was diagnosed to have CPSP.

The Judgement

The patient was well aware of alternative options to a hysterectomy. Given the material risk of CPSP as a complication following a TAH and BSO was so low, it was not incumbent upon the clinician to warn of this risk. It was ruled that even if she had been warned of the risk of CPSP, she would still have proceeded to a hysterectomy. In addition, there was a failure to apply the test of causation to the development of CPSP, hence the case was ruled in favour of the defendant.

In the case of both *Hannigan v Lanarkshire Acute hospitals NHS Trust (2012)* and *Dawn Harkin v Lancashire Teaching Hospitals NHS Foundation Trust, Preston County Court (HHJ Beech) 2017* , cases of ureteric injury were successfully defended, as adequate means to protect the ureters were taken at the time of surgery. In the case of *Hooper v Young* (QBENF 94/1654 [1998] Lloyd's Rep Med 61), an initial case of negligence was ruled in favour of the claimant but on appeal this was turned down.

Legal Commentary

Eloise Power

EG v Kettering General Hospital NHS Foundation Trust (2018) (Unreported)

This reported settlement involved an injury to the left ureter and associated loss of kidney function following a hysterectomy. The claimant would require a nephroureter-ectomy in the future. Liability was disputed, but the matter settled at a total of £500,000.

Although the case report gives little detail of the exact allegations, claims involving ureteric injury consequent upon gynaecological surgery are frequently encountered in practice, and the case of *EG* unfortunately seems typical of this category of case. The majority of cases reach settlement, but this cannot be regarded as inevitable, as demonstrated by the Court of Appeal's judgement in the case of *Hooper v Young* [1998] Lloyd's Rep Med 61.

On the facts in *Hooper*, there were three possible explanations for the ureteric damage suffered by the Claimant: (1) misplacement of an encircling suture around the ureter; (2) application of a clamp; (3) kinking of the ureter by a suture placed near, but not encircling, the ureter. The experts unanimously agreed that the first two explanations amounted to negligence. The trial judge found that the third explanation could occur with or without negligence: *"thus the burden of proof was on the plaintiff to prove that kinking had occurred as a result of negligence and to eliminate mere inadvertence by an experienced surgeon working in a confined space"*. The trial judge nevertheless found in favour of the plaintiff. His reasoning was rather unclear: *"I accept, that neither of the three possibilities would have occurred but for some error amounting to negligence on the part of the defendant"*. Stuart-Smith LJ, giving unanimous judgement for the Court of Appeal, held that the plaintiff had failed to discharge her burden of proof: *"I have come to the conclusion, albeit with some reluctance, that there was no evidence from which it could be inferred that the defendant had not followed his usual procedure or that he had placed the stitch unreasonably close to the ureter."*

Stuart-Smith LJ made some further comments in relation to the principle of *res ipsa loquitur*, which translates as "the facts speak for themselves":

> It is a pity in retrospect that the concept of res ipsa loquitur ever entered this case. It is primarily a rule of evidence. It may have been appropriate in regard to encirclement and clamping. In my view, it had no place in the kinking by a suture which could have occurred with or without negligence.

Essentially, the implication of Stuart-Smith LJ's words is that *res ipsa loquitur* will only assist claimants in clear cases, such as the textbook example of amputating the wrong limb. The principle will not assist in situations where claimants have suffered an injury which could have occurred with or without negligence. To an extent, this should hardly need spelling out – in situations where an injury could have occurred with or without negligence, the facts simply do not speak for themselves. In general terms, experts and lawyers would be well advised to explain and justify any allegation of negligence which they make rather than relying optimistically upon timeworn Latin principles.

For further discussion of *res ipsa loquitur* and the related concept of *prima facie* inferences, please see the legal commentary at Chapter 22.

Duce v Worcestershire Acute Hospitals NHS Trust [2018] EWCA Civ 1307

The Court of Appeal's judgement in *Duce* is one of the most influential decisions on causation following the landmark judgement of the Supreme Court in *Montgomery*.

The principles relating to consent in *Montgomery* are considered in more detail in Chapter 4. A point arising from the *Montgomery* judgement which is sometimes overlooked is the approach taken to causation. Lords Kerr and Reed expressed the relevant principle pithily: *"The question of causation must also be considered on the hypothesis of a discussion which is conducted without the patient's being pressurised to accept her doctor's recommendation"* [para 103]. On the facts in *Montgomery*, the evidence pointed *"clearly in one direction"*: if Mrs Montgomery had been advised of the risk of shoulder dystocia, she would have elected to have a caesarean section. Her treating obstetrician had indeed conceded this point when giving oral evidence.

In the years following the *Montgomery* judgement, there have been a number of cases in which claimants have sought to apply the approach taken by the House of Lords in the old case of *Chester v Afshar* [2004] UKHL 41 to the post-*Montgomery* framework. *Chester v Afshar* involved a neurosurgeon's failure to warn of a small but significant risk of surgery. Lord Bingham summed up the question for consideration as follows:

> whether the conventional approach to causation in negligence actions should be varied where the claim is based on a doctor's negligent failure to warn a patient of a small but unavoidable risk of surgery when, following surgery performed with due care and skill, such risk eventuates but it is not shown that, if duly warned, the patient would not have undergone surgery with the same small but unavoidable risk of mishap [para 1].

On the facts, the trial judge found that if the claimant had been properly warned about the risk, she would not have undergone surgery on the date when she did. However, there was no finding to the effect that she would not have undergone the surgery eventually. The risk was unavoidable and would have been the same regardless of when she underwent the surgery.

The majority of the House of Lords (with Lords Bingham and Hoffmann dissenting) held that the claimant's case should succeed. The conclusions of their Lordships have provoked considerable academic discussion and legal argument among practitioners over the years, and can fairly be regarded as controversial. Many claimants, including the claimant in *Duce*, have drawn optimism from the following well-known words of Lord Hope in *Chester v Afshar*:

> *To leave the patient who would find the decision difficult without a remedy, as the normal approach to causation would indicate, would render the duty useless in the cases where it may be needed most. This would discriminate against those who cannot honestly say that they would have declined the operation once and for all if they had been warned. I would find that result unacceptable. The function of the law is to enable rights to be vindicated and to provide remedies when duties have been breached. Unless this is done the duty is a hollow one, stripped of all practical force and devoid of all content. It will have lost its ability to protect the patient and thus to fulfil the only purpose which brought it into existence. On policy grounds therefore I would hold that the test of causation is satisfied in this case. The injury was intimately involved with the duty to warn. The duty was owed by the doctor who performed the surgery that Miss Chester consented to. It was the product of the very risk that she should have been warned about when she gave her consent. So I would hold that it can be regarded as having been caused, in the legal sense, by the breach of that duty [para 87].*

An attempt was made in *Duce* to rely upon Lord Hope's approach in *Chester v Afshar*. On the facts, the claimant in *Duce* had not been warned of the risk of post-operative pain. The claimant's case on the exact nature of the warnings which should have been given evolved during trial. She argued that if she had been warned about post-operative pain, she would not have proceeded to surgery on the day in question. The trial judge found that even if she had been warned about post-operative pain, she would have proceeded to surgery on the day in question. The submission made on behalf of the claimant in Duce was that the approach of Lord Hope in Chester v Afshar created an "alternative pathway" to causation in consent cases [para 51]. This submission was resoundingly rejected by the Court of Appeal. In the words of Hamblen LJ:

the majority decision in Chester does not negate the requirement for a claimant to demonstrate a "but for" causative effect of the breach of duty, as that requirement was interpreted by the majority, and specifically that the operation would not have taken place when it did.

A similar restriction upon *Chester* can be seen in the Court of Appeal's judgement in *Correia v University Hospital of North Staffordshire NHS Trust* [2017] EWCA Civ 356, where Simon LJ held as follows [para 28]:

The crucial finding in Chester v. Afshar was that, if warned of the risk, the claimant would have deferred the operation. In contrast, in the present case, it was not the appellant's case that she would not have had the operation, or would have deferred it or have gone to another surgeon. . . To some extent, the reason for this omission is the artificial nature of the appellant's argument on this part of the case. Nevertheless, it seems to me that if a claimant is to rely on the exceptional principle of causation established by Chester v. Afshar, it is necessary to plead the point and support it by evidence.

A further attempt to rely upon *Chester* failed in *Diamond v Royal Devon and Exeter NHS Foundation Trust* [2019] EWCA Civ 585, where Nicola Davies LJ, giving unanimous judgement for the Court of Appeal, considered *Montgomery, Chester v Afshar, Duce* and *Correia*. The issue in the case was whether the claimant's shock, distress and depression were caused by the failure to obtain properly informed consent for a mesh hernia repair. The Court observed that *"Montgomery lends no support for the proposition that a failure to warn of a risk or risks, without more, gives rise to a free-standing claim in damages"* [para 35]. On the facts, the Court upheld the trial judge's finding that the claimant would still have proceeded with the mesh repair even if she had been warned of the relevant risk. The claimant's appeal accordingly failed.

A recent attempt to rely upon *Chester* was made in the case of *Brint v Barking, Havering and Redbridge University Hospitals NHS Trust* [2021] EWHC 290 (QB),[1] where a claimant who suffered an extravasation injury during a CT scan argued that she should succeed in recovering damages even if she would have agreed to undergo the scan after having been warned of the risk of extravasation. HHJ Platts (sitting as a Judge of the High Court) had already found that appropriate warnings had been given, but made the *obiter* observations that the present case was not a case where the patient would find the decision difficult: *"I would therefore have concluded, had I had to decide it, that the present case can be distinguished on its facts from* Chester *and that the normal principles of causation should apply"* [para 40].

By contrast, in the first instance case of *Crossman v St George's Healthcare NHS Trust* [2016] EWHC 2878 (QB), the Court considered a situation where surgery was performed earlier than it should have been due to negligence. The claimant suffered a non-negligent complication of surgery (a nerve injury). If he had undergone the same procedure on a different date, he would have had the same chances of suffering this complication. However, the risk would have been very low, and would not have eventuated on the

---

[1] The present author acted for the defendant Trust in *Brint*.

balance of probabilities. The judge found that the claimant's case succeeded on conventional causation principles without the need for consideration of *Chester v Afshar*.

The approach taken by the Court in *Crossman* has been criticised. In *Barry v Cardiff and Vale University Local Health Board* (2018, unreported) the Court regarded the case as having been wrongly decided and declined to follow it. It is to be hoped that the higher courts will give further consideration to the issue raised in *Crossman* and *Barry*, namely the approach to be taken to cases where (a) due to negligence, a claimant has undergone surgery earlier or later than they should have done, (b) where the claimant has suffered a non-negligent complication of surgery and (c) where the likelihood of suffering the complication is unchanged due to the delay/advancement of the date for surgery. This issue is encountered in practice on a surprisingly regular basis, and clarity would be most welcome.

Clinical Commentary

Janesh K Gupta

Good Practice Guidance

Management of Abnormal Uterine Bleeding

It is important at every initial assessment to consider the patient's symptoms and their impact on quality of life and realistic expectations for outcomes following hysterectomy. When there are no obvious structural abnormalities (fibroids) and disease state such as endometriosis or adenomyosis and there is no evidence of endometrial hyperplasia or endometrial carcinoma, i.e. in a benign state, then pharmacological treatments should be offered as first-line treatment.

Medical Management

Hysterectomy for heavy menstrual bleeding (menorrhagia) is a permanent solution which should only be a last resort option, particularly when there is no obvious disease state such as fibroids, endometriosis or adenomyosis. Pharmacological methods such as levonorgestrel-releasing intrauterine system, tranexamic acid, non-steroidal anti-inflammatory drugs, combined oral contraceptives, high-dose progestogen treatment and endometrial ablation should be considered before hysterectomy is performed [1,2].

Therefore, hysterectomy should only be a second-line treatment strategy for heavy menstrual bleeding, for which women need to have tried first-line treatment strategies, and for these to be unsuccessful, before being offered a hysterectomy.

NICE guidance indicates that when discussing the route of hysterectomy (laparoscopy, laparotomy or vaginal) with the woman, an individual assessment should be carried out and her preferences taken into account [2007, amended 2018].

Hysterectomy (Total versus Subtotal)

- Vaginal
- Open (suprapubic/midline)
- Laparoscopic or laparoscopic-assisted
- Robotic

Table 18.1. Complications of hysterectomy

Infection

Bleeding and need for blood transfusion

Clots in legs and lungs (thrombosis)

Injury to bladder, bowels and ureters

Need for laparotomy if vaginal, laparoscopic or robotic hysterectomy is performed

Failure to achieve the desired result if subtotal hysterectomy is performed

Chronic pain

Sexual problems

Hernia formation (*this risk is greater with open midline surgery*)

The latest evidence from the Cochrane review published in 2015 [3] indicates that out of the four different types of hysterectomy methods – abdominal hysterectomy, vaginal hysterectomy, laparoscopic hysterectomy and robotic hysterectomy – vaginal hysterectomy has been identified to be superior to laparoscopic and abdominal hysterectomy, as this method is associated with lower complication rates and a faster return to normal activities. The main patient outcomes that are important to women are return to normal activities, patient satisfaction, quality of life, and lower surgical complications, particularly injuries to bowel, bladder and ureters. The latter surgical complications can be significant and can delay recovery and necessitate return to theatre and repeat operations (see Table 18.1).

In the context of randomised control trials, where women are recruited into one or other type of hysterectomy, usually the surgical expertise for performing such surgery, e.g. laparoscopic hysterectomy or vaginal hysterectomy, tends to be done by those deemed to be experts in these methods. In the controlled environment of randomised controlled trials, laparoscopic hysterectomy is associated with an at least two-fold increased risk of major urinary tract injuries to ureters and bladder. Therefore, it is likely that this risk will be higher when laparoscopic hysterectomy is performed by those outside randomised controlled trials, as surgical expertise is likely to be less so than in those performing randomised control trials. This also indicates the need for careful pre-operative counselling and to follow Montgomery principles that patients undergoing laparoscopic hysterectomy should be given this specific risk, that there is likely at least a two-fold increased risk of major urinary tract injuries associated with this type of surgery.

Although robotic hysterectomy has been increasing over the past few years, the evidence does not support its routine implementation into general gynaecological surgical practice. Therefore, given the current evidence, surgeon expertise and preference, there should be a careful discussion with the woman regarding the best hysterectomy method, particularly when vaginal hysterectomy is not possible. The alternative methods should then be between abdominal and laparoscopic hysterectomy. The latter method should include specific counselling regarding the at least two-fold increased risk of major urinary tract injuries [4]. It is possible that outside clinical controlled trials the risk of injury to other organs may be higher when surgery is performed by general gynaecologists.

When there is obvious surgical structural disease such as fibroids, then the option for hysteroscopic (if there are submucous fibroids) or open versus laparoscopic myomectomy can be considered, particularly if there is a need for fertility sparing. Uterine artery embolization is also an alternative option, but this tends to be specifically more successful when there are single fibroids compared to multiple fibroids, and single fibroids less than 10 cm in size compared to multiple fibroids [5].

NICE also indicates that clinicians should discuss the options of total hysterectomy (removal of the uterus and the cervix) and subtotal hysterectomy (removal of the uterus and retention of the cervix) with the woman [2007, amended 2018].

The choice between subtotal and total hysterectomy depends on the surgical disease present in the pelvis, in particular mobility of the cervix, which may be restricted by previous surgery but more so due to endometriosis. This can make the surgical planes difficult and increases the risk of complications, in particular injury to bowel, ureters and bladder. Depending on the surgical expertise, a decision must be made as to whether retention of the cervix is safer when there is no obvious disease in the pelvis and the surgical planes are normal. The decision between subtotal hysterectomy and total hysterectomy should be discussed with the woman. The evidence does not suggest that subtotal hysterectomy improves outcomes for sexual, urinary or bowel function compared to total abdominal hysterectomy. It was previously thought that avoiding the disruption of the pelvic nerves and not performing bladder dissection would result in less risk of urinary dysfunction. However, the evidence indicates that women are more likely to experience ongoing cyclical vaginal bleeding due to retention of the cervical stump; this can continue for up to one year and there may be a need for future removal of the cervical stump [6].

Referral to Subspecialist

If a hysterectomy is desired, it should be in the context that this a permanent non-reversible solution and referral to subspecialists should occur when a woman desires a laparoscopic/robotic hysterectomy. This is on the premise that such procedures are associated with quicker discharge from hospital, but may be associated with a higher risk of major urinary tract injuries such as to bladder and ureters [3, 4]. If there is significant pelvic disease due to endometriosis, then this may also need a referral to a specialist centre, with the possibility of colorectal surgeons performing the joint operation.

Training of Clinicians

In the United Kingdom there are specific training programmes for advanced laparoscopic surgical skills. This is performed through a form of mentorship with a consultant who is a recognised trainer.[2]

This is reinforced through NICE guidance that suggests that advanced laparoscopic skills are required for these procedures, and clinicians should undergo special training and mentorship. The Royal College of Obstetricians and Gynaecologists has developed an Advanced Training Skills Module, 'Benign Gynaecological Surgery: Laparoscopy'.

---

[2] See www.bsge.org.uk/ for details.

This would need to be supplemented by further training in order to achieve the skills required for total laparoscopic hysterectomy.[3]

1. Current evidence on the safety and efficacy of laparoscopic techniques for hysterectomy (including laparoscopically assisted vaginal hysterectomy [LAVH], laparoscopic hysterectomy [LH], laparoscopic supracervical hysterectomy [LSH] and total laparoscopic hysterectomy [TLH]) appears adequate to support their use, provided that normal arrangements are in place for consent, audit and clinical governance.

2. Clinicians should advise women that there is a higher risk of urinary tract injury and of severe bleeding associated with these procedures, in comparison with open surgery.

Causes of Litigation

The reasons for litigation include the following:

- Failure to adhere to national guidance issued by NICE
- Preoperative counselling/choices provided
- This is particularly so for LH where there should be a specific discussion detailing the at least two-fold increased risk of major urinary tract injuries
- Consent and discussion of complications
- Lack of adequate training of surgeon
- Complications during/arising from the procedure and failure to advise of these complications
- Failure to adequately select patients
- Failure to adhere to the principles of safe laparoscopic entry as recommended by National Bodies (see below)
- Failure to detect bowel injury at the time of surgery
- Failure to detect bowel injury in the early postoperative period
- Failure to convert to a laparotomy when bowel injury is suspected
- Failure to call a bowel surgeon when bowel injury is suspected/occurs
- Attempting repair of bowel injury in the absence of an adequate case load as a gynaecologist

Avoidance of Litigation

To avoid litigation when performing continence surgery, ensure the following have been taken into account:

- Ensure medical treatments are considered where appropriate
- Patients should be given adequate time to consider their options
- All risks and complications of the various options should be discussed, as well as the option of no treatment
- Patient information leaflets should be provided for all types of hysterectomy

---

[3] See www.nice.org.uk/guidance/ipg239/resources/laparoscopic-techniques-for-hysterectomy-pdf-1899865344377797 for details.

- Clinicians undertaking these procedures should be able to demonstrate they have had the training and maintain their caseload. Data for this surgery should be entered on a registry/database

References

1. Gupta, J, Kai, J, Middleton, L, Pattison, H, Gray, R, Daniels, J, et al. Levonorgestrel intrauterine system versus medical therapy for menorrhagia. *N Engl J Med* 2013; 368(2): 128–37.

2. National Institute for Health and Care Excellence (NICE). Heavy menstrual bleeding: assessment and management NICE guideline [NG88]. 2020. Available from: www.nice.org.uk/guidance/ng88

3. Aarts, JW, Nieboer, TE, Johnson, N, Tavender, E, Garry, R, Mol, BW, et al. Surgical approach to hysterectomy for benign gynaecological disease. *Cochrane Database Syst Rev* (Online) 2015; (8): CD003677.

4. Gupta, J. Vaginal hysterectomy is the best minimal access method for hysterectomy. *Evid Based Med* 2015; 20(6): 210.

5. Gupta, JK, Sinha, A, Lumsden, MA, Hickey, M. Uterine artery embolization for symptomatic uterine fibroids. *Cochrane Database Syst Rev* (Online) 2014; (12): CD005073.

6. Lethaby, A, Mukhopadhyay, A, Naik, R. Total versus subtotal hysterectomy for benign gynaecological conditions. *Cochrane Database Syst Rev* (Online) 2012; (4): CD004993.

Chapter 19

Endometriosis

Alfred Cutner, Martin Hirsch

CASE COMMENTARY

Swati Jha

Successful Claim

FB v Nottingham Hospitals NHS Trust (2020)

The Claim

The claimant presented with abdominal pain from the age of 18 years through to the age of 36 years. When she finally underwent a laparoscopy, she was found to have grade 4 endometriosis which had spread around her ovaries, colon and the wall of the abdomen. She underwent treatment, but as the endometriosis was so far advanced it could not be fully treated and it was alleged: i) it had been negligent to consider her symptoms to be related to irritable bowel syndrome (IBS) alone; ii) there had been a failure to consider a diagnosis of endometriosis earlier; iii) there had been a failure to perform a laparoscopy earlier, even though her symptoms remained unchanged after treatment.

The Summary

The claimant repeatedly visited her GP from the age of 18 with severe period pains and was initially given the contraceptive pill. As the pain persisted, following several further attendances at A & E as well as the GP practice, she was referred to see a gynaecologist. At the first appointment with the gynaecologist, as her symptoms were not suggestive of endometriosis, she was discharged back to the GP. Following multiple further visits she was referred back to the gynaecologist aged 22 years and underwent an ultrasound scan which was normal. She was again discharged with a diagnosis of IBS. She continued to be treated for IBS for the next 13 years, but when she came off her contraceptive pill and started to have severe pain, she was finally booked for a laparoscopy which revealed grade 4 endometriosis. The claimant alleged that had a laparoscopy been performed earlier, the diagnosis would have been made and treatment with surgery or hormonal treatment would have treated her pain and prevented progression of the endometriosis to such a severity. It was conceded that the claimant should have undergone a laparoscopy when she was seen aged 22 years. The severe endometriosis rendered her infertile, requiring IVF to conceive. She also suffered premature ovarian failure which reduced her life expectancy by two years. She suffered from *"severe pain, urgency to defecate, excessive vaginal bleeding, severe dyspareunia and a mild to moderate depressive illness and would require a hysterectomy."* Ongoing pain meant she had to end her career as a full-time teacher and work in the role of a supply teacher instead. She also suffered a depressive illness for which she required treatment.

The Judgement

The case was settled out of court in favour of the claimant, in view of the delayed diagnosis, with total damages amounting to £500,000. Of this, the pain, suffering and loss of amenity (PSLA) pay out was £120,000 and loss of future earnings amounted to £55,000, with a pension loss of £150,200.

Unsuccessful Claim

Weeks v Wright [2013] EWHC 4744 (QB)

The Claim

The claimant was referred by her GP at the age of 25 for abdominal pain affecting her day-to-day activities. The possibility of endometriosis with involvement of the rectum was raised and confirmed on an ultrasound scan performed preoperatively. The claimant underwent laparoscopic surgery with excision of a rectovaginal nodule of endometriosis and was discharged from hospital the next day. Six days after her initial surgery, she was readmitted with pain and underwent a laparotomy. At surgery, a 2 cm perforation of the rectum was detected and repaired. The patient required a loop sigmoid colostomy which was later reversed. It was claimed that: i) the rectal probe had not been adequately used to identify and delineate the rectum; ii) the diathermy instrument had been used to directly apply current to the rectal tissue, causing damage. Indirect heat causing damage to rectal tissue was not a recognised complication of the procedure.

The Summary

The procedure was recorded at the time, so this could be used to assess the surgical techniques adopted. The first issue was the manner in which the rectal probe was used to delineate the rectum and whether this was the only means of delineating the rectal wall. The expert for the defendant highlighted that there is no strict guidance on how the rectal probe should be used and different clinicians use it differently, whereas some prefer not to use it at all. The important factor is that delineation should take place by some means at the time of surgery, and in this case was performed appropriately using a combination of visual appearances, the probe, touch and experience. The second issue of discussion was the use of diathermy and whether the damage occurred due to the direct application of diathermy to the rectal tissue or by heat spread from application of diathermy to neighbouring tissues. Whereas the claimant presented the view that injury to viscera from heat spread was not a known complication of using monopolar diathermy, the defendant took an opposing view.

The Judgement

The expert for the defendant was another endometriosis expert, whereas the expert for the claimant was not an endometriosis specialist and was felt to be more convincing by virtue of their personal experience of dealing with endometriosis. The defendant's expert was therefore considered more reliable and their evidence preferred by the judge.

The complication of heat spread from the application of diathermy to neighbouring tissues could result in inadvertent heat damage to the tissue of the rectal wall, leading to necrosis and subsequent perforation several days later. Secondly, this is a recognised risk of the procedure and can occur without any negligent act. The judgement was in favour of the defendant.

Legal Commentary

Eloise Power

Valuing Pain, Suffering and Loss of Amenity in Gynaecological Cases (with Reference to FB v Nottingham Hospitals NHS Trust)

The task of valuing the pain, suffering and loss of amenity (PSLA) aspect of gynaecological claims can present difficulties, particularly where the injuries include dyspareunia or apareunia, or where there are multiple injuries.

In general, valuing PSLA in any clinical negligence or personal injury case requires professional judgement. Judges and practitioners have access to the following materials in arriving at an appropriate judgement:

(a) The Judicial College (JC) Guidelines (which were formerly known as the Judicial Studies Board Guidelines): the JC Guidelines cover a range of injuries, are regularly updated and are invariably used by courts and practitioners. At the time of writing, the JC Guidelines are in their fifteenth edition. Unfortunately, the JC Guidelines provide little assistance in valuing gynaecological claims which do not relate to fertility. This important issue – which raises crucial Human Rights Act implications – is discussed in more detail below.

(b) Reports of court judgements: courts and practitioners have access to wide legal databases covering a range of reported cases. The facts relating to every injury are different, and the PSLA awards set out in the court judgements should consequently be regarded as guidance rather than as binding authority. Practitioners will typically argue that the facts of the case they are dealing with are more (or less) serious than the facts of the reported judgement.

(c) Reports of settlements: particular care must be taken when relying on reports of settled cases. Some cases settle at an undervalue (or indeed at an overvalue) for sound reasons: claimant lawyers may have concerns about the underlying merits, or defendant lawyers may have commercial reasons for achieving an early settlement rather than incurring the costs of proceeding. Having said that, there is sometimes no alternative to relying on reports of settlements, particularly in circumstances where cases involve an unusual injury or an unusual combination of injuries. At the very least, these reports – such as the report in the case of *FB v Nottingham Hospitals NHS Trust* – provide information about real-world outcomes and can provide a useful starting point or point of reference.

Where cases involve multiple injuries, the Court of Appeal has set out an important point of principle in *Sadler v Filipiak* [2011] 10 WLUK 190. Etherton LJ (with whom the other Court of Appeal judges agreed) held that the Court should first consider the various injuries and fix a particular figure as reasonable for each, and secondly stand back and have a look at what would be the global aggregate figure and ask whether it was reasonable compensation for the totality of the injury. These are important principles to bear in mind when valuing gynaecological cases: such cases frequently involve multiple areas of injury such as loss of fertility, dyspareunia/apareunia, chronic pain, bowel symptoms and bladder symptoms.

The JC Guidelines on the female reproductive system provide helpful assistance in cases involving loss of fertility but provide no meaningful assistance in cases involving the loss of sexual function. (Separate guidelines exist for cases involving bladder and bowel injuries and for chronic pain). The current edition of the guidelines on the female reproductive system provide as follows:

The level of awards in this area will typically depend on:

- whether or not the affected woman already has children and/or whether the intended family was complete;

- scarring;

- depression or psychological scarring;

- whether a foetus was aborted.

(a) *Infertility whether by reason of injury or disease, with severe depression and anxiety, pain, and scarring: £107,810 to £158,970[1]*

(b) *Infertility resulting from failure to diagnose ectopic pregnancy not included in section (a) above but where there are resulting medical complications. The upper end of the bracket will be appropriate where those medical complications are significant: £31,950 to £95,850*

(c) *Infertility without any medical complication and where the injured person already has children. The upper end of the bracket is appropriate in cases where there is significant psychological damage: £16,860 to £34,480*

(d) *Infertility where the injured person would not have had children in any event (for example, because of age): £6,190 to £11,820*

(e) *Failed sterilisation leading to unwanted pregnancy where there is no serious psychological impact or depression: in the region of £9,570*

(f) *Where there is a delay in diagnosing ectopic pregnancy but fertility is not affected. Award dependent on extent of pain, suffering, bleeding, whether blood transfusion is required, anxiety and adjustment disorder, and whether there is resultant removal of one of the fallopian tubes: £3,180 to £19,170*

It is the present author's view that the focus on fertility alone, with no consideration of sexual function, is incomplete, outdated and potentially discriminatory. In practice, many cases will fall outside the scope of the JC Guidelines on the female reproductive system. A few examples from the present author's recent practice include a case involving unnecessarily radical surgery, resulting in the removal of the claimant's clitoris and causing a complete loss of sexual function; a case of total apareunia resulting from the use of trans-vaginal mesh in a young woman; a case of dyspareunia resulting from an unnecessary anterior and posterior repair which led to the need for further surgery.

In marked contrast with the JC Guidelines on the female reproductive system, the JC Guidelines on the *male* reproductive system include clear guidance on cases involving loss of sexual function (in addition to guidance on cases involving loss of fertility):

---

[1] For simplicity, only the up-to-date bracket has been provided (incorporating a 10% uplift applicable from 1 April 2013 onwards).

(i) Total impotence and loss of sexual function and sterility in the case of a young man. The level of the award will depend on: age; psychological reaction and the effect on social and domestic life: in the region of £139,210

(ii) Impotence which is likely to be permanent, in the case of a middle-aged man with children: £40,370 to £73,580.

In the case of *Carvalho Pinto De Sousa Morais v Portugal* [2017] 7 WLUK 551, the European Court of Human Rights held that Portugal should not have discriminated between men and women in relation to damages recoverable for the enjoyment of sexual activity:

The question at issue here is not considerations of age or sex as such, but rather the assumption that sexuality is not as important for a fifty-year-old woman and mother of two children as for someone of a younger age. That assumption reflects a traditional idea of female sexuality as being essentially linked to child-bearing purposes and thus ignores its physical and psychological relevance for the self-fulfilment of women as people.

The principle in *Carvalho Pinto De Sousa Morais v Portugal* appears not as yet to have been tested in the British courts. In practical terms and pending any future legal developments, it is the practice of the present author to value cases involving apareunia and dyspareunia in women by reference to the JC Guidelines on the male legal system.

Looking at the settlement which was achieved in the case of *FB v Nottingham Hospitals NHS Trust*, it can be inferred that the parties placed the matter within bracket (a) of the JC Guidelines on the female reproductive system. Bracket (a) does not make reference to sexual function. It is very much to be hoped that future authors of the JC Guidelines will take the principle in *Carvalho Pinto De Sousa Morais v Portugal* into account when revising the section on the female reproductive system.

Selecting the Right Expert (with Reference to Weeks v Wright)

The judgement of HHJ Forster QC (sitting as a Deputy High Court Judge) in *Weeks v Wright* serves as a salutary reminder of the importance of careful expert selection in clinical negligence cases. This issue is covered in more detail in Chapter 3.

The key issue in *Weeks v Wright* was whether the claimant's diathermy burns had been caused negligently or whether this amounted to a recognised risk of a laparoscopic procedure for the excision of a rectovaginal nodule of endometriosis. At paragraph 27 of the judgement, HHJ Forster QC held as follows:

Having carefully considered the evidence, I find the answer to the dispute in the oral evidence of Mr Kettner. I find his evidence to be direct, focused and the most persuasive. I accept his evidence that inadvertent heat damage to the tissue of the rectal wall is a recognised complication. Mr Gilmer does not have the same immediate experience of the procedure.

A similar point was considered in *Toth v Jarman* [2006] EWCA Civ 1028, which is a well-known Court of Appeal judgement on duties of experts and conflicts of interest. Sir Mark Potter, giving judgement on behalf of the unanimous Court of Appeal, upheld the trial judge's judgement in a case involving nervous shock consequent upon a child's brain injury and death. The judgement includes the following observation [para 95]:

As already made clear, the judge's preference for the expertise of Professor Hull was based less upon his research background than his practical experience in the treatment of hypoglycaemic children and their response to IV and/or IG administration of glucose.

Although the approach of the Court to expert witnesses will be fact-specific, those acting for claimants and defendants in cases involving a particular medical procedure would be well advised to ensure that wherever possible, expert witnesses are able to draw upon their own practical experience of the procedure as well as invoking the medical literature.

Clinical Commentary

Alfred Cutner and Martin Hirsch

Good Practice Guidance

When considering how to manage patients with severe endometriosis, the following considerations need to be taken into account:

- Presenting symptoms and aims of treatment
- Multidisciplinary referral and management
- Pre-operative preparation
- Performance of surgery
- Post-operative care
- Long-term management

Presenting Symptoms and Aims of Treatment

Most patients present either due to pain symptoms or difficulty falling pregnant. They may present with a combination of both and then it is important to determine the main priority of treatment.

The most common pain symptom is pain with menstruation. The patient may also complain of pain with intercourse, pain opening her bowels and bladder pain. In addition, the pain may occur during ovulation. The pain may become non-cyclical in nature. Loin pain should raise awareness of potential ureteric involvement and cyclical shoulder pain may indicate diaphragmatic involvement. Rarely bowel obstruction may develop due to progressive disease and the clinician must be aware of the possibility of silent obstruction of the ureter resulting in loss of renal function. Where there is a large cyst, she may present due to an abdominal mass. Lung endometriosis is recognised but cyclical haemoptysis or pneumothoraxes due to endometriosis are very uncommon [1].

The level of urgency and the requirement for treatment will depend on an assessment of the risks and benefits. Where there is a large abdominal mass causing pressure symptoms or a nodule causing bowel obstruction or ureteric compromise, treatment will be urgent and necessary. Where the treatment is for pain or fertility, time must be taken to fully consider all the options and the implications of the various options.

There is no evidence to suggest earlier diagnosis improves long-term prognosis. However, a diagnosis enables access to secondary- or tertiary-level care, support groups, and consideration of the different treatment options. A clinician could be considered negligent for not considering appropriate investigations, referral or treatment for patients with symptoms of endometriosis where initial empirical treatment has been ineffective [2].

Whilst endometriosis is a common cause for pain, clinicians must consider other causes for pain, particularly in circumstances where previous endometriosis treatments have been unsuccessful. An unnecessary or a repeat surgical procedure without consideration of other causes, resulting in a complication, would be considered a breach of duty. In addition, a delay in effective treatment may result in a prolonged period of suffering having a negative impact on quality of life.

Other common causes for pain that should be considered include: adenomyosis, bladder pain syndrome, irritable bowel syndrome, inflammatory bowel disease, renal colic, appendicitis, ovarian torsion and pelvic inflammatory disease. A careful history, examination, and appropriate imaging can help rule in or out these diagnoses. Where a patient presents with new or recently enhanced symptoms, the clinician should be cautious not to miss potentially serious acute conditions in patients with a history of endometriosis. The incidence of acute events such as appendicitis and pelvic inflammatory disease will be comparable if not greater amongst this cohort, and vigilance not to dismiss symptoms and ignore common signs is essential.

Multidisciplinary Referral and Management

The majority of patients presenting with symptoms of endometriosis will have tried empirical treatment via their general practitioner. In secondary care, it is important to make a diagnosis and then triage to appropriate care.

Clinical examination may help rule in the condition, with findings such as an adnexal mass or painful induration or nodularity in the rectovaginal space highly suggestive of endometriosis. The absence of these findings does not exclude endometriosis [3].

Imaging modalities have a varied sensitivity and specificity depending on the skill of the investigator and the disease type. Transvaginal ultrasound has a high level of accuracy for the detection of deep rectovaginal endometriosis, bowel endometriosis, and ovarian endometriosis, but not peritoneal or superficial disease. This is mirrored for magnetic resonance imaging (MRI). There are no blood serum, menstrual, or urine biomarkers currently recommended for the non-invasive diagnosis or monitoring of endometriosis [2,3]. However, a mildly raised CA125 is associated with endometriosis and, where consistent with other findings suggestive of endometriosis, should not prompt an oncological referral [4].

Patients with an ultrasound diagnosis suggestive of severe disease and requesting consideration of surgical care should be referred to an endometriosis centre [2,5]. In addition, some patients will be identified due to an initial laparoscopy to either diagnose the cause of pain or fertility or after planned surgery for presumed non-severe disease in secondary care.

Endometriosis centres consist of a multidisciplinary group of clinicians to enable consideration of all aspects of care. The make-up of a service includes:

- Gynaecologist
- Colorectal surgeon
- Urologist
- Nurse specialist
- Pain management access
- Links to fertility services
- Appropriate radiology

Such centres of excellence are supported by The British Society of Gynaecological Endoscopy (BSGE) [4] and The National Institute for Health and Care Excellence (NICE) [2].

Pre-operative Preparation

Local secondary-care gynaecological services manage the majority of endometriosis patients. The cohort of patients with severe endometriosis represent 5–30% of all those with endometriosis which are recommended to have their care managed at a specialist endometriosis centre. Based on United Kingdom population statistics, it is estimated that there are 0.3–1.0 million patients with endometriosis, of which 15,000–300,000 suffer with severe endometriosis, with an estimated 5,000 new cases annually [5].

A large proportion of patients with endometriosis will be successfully managed long term with simple hormonal treatments such as the combined contraceptive pill, progesterone-only pill, or Mirena intra-uterine system (IUS). A percentage will require surgical treatment and of these, some will require repeat surgery due to recurrent or persistent endometriosis-associated pain. In the majority of patients, surgery will be undertaken to enhance quality of life after having failed or declined medical treatment options. The common reasons include improvement of pain symptoms or to enhance conception, either spontaneously or with assisted reproduction such as in-vitro fertilisation (IVF). A small proportion of patients will require surgery to preserve organ integrity. Amongst this small cohort, the commonest reason would be to relieve an obstructive endometriotic process on the ureter causing hydroureter or hydronephrosis. In rare circumstances, patients with bowel endometriosis develop a progressive stricture culminating in bowel obstruction.

The benign nature of the disease requires a symptom-focused treatment strategy, led by the patient with guidance from the clinician. The focus of discussion centres on the benefits and risks of the treatment options available and how they will impact on the principal symptom of concern. Treatment options broadly include doing nothing, conservative measures (e.g. dietary modifications), medical treatments including pain management services and hormone manipulation, and surgical treatment. Surgery for the treatment of endometriosis carries the greatest risk of all interventions. The major complication rate associated with surgery for severe endometriosis is 7% [6].

Patients who are at increased risk from surgery or who are keen to have a non-surgical solution could consider the option of long-term gonadotropin-releasing hormone agonists (GnRHa). These products are licenced for six months use in patients with endometriosis-associated pain without strong evidence to suggest dosage and duration [3]. The prolonged use of these products is associated with reducing bone mineral density and the potential long-term harms associated with a hypoestrogenic state such as cardiovascular disease, including stroke. The addition of addback hormone replacement therapy (HRT) reduces these risks. The off-licence usage and risks need to be discussed carefully in direct comparison with the risks associated with alternative interventions.

In line with recent general medical council (GMC) consent guidance, a detailed discussion of the following should take place in relation to the patients' individual circumstances:

a. Diagnosis and prognosis.
b. Uncertainties about the diagnosis or prognosis, including options for further investigation.

c. Options for treating or managing the condition, including the option to take no action.

d. The nature of each option, what would be involved, and the desired outcome.

e. The potential benefits, risks of harm, uncertainties about and likelihood of success for each option, including the option to take no action. Harm is defined as any potential negative outcome, including a side effect or complication [7].

A multidisciplinary meeting should be considered where there are uncertainties as to the benefit or the risks of surgery, or the surgery to be undertaken is complex with potential serious risks. All aspects of care, from decision-making, surgical route, operative technique and appropriate surgical skill set required (including colorectal surgeons, urological surgeons) lend themselves to discussion in a multidisciplinary meeting. This shared decision-making forum helps guide the patient to make the correct choice and reduces the risk of criticism to an individual clinician should a retrospective claim be made regarding decision-making.

In patients who suffer complications from surgery it is not uncommon for claimants to argue that had they been offered more conservative therapies they would have accepted that option and could therefore have avoided surgery. It is therefore common practice that clinicians discuss and document all treatment options, including more conservative medical treatments, unless there are individual circumstances requiring immediate recourse to surgical intervention.

For those patients with rectovaginal endometriosis scheduled for a combined operating list with colorectal surgeons, it is best practice for the risks to be discussed with a consultant trained in the specific procedure she may undergo. For those patients with pre-operative hydronephrosis or hydroureter, the risk of requiring urological surgery is increased. A gynaecologist is not best placed to consent a patient for the risks associated with a colorectal or urological procedure that she or he is not trained in. A pre-operative outpatient consultation with clear discussion and documentation of the risks of these procedures with trained colorectal or urological specialists is best practice. Where these complex procedures become more common within a specialist unit, it would be appropriate for the gynaecologists to counsel fully regards these other aspects of care.

The GMC recommend that patients have access to decision aids offered by their clinician to read, watch, or listen. These are not a substitute for consent and form an additional source of information that the patient can access when away from the clinical consultation to guide the decision-making process. The giving of an information leaflet does not ensure that the information has been imparted. Giving an information leaflet and then confirming on a second occasion that she fully understands the content and has no further questions would be best practice.

The risk of surgical complications is greater in patients with medical comorbidities including raised body mass index (BMI), smoking, drug use, and excessive alcohol consumption. Laparoscopic pelvic surgery for patients with a raised BMI can be very difficult as the angulation of Trendelenburg (30 degrees) required to visualise and operate in the pelvis may be limited by anaesthetic ventilatory pressures. The risk of infection and thromboembolism rises with a raised BMI. The optimisation of medical conditions and communication with appropriate consultant specialists ahead of instigating treatments should be considered as routine practice. In addition, informing a patient of her increased risks and giving her an opportunity to reduce these risks (where appropriate) should form part of the counselling process.

Performance of Surgery

The pre-operative discussion and consent will form the basis for the operative approach and technique used to treat endometriosis. The fibrotic nature of the disease results in significant distortion of the normal anatomy and the appropriate case selection for the surgeon is paramount. Many centres nationally use a pooled surgical list where patients seen in clinic by Surgeon A are scheduled on the theatre list of Surgeon B due to waiting list pressures. Surgeons intending to perform laparoscopic surgery for the management of severe endometriosis should have the appropriate training, supervision, and experience [8].

The excision of deep endometriosis is associated with risk, but it is a recommended treatment to improve pain and quality of life. There is an international recommendation for this surgery to be performed at a centre of expertise that offers all treatments in the context of a multidisciplinary team [3]. Among patients who have completed their family or failed more conservative measures, this surgery could be considered in conjunction with a hysterectomy and removal of ovaries [2,3]. Expert opinion recommends that pre-operative GnRHa analogues should be considered for 12 weeks prior to the excision of rectovaginal endometriosis [2,3].

The management of pain associated with ovarian endometriomas and hydrosalpinges requires caution and discussion regarding past, current and future fertility desires. The removal (cystectomy) of an ovarian endometrioma is associated with both a greater reduction in pain but also a fall in surrogate markers of ovarian reserve. This is more pronounced with bilaterality, increasing endometrioma size, and with previous ovarian surgery. The alternative procedure, ovarian cyst drainage with ablation of the cyst wall, is associated with a higher rate of recurrence while conveying a lower risk of reducing these markers of ovarian reserve [3]. It is important that this information has been relayed to the patient and documented in advance of the consent process. Consideration of egg storage or embryo storage (where appropriate) prior to surgery should be discussed with the patient at high risk of reduced ovarian function.

Surgery for severe endometriosis should be carried out in an appropriately equipped theatre with the correct level of skills of the surgeon, assistant, and support team [5].

The performance of surgery and safe entry techniques for laparoscopy are easily accessible in the Royal College of Obstetricians and Gynaecologists Green-top Guideline No.49 [9]. Entry-related injuries contribute a significant proportion of all injuries, and it is imperative that the most appropriate entry method and location is used depending on the individual patient's risk factors. The clinician must be competent at different entry techniques. The chosen method should be individualised according to the patient's weight, extent of disease, and previous surgical history.

Following generation of the pneumoperitoneum, a surgeon should be able to perform the procedure required and be cognisant of the possibility of an injury occurring without them being aware. The surgeon should be familiar with their equipment, instrumentation, and energy sources. They should be aware of the risks of the energy source being used.

In cases of rectal endometriosis where there has been significant dissection in the recto-vaginal space, a rectal integrity test is required. A bladder syringe of air used to be commonly employed, but most clinicians now recommend using a sigmoidoscope to ensure an adequate pressure is achieved. In patients undergoing excessive anterior pelvic dissection, a bladder integrity test is recommended. Where required, appropriate repair methods should be undertaken by a surgeon with the correct expertise.

There remains uncertainty regarding the involvement of allied urological and colorectal specialists at the time of surgery for severe endometriosis. This is compounded by the diagnostic difficulties clinicians have in making accurate pre-operate prediction of the complexity that they will encounter at the time of surgery. This subsequently leads to poor prediction modelling to identify which cases require the presence of urological and colorectal colleagues from the start of the case rather than availability. The presence of bowel endometriosis with increasing nodule size and rectal muscularis invasion are predictive of the requirement for invasive colorectal procedures from a rectal shave, disc resection, and segmental bowel resection. Where there is a high probability of requiring colorectal support during the operation then it would be considered best practice for them to be present from the start to enable appropriate joint decision-making. Local arrangements would depend on the experience of the endometriosis team. Where the findings are greater than that expected and the patient has not been fully counselled or the appropriate support from other specialties is not available, the operation should be abandoned, and arrangement made for a second procedure on another occasion.

The presence of hydronephrosis would warrant a pre-operative urological assessment with imaging modalities including computed tomography (CT), a renal perfusion scan (MAG3) and blood tests helping to determine the extent of obstruction and function. The use of ureteric dissection is commonly undertaken to identify and lateralise the ureters during excisional surgery. The use of ureteric stenting with JJ stents should be considered where there is excessive or repeat ureterolysis to protect the kidneys should a stricture occur. A concomitant bowel resection or hysterectomy raises the relative indication for JJ stents [10].

The uncertain nature of whether a patient will undergo excessive ureterolysis requires close liaison and availability of urological colleagues to site JJ stents. The routine usage and insertion of ureteric catheters aids identification and dissection of the ureters during surgery. This is a mandatory skill for those completing the advanced training skills module in the laparoscopic excision of benign gynaecological disease [8]. When they are used will depend on local experience but should be considered in more complex cases.

Post-operative Care

Patients with endometriosis-associated pain are often using analgesics prior to surgery and will develop a level of tolerance. The acute insult of surgery often leads to acute on chronic pain that can be difficult to manage with routine analgesia. The input of specialist acute pain services is recommended while excluding operative complications as a cause for immediate post-operative pain.

Severe endometriosis often runs in close proximity to the bowel, bladder, ureters, hypogastric nerve, and blood vessels. Injuries to these structures are reported widely and surgeons should be vigilant for these.

The group of patients undergoing surgery are often fit and healthy reproductive-age patients with limited medical co-morbidities. The development of a temperature or tachycardia following this complex surgery should raise suspicions of possible infective morbidity or visceral injury. Use of inflammatory markers such as CRP may raise concern. Computed tomography (CT) can, with a single imaging modality, assess the integrity of the bowel, bladder, ureters, and assess for pelvic collections. The addition of a delayed urographic phase allows for the assessment of ureteric or bladder injuries. Patients should get better quickly from laparoscopic surgery, and early recourse to imaging such as CT should be considered where there are concerns of an abdominal complication. In addition, opinions of appropriate colleagues should be sought where there is any concern.

Long-Term Management

The long-term management of endometriosis requires an individualised approach. For those patients who undergo surgery, it is recommended to use hormonal therapy as secondary prevention until they wish to conceive or reach the age of menopause. For those not wishing for surgery and opting for either conservative or medical therapy, monitoring can be considered based on symptoms, however there is no clear guidance on monitoring asymptomatic disease. Patients with severe disease and a large recto-vaginal nodule who decline surgery, should be considered for follow-up [2]. Most clinicians would recommend a follow-up scan to exclude extension of the nodule resulting in ureteric compromise. There is no guidance on the number and time scale of follow-up scans. However, as a minimum, a scan one year after initial diagnosis should be carried out. Assuming that there is no significant progression, further scans will be driven by symptom progression.

Causes of Litigation

Pre-intervention

- Failure to adhere to local/national guidance (NICE)/International Guidance (ESHRE)
- Preoperative counselling/failure to document choices or alternatives
- Failure to counsel and consent for common or serious complications
- Lack of adequate training of surgeon taking consent
- Lack of appropriate/timely imaging or intervention

Intra-operative

- Lack of adequate training of surgeon performing the procedure
- Lack of appropriate support/infrastructure to perform procedure
- Failure to adhere to the principles of safe laparoscopic entry as recommended by National Bodies (see below)
- Failure to detect bowel injury at the time of surgery
- Failure to detect urinary tract injury
- Failure to call appropriate specialist when an injury is suspected/occurs

Post-operative

- Failure to detect bowel injury in the early postoperative period
- Failure to detect urinary tract injury in the early postoperative period
- Failure to call appropriate specialist when an injury is suspected/occurs
- Failure to arrange appropriate post-operative treatment/investigations/follow-up

Avoidance of Litigation

To avoid litigation when performing endometriosis surgery, ensure the following have been taken into account:

- Ensure treatment recommendations are in line with local/national/international guidance
- Ensure all treatment options are discussed in line with GMC consent guidance 2020
- Patients should be given adequate time to consider their options
- All risks and complications of the various options should be discussed and the patient offered time to consider these options
- Patients should have confirmed that they understand all aspects of proposed surgery and risks and options before admission
- Appropriate information should be provided for endometriosis surgery
- Clinicians undertaking these procedures should be able to demonstrate they have had the training and caseload to justify their practice
- Clinicians should be able to produce a record of their outcomes

References

1. Hirsch, M, Berg, L, Gamaledin, I, Vyas, S, Vashihst, A. The management of women with thoracic endometriosis: a national survey of British gynaecological endoscopists. *Facts Views Vis Obgyn* 2020; 12(4): 291–8.

2. National Institute for Health and Care Excellence (NICE). Endometriosis: diagnosis and management. NICE Guideline [NG73]. 2017. Available at: www.nice.org.uk/guidance/ng73/documents/draft-guideline

3. Dunselman, GAJ, et al. ESHRE guideline: management of women with endometriosis. *Hum Reprod* 2014; 29(3): 400–12.

4. Hirsch, M, Duffy, JMN, Davis, CJ, Nieves Plana, M, Khan, KS. Diagnostic accuracy of cancer antigen 125 for endometriosis: a systematic review and meta-analysis. *BJOG* 2016; 123(11): 1761–8.

5. NHS England. "NHS Standard Contract for Complex Gynaecology – Severe Endometriosis. Schedule 2 – The Services A. Service Specifications 2013. Available at: www.england.nhs.uk/wp-content/uploads/2018/08/Complex-gynaecology-severe-endometriosis.pdf

6. Byrne, D, Curnow, T, Smith, P, Cutner, A, Saridogan, E, Clark, TJ. Laparoscopic excision of deep rectovaginal endometriosis in BSGE endometriosis centres: a multicentre prospective cohort study. *BMJ Open* 2018; (8); e018924–e018924.

7. General Medical Council (GMC). Guidance on professional standards and ethics for doctors: decision making and consent. 2020. [Online]. Available at: www.gmc-uk.org/-/media/documents/updated-decision-making-and-consent-guidance_pdf-84160128.pdf

8. Royal College of Obstetricians and Gynaecologists (RCOG). Advanced training skills module: advanced laparoscopic surgery for the excision of benign gynaecological disease. 2010. [Online]. Available at: www.rcog.org.uk/globalassets/documents/careers-and-training/atsms/atsm_advancedlaparoscopic_curriculum.pdf

9. Royal College of Obstetricians and Gynaecologists (RCOG). Preventing Entry-related Gynaecological Laparoscopic Injuries. Green-top Guideline No. 49. 2008. [Online]. Available at: https://mk0britishsociep8d9m.kinstacdn.com/wp-content/uploads/2016/03/GtG-no-49-Laparoscopic-Injury-2008.pdf

10. Fisher, G, Smith, RD, Saridogan, E, Vashisht, A, Allen, S, Arumuham, V, et al. Case selection for urological input in planned laparoscopic rectovaginal endometriosis surgery. *Facts, Views & Vision in ObGyn* 2019; 11(2): 111–17.

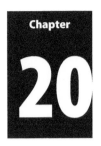

Miscarriage and Ectopic Pregnancy

Stephen Porter

CASE COMMENTARY

Swati Jha

Successful Claim

Rathore v Bedford Hospitals NHS Trust [2017] EWHC 863 (QB), 2017 WL 01435526

The Claim

The patient had an ectopic pregnancy following a failure to treat a chlamydia infection the preceding year. In addition to the ectopic pregnancy, it was claimed she endured a year of unnecessary pain and suffering, a higher chance of suffering a future ectopic pregnancy, extreme stress owing to this, and as a consequence had developed a stress-related skin condition. Claims were also made for voluntary care, medication charges and loss of future earnings.

The Summary

The claimant was admitted to hospital two weeks after the birth of her second child with secondary postpartum bleeding. Vaginal swabs were taken and she was discharged home. The results were positive for chlamydia but she was not informed and the infection was not treated. A year later she was found to have an ectopic pregnancy and it was identified that she had an untreated chlamydia infection which was subsequently treated. Her husband was also treated and subsequent swabs were negative.

However, she went on to develop chronic pain syndromes of a somatoform nature and was also involved in a road traffic accident which subsequently led to her inability to work permanently.

The Judgement

It was conceded by the defendant that a failure to treat the chlamydia had resulted in the ectopic pregnancy and the pain and suffering arising from this. The judge also agreed that the initial effects of the stress, including facial rash and the somatoform disorder in the early stages following the ectopic pregnancy, were related to a failure to detect and promptly treat the chlamydia, but subsequent psychological problems, marital break-down and future loss of earnings were unrelated.

Unsuccessful Claim

Laycock v Gaughan and Others [2011] IEHC 52

The Claim

The claimant underwent a laparoscopy for an ectopic and due to bleeding ended up as a laparotomy. She claimed that the surgery should have been performed laparoscopically and due to open surgery she had been left with an unnecessary scar resulting in post-operative pain, discomfort and distress. She also claimed that there had been a delay in the diagnosis of the ectopic and she had been inadequately monitored, which exposed her to the risk of life-threatening injury. She also claimed that a previous diagnostic laparoscopy, done months before the ectopic pregnancy, was performed negligently.

The Summary

The claimant underwent a diagnostic laparoscopy, three months preceding the ectopic pregnancy, for chronic pelvic pain. She suffered significant bruising to her abdomen and claimed this was due to injury to the inferior epigastric blood vessels at the time of placement of the secondary ports.

Subsequently, she presented with an ectopic pregnancy and was monitored in the early pregnancy assessment unit. No pregnancy was identified inside the uterus on a scan and a pregnancy hormone test was performed, with another one planned a week later. Following the second hormone test, an ectopic was diagnosed, for which a laparoscopy was performed, but due to the presence of blood in the abdomen obstructing the view, it was converted to an open laparotomy and a salpingectomy was performed.

The Judgement

In relation to the bruising following the diagnostic laparoscopy, injury to the inferior epigastric was dismissed, as this would have been detected at the time of surgery due to the extent of bleeding. The bruising therefore ensued due to injury to one of the smaller blood vessels of the abdomen, which is a known complication of secondary port insertion.

In relation to the management of the ectopic, it was felt the monitoring and management with a salpingectomy were appropriate. In relation to the need to convert from a laparoscopy to a laparotomy, the defendant chose to take the safest course from the patient's viewpoint. It would have been unreasonable to continue laparoscopically if it was unsafe to do so or to look for an alternative surgeon who could have performed the operation laparoscopically, as the patient required urgent management which could not be deferred. It was therefore reasonable to convert to a laparotomy.

The case was dismissed on both counts.

Legal Commentary

Eloise Power

Rathore v Bedford Hospitals NHS Trust [2017] EWHC 863 (QB)

Sadly, the development of long-term pain is a feature of many gynaecological and obstetric cases, both in relation to ectopic pregnancies and in relation to other areas.

Pain cases can present particular difficulties for the Courts: the available evidence is typically of a subjective nature, and expert witnesses may have little to go on beyond the information provided by the claimant. Where credibility is in issue, this presents obvious problems. These problems can be compounded by the high monetary value of some schedules in pain cases, particularly where it is alleged that pain has prevented a claimant from working or attending to normal domestic responsibilities.

The case of *Rathore* posed some particularly knotty evidential questions in relation to the causation of the claimant's pain condition. The exact diagnosis of the pain condition was in itself an issue in the case: the Court described the claimant's condition as chronic widespread pain (CWP) resulting from persistent somatoform pain disorder (PSPD)/ somatic symptom disorder (SSD) and leading to opiate dependency. It was the claimant's case that her CWP resulted from the ectopic pregnancy, laparoscopy and salpingectomy, which she had suffered as a result of the defendant's negligence (breach of duty was admitted). The defendant denied that these events had caused the pain condition, and also denied that the claimant's symptoms were as severe as she had claimed. The claimant served a schedule of loss which exceeded £3 million, on the basis of causation of a disabling and permanent pain condition.

In the course of evaluating the evidence, Blake J observed that:

> Pain is a subjective experience that cannot be objectively identified and assessed by this court or treating or forensic professionals. Her account of when, where and how she suffered pain and the intensity of the pain she suffered is thus the foundation of the assessment made by experts: gynaecologists, psychiatrists, pain treatment consultants and care experts... *On any view the claimant's evidence is central to the determination of the central issues in dispute*... [para 36, emphasis added].

Given the importance of the claimant's own evidence in relation to pain, the Court proceeded to assess her account against other contemporaneous documents in the case, including benefits records, Social Services records relating to her children, diary entries, social media and employment records. These documents contained multiple points which contradicted the claimant's evidence: for example, the benefits records and employment records established that the claimant had developed significant mobility problems after an unrelated road traffic accident in 2011.

In *Rathore*, the approach to the claimant's social media account (which had been accessed on behalf of the defendant) is of interest. The Court observed as follows:

> I recognise that reliance on individual posts showing the claimant in glamorous clothing, attending social events with others, including her husband, should be treated with considerable caution [para 46].

On the other hand, the Court clearly placed some weight upon the social media evidence when taken as a whole and evaluated in conjunction with other sources of evidence:

> Although no single entry or photograph presents a knockout blow to the claimant's credibility, and I take into account that in Facebook the claimant may be presenting a positive image of herself, I am satisfied that her social life and her mobility was considerably greater than she claimed for the purposes of the present case and the DLA application. Her unreliability on these issues is not a problem of recollection of the trajectory of her illness as seen through the spectrum of someone with a psychiatric condition, rather she has given exaggerated or untruthful accounts of her social life at a time when she claims to have undergone a significant deterioration in her condition and was making a number of different claims for compensation [para 94].

Based upon the approach taken by Blake J, defendants would be well advised to review claimants' public social media accounts and to invite the Court to take them into account as part of the overall picture, but it is unlikely to make sense (except in the clearest of cases) to rely solely upon such material.

The Court found that causation was only established in respect of a relatively short period following the ectopic pregnancy (between October 2005 and the autumn of 2009): *"by the autumn of 2009, any lingering causal contribution made to the claimant's psychological disorders was negligible or non-existent"* [para 182]. Damages were assessed in the sum of £68,742.38, a tiny fraction of the sum of over £3 million which the Claimant had sought. A similar causation issue was recently considered by the Court in *Brint v Barking, Havering and Redbridge University Hospitals NHS Trust* [2021] EWHC 290 (QB), 2021 WL 00540059, where the Court considered the history of a claimant with a *"long history of presenting with complaints that have no obvious organic cause"* and concluded that a claimant's symptoms were only related to the index events for a short-term period. These comments were obiter dicta, as the claim failed on breach of duty. These cases underline the importance of ensuring that the expert evidence clearly demarcates the causation flowing from the alleged breach of duty.

As a general observation, claimants and defendants in pain cases would be well advised to obtain all relevant contemporaneous documents at the earliest possible point. Crucial documents in many cases will include benefits records, Blue Badge records, other official documents and employment records. These records should be made available to expert witnesses at the earliest opportunity. From the viewpoint of claimants, this will enable the value of their case to be assessed more accurately. Depending on the facts, the provision of relevant contemporaneous records can assist in managing expectations and avoiding disappointing outcomes and Pyrrhic victories, such as the outcome in *Rathore*. From the viewpoint of defendants, the provision of contemporaneous documents will assist in arriving at realistic settlement figures. In the well-known words of Lord Pearce in *Onassis v Vergottis* [1968] 2 Lloyds Rep 403:

> It is a truism, often used in accident cases, that with every day that passes the memory becomes fainter and the imagination becomes more active. For that reason a witness, however honest, rarely persuades a Judge that his present recollection is preferable to that which was taken down in writing immediately after the accident occurred. Therefore, contemporary documents are always of the utmost importance.

These words apply as much to quantum as to primary liability.

Laycock v Gaughan and Others [2011] IEHC 52

This case was decided by the High Court of Ireland. Clinical negligence cases in Ireland are governed by legal principles which are similar to *Bolam*, set out by the Supreme Court of Ireland in *Dunne v National Maternity Hospital* [1989] IR 91. A key area of interest in the case is the approach which the Court took to "gold standard" surgery. On the facts, laparoscopic surgery for ectopic pregnancy was regarded as the "gold standard". The Court heard evidence to the effect that at the material time (2004), some 37% of ectopic pregnancies diagnosed in the National Maternity Hospital, Ireland, were treated by way of laparotomy. The doctor who treated the plaintiff was not trained or experienced in laparoscopic surgery. On the facts, the Court accepted the position that it would not have been reasonable or appropriate for the doctor to have taken the time to search for laparoscopically skilled practitioners *"at a time when the plaintiff required immediate surgical intervention to stop bleeding which was compromising her health and wellbeing."*

The Court observed that: *"evidence of failure on the part of a medical practitioner to provide a patient with the most advanced and technically perfect treatment available is not necessarily evidence of negligence by the practitioner."*

It is interesting to consider how this case would be approached if it were heard today under the English/Welsh jurisdiction. The judgement in *Laycock* made reference to the RCOG Guideline No. 21 of May 2004, which established that where possible, surgery should be undertaken laparoscopically. Understandably, this was given little weight: the relevant events in *Laycock* predated the May 2004 Guideline, and the Guideline did not apply to Ireland in any event. The May 2004 Guideline has now been superseded by "Diagnosis and Management of Ectopic Pregnancy (Green-top Guideline No. 21), published 4 November 2016 as a joint guideline by the RCOG and the Association of Early Pregnancy Units (AEPU).[1] This Guideline provides as follows: *"A laparoscopic surgical approach is preferable to an open approach"*. The grade of recommendation is A, which is the highest available grade of recommendation.[2] Clearly, the concept of a reasonable standard of care can change over time, and one generation's "gold standard" can be another generation's reasonable standard (see Chapter 6 for further discussion of this issue).

Clinical Commentary

Stephen Porter

Good Practice Guidance

General Principles of Early Pregnancy Care and Initial Assessment

Complications of early pregnancy can cause an enormous amount of distress to some women and their partners. It is therefore vital that healthcare workers and the system within which they work provide an environment of sensitivity, respect and dignity to women and their families. Within this framework a thorough gynaecological and obstetric history, as well as the details of the present pregnancy, should be obtained. An examination based on the history should include a basic set of observations, abdominal and pelvic assessment.

The initial objective, once it has been determined that the patient is haemodynamically stable, is to ascertain whether the pregnancy is intrauterine, extrauterine, viable or non-viable. It is not unusual for it to take several days or weeks before the diagnosis can be made with certainty. Honest, clear and sensitive communication is therefore essential.

Women should ideally be treated in a dedicated early pregnancy assessment unit. Care should be courteous, professional and informed by the best available evidence.

---

[1] https://doi.org/10.1111/1471-0528.14189
[2] See Appendix 1 of the Guideline for a full description of the classification of evidence levels and grades of recommendations.

All management options should be discussed, documented and supported by written information. The potential impact that each option has on future fertility should be discussed. Women managed expectantly or medically should be informed of symptoms which will require prompt medical attention. They should also be given details of how to access medical care 24 hours a day. Women who are managed surgically should be informed of what to expect during the post-operative period and where and how to seek help. Rhesus negative patients who have been managed surgically should also be given 250iu of anti-D.

Follow-up should be offered to all women if more time is needed to debrief following a complication of early pregnancy.

Patients should be signposted to support organisations and groups.

Miscarriage

Diagnosis

Vaginal bleeding and pain in early pregnancy are not uncommon and should be regarded as a continuum. The initial approach aims to determine whether the pregnancy is viable or non-viable.

A pelvic examination including a speculum, although not harmful to the pregnancy [1], is rarely conclusive. The investigations of choice are transvaginal ultrasound and serum β-hCG. In the presence of a β-hCG of 1500iu/l, transvaginal ultrasound performed by a sonographer or a suitably trained clinician is the key investigation in the diagnosis of miscarriage [2,3].

A miscarriage should be considered when:

o The mean gestational sac diameter is 25 mm or over and the sac does not contain a visible fetal pole or yoke sac [4].

o If the crown rump length is 7 mm or more in the absence of fetal heart pulsations [5].

It is important to bear in mind and to inform patients that a diagnosis of miscarriage on the basis of one transvaginal scan (TVS) is not 100% accurate, particularly at early gestation.

If the scan at presentation demonstrates an empty uterus:

o Serum β-hCG should be measured

   o If the level is over 1500iu/ml – suspect an ectopic pregnancy – repeat β-hCG in 48 hours

   o If the level is less than 1500iu/ml – repeat β-hCG in 48 hours and the TVS in seven days [4].

If the scan at presentation demonstrates an intrauterine pregnancy but cannot confirm viability:

o Repeat the scan in seven days and perform serial β-hCG until viability or non-viability is clearly established

A fall of over 50% of β-hCG in 48 hours in the presence of pain and bleeding suggests a failing pregnancy. It should be borne in mind that a declining β-hCG may also occur with an ectopic pregnancy and levels should be correlated with scan findings.

Management of Miscarriage

Women with a confirmed miscarriage who are haemodynamically stable have the option of expectant, medical or surgical management. In those who are unstable, acute management and resuscitation should include a speculum examination in order to remove products which may be at the os [1]. Those managed expectantly or medically should be provided with written information which contains information on the avoidance of the use of tampons, the likely timescale of completion of pregnancy loss and details of how to access medical care.

Expectant Management

Expectant management over a 7–14-day timeframe should not be offered to women:

o with signs of infection

o who are at increased risk of bleeding

o who have a history of a previously traumatic pregnancy.

If the bleeding and pain resolve within 7–14 days of expectant management, the woman should be advised to perform a urine pregnancy test and return for review if it is positive. If bleeding and pain has either not started after 7–14 days of expectant management or has not stopped, an ultrasound should be done, and the patient offered medical or surgical treatment.

Medical Management

Medical management of a confirmed miscarriage involves a vaginal or oral dose of misoprostol of between 600–800 micrograms. Women should be informed that bleeding is likely to occur within 24 hours and that complete miscarriage occurs in 70% by two weeks and in 80% by four weeks [6]. The National Institute of Health and Clinical Excellence (NICE) advises against use of mifepristone [4]. Women should be given analgesics. Arrangements should be in place for the woman to contact the early pregnancy assessment unit if bleeding has not started after 24 hours. The options at that point are a further dose of misoprostol or surgical management.

Surgical Management

Surgical management is either via manual evacuation under local anaesthesia or surgical evacuation in theatre. Care should be taken to avoid uterine perforation or incomplete evacuation of products of conception. Anti-D should be offered to all Rhesus negative patients. Antibiotics should be given to women with overt signs of clinical infection and considered in cases of incomplete miscarriage [7].

Recurrent Miscarriage

The immediate management of women who are having their third consecutive miscarriage is the same as outlined above. In addition, a number of specific investigations are recommended as outlined in Table 20.1 [8].

Treatment of Recurrent Miscarriage

Women should be given written information, counselling and support. Where available, management should be in a specialist recurrent miscarriage clinic. In addition to specific measures related to any identifiable cause, early access to regular first trimester scanning should also be offered.

The use of low-dose aspirin and unfractionated heparin has been shown to significantly improve live births in women with an acquired thrombophilia [9]. The data

Table 20.1. Investigations for recurrent miscarriage

Test	Timing	Additional measures
Acquired thrombophilia (anti-phospholipid antibodies)	Two samples taken outside of pregnancy at least 12 weeks apart	Lupus anticoagulant and anti-cardiolipin (IgG and/or IgM) in medium or high titre >40 mg/l or above 99 centile
Cytogenetic analysis	Product of conception sent (dry) following miscarriage	Parental peripheral blood karyotyping if unbalanced structural chromosomal anomaly identified
Imaging	An ultrasound scan of the pelvis in the non-gravid state	If suspected anomaly identified, further evaluation with hysteroscopy, laparoscopy or 3D pelvic imaging.
Inherited thrombophilias Factor V Leiden, Protein S, factor II (prothrombin) gene mutation	To be performed at least six weeks post miscarriage	

suggesting improved pregnancy outcome with heparin for those with inherited thrombophilias is less robust [8]. With the exception of cervical cerclage, there is little data that points to benefit from correction of anatomical anomalies [8]. Couples who have unbalanced translocations should be referred for genetic counselling and consideration for preimplantation genetic diagnosis.

Ectopic Pregnancy

Diagnosis

Although the classical presentation of six to eight weeks of amenorrhoea followed by bleeding and pain is well documented [10], up to one third of women with ectopic pregnancy have no clinical signs and 9% have no symptoms [11,12]. Transvaginal ultrasound and serum β-hCG therefore form the cornerstone of initial assessment and may be all that is required for diagnosis. In some cases of pregnancy of unknown location (PUL), the diagnosis is made at laparoscopy.

Transvaginal Ultrasound –– Transvaginal ultrasonography (TVS) may positively identify an ectopic pregnancy or a viable intrauterine pregnancy. In instances when TVS fails to identify the location of a pregnancy, a pregnancy of unknown location is diagnosed (PUL).

The majority of PULs will be diagnosed as failed or viable intrauterine pregnancies. Up to 20% however will subsequently be found to be an ectopic pregnancy [13].

Transvaginal ultrasonography will identify a normal intrauterine pregnancy at 5.5 weeks [14].

o A pseudo sac, which is a central collection of fluid within the endometrial cavity, does not contain a yolk sac or an embryo. Within the usually eccentrically placed gestation sac, cardiac activity should be visible at six weeks.

A tubal ectopic pregnancy is suggested when a transvaginal ultrasound scan shows:

o   the absence of an intrauterine pregnancy

o   the positive identification of an adnexal mass, usually on the side of the corpus luteal cyst that moves separately form the ovary, and

o   the presence of free fluid in the Pouch of Douglas.

Ultrasound features of ectopic pregnancies are included in Table 20.2 [15].

Measurement of Serum β-hCG -- Serial β-hCG measurements are indicated when there is diagnostic uncertainty or a pregnancy of unknown location (PUL). Samples should be taken as close to 48 hours apart as possible. Although many normal IUPs will show a doubling of β-hCG over this time frame [16], a more conservative rise of 50% in two days is used in many units [17].

In the absence of ultrasound visualisation, however, a rise of over 50% in isolation should not be taken as diagnostic of an IUP, as some non-viable intrauterine and ectopic pregnancies will demonstrate an exponential rise in β-hCG.

- A rise of less than 50% in 48 hours suggests pregnancy failure.
- A fall of 21–35% or greater in 48 hours indicates either a failing intrauterine or resolving ectopic pregnancy. The rate of hCG decline in spontaneous abortions is described by a quadratic profile, with a faster decline in hCG value with higher presentation levels [18].
- Just over two thirds of ectopic pregnancies have serum β-hCG levels that show an attenuated rise and fall compared to viable intrauterine and failing intrauterine pregnancies respectively [19].
- If serial β-hCG measurements and TVS are incompatible with a viable or failing intrauterine pregnancy, the diagnosis is an ectopic pregnancy. The management options are surgical, medical or conservative.

Serum Progesterone -- Serum progesterone has no place in the diagnosis of ectopic pregnancy [15]

Laparoscopy -- Although laparoscopy is no longer regarded as the gold standard for diagnosis, in some cases of PUL it may be necessary. A degree of clinical judgement is required. If performed too early, an ectopic may be missed; if performed too late, rupture and haemorrhage may occur.

Management of Ectopic Pregnancy

Surgery -- Although the management of ectopic pregnancy is tailored to the patient according to their presentation, clinical condition, suitability for various options and preference, there are a few principles which a should be adhered to:

o   Those who are stable with unruptured ectopic pregnancy or PUL may be suitable for surgical, medical or expectant management.

o   Surgery is the treatment of choice for all cases of ruptured ectopic pregnancy.

o   Patients who are unstable haemodynamically should have a laparotomy. Otherwise, a laparoscopic approach is preferable.

o   At laparoscopy or laparotomy, if the contralateral tube is normal, salpingectomy should be performed. In the presence of an absent or diseased contralateral tube, a salpingotomy may be considered [4].

Table 20.2. Ultrasound features of ectopic pregnancy

Site	Ultrasound features
Tubal	o A non-cystic adnexal mass/an empty extrauterine sac which may contain a yolk sac or a fetal pole. o Endometrium may or may not contain a pseudo-sac o Fluid in the pouch may be present echogenic shadows
Cervical	o Barrel-shaped cervix o Empty uterine cavity o Gestational sac below the level of the internal os o Blood flow around the gestational sac using colour Doppler o Absence of "sliding" of the gestational sac along the endocervical canal when pressure applied to the cervix with the ultrasound probe
Caesarean scar	o Empty uterine cavity o Empty endocervical canal o Gestational sac or trophoblastic mass with evidence of circulation identified in caesarean scar o Thin or absent layer of myometrium between gestation sac and bladder
Interstitial	o Products of conception/gestational sac located in the intramural part of the tube and surrounded by less than 5 mm of myometrium in all imaging planes o The presence of a thin echogenic line extending from the uterine cavity to the interstitial sac, the "interstitial line sign" o Empty uterine cavity
Ovarian	o No specific ultrasound criteria o Empty uterus and a wide echogenic ring with an internal anechoic area on the ovary o Corpus luteum should be identified separate from the suspected ovarian pregnancy
Abdominal	o Absence of an intrauterine gestational sac o Absence of both an evident dilated tube and a complex adnexal mass o A gestational cavity surrounded by loops of bowel and separated from them by peritoneum o A wide mobility similar to fluctuation of the sac, particularly evident with pressure of the transvaginal probe toward the posterior cul-de-sac
Heterotopic	o Intrauterine pregnancy o A non-cystic adnexal mass/an empty extrauterine sac which may contain a yolk sac or a fetal pole o Fluid in the pouch may be present echogenic shadows

Women should be informed that subsequent intrauterine pregnancy and repeat ectopic pregnancy rates following salpingectomy are similar to those following salpingotomy [20]. All Rhesus negative women treated surgically should be offered 250iu of Anti-D.

Following salpingectomy, women should be advised to perform a urine hCG after three weeks and seek medical advice if it is positive [4]. Serum β-hCG on day 1 and 7 following salpingotomy should be repeated weekly until levels return to normal, in order to detect persistent trophoblast. Persistent trophoblast, detected by failure of β-hCG to fall, is treated with systemic methotrexate.

Table 20.3. Criteria for medical management of ectopic pregnancy

Criteria category	Features compatible with methotrexate treatment
Clinical features	o Haemodynamically stable o Minimal abdominal pain
Serum beta-human chorionic gonadotrophin (β-hCG) concentrations	o <5000 iu/l prior to treatment
Ultrasound scan findings	o Unruptured ectopic pregnancy <35 mm diameter o No fetal heart activity or clear yolk sac in adnexal mass o No or very little free fluid in pouch of Douglas o Unlikely to be early intrauterine pregnancy failure
Patient characteristics	o Prefers medical option o Willing and able to attend follow-up for up to six weeks o Willing to abstain from alcohol for seven days following the treatment
Medical history	o No active peptic ulcer disease o No renal disease, hepatic disease, severe anaemia, leucopenia or thrombocytopenia
Concurrent medication	Should not be on: o Non-steroidal anti-inflammatory agents (NSAIDs), aspirin, penicillins, sulphonamides, trimethoprim, tetracyclines, diuretics, phenytoin, antimalarials, ciclosporin, retinoids, probenecid, folic acid, hypoglycaemics, live vaccines, nephrotoxic or hepatotoxic drugs

Medical Treatment --Intramuscular methotrexate is a suitable option for patients with unruptured ectopic pregnancy who are haemodynamically stable and have the characteristics in Table 20.3.

A single methotrexate dose of 50mg/m^2 should be followed by serum β-hCG measurements on days 4 and 7.

o If there is a fall of more than 15%, measurements are repeated weekly until they are less than 15iu/l.

o If β-hCG levels fall by less than 15%, a TVS should be performed to exclude fetal heart activity and evidence of rupture [21]. Consideration can then be given to either a further dose of methotrexate or surgery.

Rupture remains a risk during treatment and may be heralded by increased pain or collapse.

Expectant Management -- Some ectopic pregnancies will resolve spontaneously and can be managed with assessment and observation.

Expectant management is an option when the following criteria are met:

o Patient clinically stable with minimal symptoms
o Initial β-hCG <1000iu/l
o Rapidly declining β-hCG
o Patient able to attend for regular follow-up

The National Institute for Health and Care Excellence recommends that women managed expectantly should have β-hCG levels measured on days 2, 4 and 7 following the initial measurement. If levels fall by 15% or more from the previous value on days 2, 4 and 7, they recommend that repeat measurements should be taken weekly until a negative result of less than 20 iu/l is obtained [4]. If β-hCG levels do not fall by more than 15% between samples, consideration should be given to methotrexate.

Causes of Litigation

o Missed diagnosis/delayed diagnosis – Failure to diagnose ectopic pregnancy. This occurs when the patient is diagnosed as having had a "complete miscarriage" but then goes on to present acutely with a ruptured ectopic pregnancy
o Wrong site surgery – removal of wrong fallopian tube
o Loss of fertility
o Surgical complications

  o Laparotomy – this may have become necessary as a result of delayed diagnosis and clinical deterioration
  o Delayed recognition of surgical injury
  o Uterine perforation at evacuation

o Expectant management

It is critical to point out that despite a decline in hCG, a resolving ectopic pregnancy may rupture. There have been cases reported where an ectopic pregnancy has ruptured despite continuously declining hCG values [22].

Avoidance of Litigation

Good Communication

Many claims are rooted in poor communication. Early pregnancy complications can exert a considerable toll on the patient and her family. When there is an unexpected or poor clinical outcome, poor communication may add to the distress experienced and result in the desire for legal redress. From presentation to discharge, communication should therefore be:

o Courteous and sensitive – for the patient and her family; complications of early pregnancy are very distressing. Clinical and non-clinical staff should be cognisant of this during every interaction with the patient and her family.
o Honest – Clinicians should be honest about the diagnostic uncertainty of PUL, honest about the options available and potential implications for future fertility and honest enough to say sorry when things have gone wrong (duty of candour).

o Supported by evidenced-based written information – Where possible oral communication about management, symptoms to look out for, and details of how to access medical care should be supported by written information leaflets.

o Ongoing – The clinical picture may evolve over a period of days or weeks. Systems need to be in place to ensure that each development is followed up with the patient.

o Consistent – Thorough hand-over between shifts will ensure that patients are not given conflicting information.

Documentation

o Communication – The date, time and content of all conversations, including those conducted by phone, should be clearly recorded in the patient's notes.

o Contemporaneous notes/results – All notes and results should be recorded contemporaneously. If entries are recorded retrospectively, the date and time of entry should be explicitly recorded.

o Surgical findings – All surgical findings, including normal findings, should be clearly recorded in the patient records and where possible supported by photographic evidence.

Access to Medical Services: Patients Should Have Easy Access to Investigations and Medical Personnel

o Scanning and β-hCG – It is important that early pregnancy assessment units provide access to scanning services and serum β-hCG. Clear protocols should be in place for weekends, in order to ensure that services can be safely accessed.

o Assessment unit – Dedicated unit with well trained staff and evidenced-based guidelines.

o **Training** – clinicians undertaking surgical management of miscarriage and ectopic pregnancy should have the training and experience to do so.

Follow-up

o Debrief – Patients should be given the opportunity to have a face to face or virtual debrief several weeks after pregnancy loss. This gives them the opportunity to discuss issues that may not have been addressed previously or have arisen in the aftermath of the lost pregnancy.

o Signposting to support groups – This can be done immediately following treatment and following debrief.

References

1. Hoey, R, Allan, K. Does speculum examination have a role in assessing bleeding in early pregnancy? *Emerg Med J* 2004; 21(4): 461–3.

2. Barnhart, KT, Simhan, H, Kamelle, SA. Diagnostic accuracy of ultrasound above and below the beta-hCG discriminatory zone. *Obstet Gynecol* 1999; 94(4): 583–7.

3. Condous, G, Okaro, E, Bourne, T. The conservative management of early pregnancy complications: a review of the literature. *Ultrasound Obstet Gynecol* 2003; 22(4): 420–30.

4. National Institute for Health and Care Excellence (NICE). Ectopic pregnancy and miscarriage: diagnosis and initial management. NICE Guideline [CG126]. 2019. Available at: www.nice.org.uk/guidance/ng126

5. Bourne, T, Bottomley, C. When is a pregnancy nonviable and what criteria should be used to define miscarriage? *Fertil Steril* 2012; 98(5): 1091–6.

6. Graziosi, GCM, Mol, BW, Ankum, WM, Bruinse, HW. Management of early pregnancy loss. *Int J Gynaecol Obstet* 2004; 86(3): 337–46.

7. May, W, Gülmezoglu, AM, Ba-Thike, K. Antibiotics for incomplete abortion. *Cochrane Database Syst Rev* 2007; 17(4): CD001779.

8. Royal College of Obstetricians and Gynaecologists (RCOG). The investigation and treatment of couples with recurrent first-trimester and second-trimester miscarriage. Green-top Guideline No. 17. 2011. Available at: www.rcog.org.uk/en/guidelines-research-services/guidelines/gtg17/#:~:text=%20Recurrent%20Miscarriage%2C%20Investigation%20and%20Treatment%20of%20Couples,Investigation%20and%20Treatment%20of%20Couples%20with%20Recurrent%20Miscarriage

9. Empson, M, Lassere, M, Craig, J, Scott, J. Therapy for miscarriage associated with antiphospholipid antibody or lupus anticoagulant. *Cochrane Database Syst Rev* 2000.

10. Walker, JJ. Ectopic pregnancy. *Clin Obstet Gynecol* 2007; 50(1): 89–99.

11. Kaplan, BC, et al. Ectopic pregnancy: prospective study with improved diagnostic accuracy. *Ann Emerg Med* 1996; 28(1): 10–17.

12. Lewis, G, Drife, J. Why mothers die 1997–1999. Fifth Report. Confidential Enquiry into Maternal Deaths United Kingdom, 2001. Available at: https://elearning.rcog.org.uk/sites/default/files/Gynaecological%20emergencies/CEMACH_Why_Mothers_Die_00-02_2004.pdf

13. Sivalingam, VN, Duncan, WC, Kirk, E, Shephard, LA, Horne, AW. Diagnosis and management of ectopic pregnancy. *J Fam Plann Reprod Health Care* 2011; 37(4): 231–40.

14. Morin, L, et al. Ultrasound evaluation of first trimester pregnancy complications. *J Obstet Gynaecol Canada* 2005; 27(6): 2005.

15. Elson, CJ, Salim, R, Potdar, N, Chetty, M, Ross, JA, Kirk, EJ. Diagnosis and management of ectopic pregnancy. *BJOG* 2016; 123(13): e15–e55.

16. Horne, AW, McBride, R, Denison, FC. Normally rising hCG does not predict live birth in women presenting with pain and bleeding in early pregnancy. *Eur J Obstet Gynaecol Reprod Biol* 2011; 156(1); 120–1.

17. Stovall, TG, Kellerman, AL, Ling, FW, Buster, JE. Emergency department diagnosis of ectopic pregnancy. *Ann Emerg Med* 1990; 19(10): 1098–103.

18. Sammel, MD, Chung, K, Zhou, L, Guo, W. Decline of serum human chorionic gonadotropin and spontaneous complete abortion: defining the normal curve. *Obstet Gynecol* 2004; 104(5): 975–81.

19. Nama, V, Manyonda, I. Tubal ectopic pregnancy: diagnosis and management. *Arch Gynaecol Obstet* 2009; 279(4): 443–53.

20. Cheng, X, et al. Comparison of the fertility outcome of salpingotomy and salpingectomy in women with tubal pregnancy: a systematic review and meta-analysis. *PLoS One* 2016; 11(3): e0152343.

21. Elson, CJ, Salim, R, Potdar, N, Chetty, M, Ross, JA Kirk, EJ. Diagnosis and management of ectopic pregnancy. *Int J Obstet Gynaecol* 2016; 123(13): e15–e55.

22. Irvine, LM, Padwick, ML. Serial serum HCG measurements in a patient with an ectopic pregnancy: a case for caution. *Hum Reprod* 2000; 15(7): 1646–7.

Ovarian Surgery, Menopause Hormone Therapy and Contraception

Peter J O'Donovan, Charles P O'Donovan

CASE COMMENTARY

Swati Jha

Successful Claim

JS v Morey (Out of Court settlement) 1 July 2020

The Claim

The claimant made the case that it was substandard care and a breach of duty to start her on the combined oral contraceptive (COC) pill as she had a clear family history of vascular disease. Because of this breach, the claimant suffered a DVT with its consequent effects.

The Summary

The claimant was 16 years old when she attended to see her GP. She was accompanied by her mother. The claimant's mother made the GP aware that she herself had suffered a DVT at the age of 19 and her father (the claimant's grandfather) had also suffered a DVT previously. The defendant denied that this information had been given by the claimant or her mother. A claim was brought against the practice nurse and GPs at the practice (all seven) as it was not possible to see who had signed off the prescription. The claimant developed a large DVT in her left leg eight months after commencement of the COC pill. As a result, she had to undergo venography, thrombectomy, and thrombolysis of her affected leg, with stenting of the iliac vein, ongoing medication and permanent pain due to post-thrombotic syndrome. She also suffered PTSD due to the surgical treatment required and was under the care of the mental health team. It was also claimed she would be unable to fulfil her career ambitions of being a social worker and maintain employment owing to her pain, as she would only be able to undertake a sedentary part-time job.

The Judgement

The case was settled out of court, with evidence presented she was additionally at risk of ulceration of her leg. The settlement agreed was for £1 million. This was initially pleaded on provisional damages but was subsequently settled on a full and final basis when the claimant was expecting her second child.

In the case of Melissa v Guy's and St Thomas' NHS Foundation Trust, the claimant went into hospital for a total abdominal hysterectomy for fibroids and she was informed her ovaries would not be removed as she was only 38 years old at the time of surgery. She had her ovaries removed as part of the surgery following discussion on the day of surgery and subsequently suffered psychological and physical effects from the oophorectomy and required long-term HRT with the added risks of breast cancer and thromboembolic disease.

Unsuccessful Claim

Joanne Lloyd v Liverpool Women's NHS Foundation Trust

The Claim

The claimant underwent a right salpingo-oopherectomy, but it was later identified there was still a remnant of ovarian tissue in situ post-surgery. It was claimed there had been a breach of duty in failing to ensure that the ovary was completely removed, and failing to identify that the ongoing problems were due to the remaining ovary.

The Summary

The claimant presented with acute abdominal pain and on an ultrasound scan was found to have a large ovarian cyst on the right side. She had a past history of removal of the left ovary for torsion and twisting. A plan was made for an elective laparoscopic removal of the cyst. The risks of the procedure were duly discussed. At the time of surgery, due to technical complexity, the procedure was converted from a laparoscopic to an open laparotomy and a removal of the right tube and ovary performed. There were significant adhesions noted at the time of the surgery, making it unsafe to proceed with laparoscopic removal of the ovary/cyst. The claimant subsequently presented to her GP five months after the removal with a further ovarian cyst on the same side. She also continued to have periods, suggestive of some degree of active ovarian tissue, and went on to have a hysterectomy with removal of the remnants of the ovarian tissue. This was a technically very difficult operation and the consultant performing surgery had to ask for the assistance of another gynaecologist, due to adhesions, to check there was no ovarian tissue buried within the adhesions. A very small portion of ovarian tissue was identified within the ovarian ligament itself following microscopic histological investigation.

The defendant made the case that this remnant of ovarian tissue was of embryogenic origin whereas it was the claimant's case that ovarian tissue had been left behind at the time of surgery, i.e. inadequate primary removal, and that instead of an oophorectomy, an ovarian cystectomy with peeling of the ovarian cyst had been performed instead.

The Judgement

It was accepted in judgement that there were significant adhesions encountered during surgery, especially in the pelvic area, making surgery technically difficult, even though this was not documented. This was based on the grounds that surgery had to be converted to an open laparotomy. This was a mitigating factor in the initial surgery. It was also ruled that the claimant had not reviewed the histology report adequately, as this revealed ovarian tissue only microscopically. It was admitted that when there were significant adhesions it may not be possible to know if all the ovarian tissue has been removed. In this case the remnant ovary was either due to a remnant ovary syndrome or failure to remove the entire ovary due to dense pelvic adhesions, neither of which was a breach of duty. There was also criticism of the expert witness for the defendant and their lack of rigour while preparing their report.

The judgement was in favour of the defendant.

Legal Commentary

Eloise Power

JS v Morey (Unreported, Lawtel AM0203698, 5 September 2019)

This case involved a claimant who was aged 16 at the date of injury and who suffered a large DVT in her left leg after prescription of the combined contraceptive pill, notwithstanding a strong family history of vascular disease which (on the claimant's case) had been provided to the prescriber.

The risk of vascular disease consequent upon the use of the contraceptive pill is well-known and has been the subject of high-profile product liability litigation in *XYZ and others v Schering Health Care Limited and others* [2002] EWHC 1420, where Mackay J held that the claimants had failed to establish that any of the "third generation" combined oral contraceptives presented any increased relative risk of venous thromboembolism in comparison with "second generation" products. As the Court observed in *XYZ*: *"There exist alternatives to oral contraception. Almost from the outset it was recognised as carrying risks accompanying the benefits it brought to those who took it. There has been a more or less continuous debate for 40 years in medical circles as to the nature and degree of those risks"* [para 6] and, in relation to the epidemiological evidence: *"science has failed to give women clear advice spoken with one voice"* [para 33].

In the light of the judgement in *XYZ*, claims arising from the use of oral contraceptives are more likely to be brought on the basis of unsuitable patient selection/a failure to warn about individual patients' increased risk (as seen in the case of *JS v Morey*) than on the basis of alleged generic defects in the products themselves.

In the case of *JS v Morey*, the issue of the future risk of ulceration of the leg fell for consideration. The expert haematologists and vascular surgeons reached agreement as to the future risk of ulceration, and the claimant indicated that the Particulars of Claim would be amended to plead provisional damages. Under section 32A of the Senior Courts Act 1981 (or section 51 of the County Courts Act 1984) the Court has the power to make an order that future damages should be awarded at a future date in the event that a claimant develops *"some serious disease"* or suffers *"some serious deterioration in his physical or mental condition"* as a result of the tort which gave rise to the cause of action. Essentially, this means that the claimant can come back for further damages if a specified risk eventuates.

The circumstances which may justify an award of provisional damages have been considered in various cases. In *Wilson v Ministry of Defence* [1991] 1 All ER 638, the Court refused to exercise its discretion in favour of a provisional damages order in circumstances where the risk faced by the claimant amounted to an ordinary continuing deterioration (osteoarthritis) rather than a *"clear and severable risk"*. Although a risk which gives rise to a provisional damages award has to be measurable rather than fanciful, it does not have to be a high probability risk: in *Mitchell v Royal Liverpool and Broadgreen University Hospitals NHS Trust*, Lawtel 11 September 2008 (unreported), a risk of serious complications of syringomyelia assessed at 0.15% was held to be measurable rather than fanciful, and the Court permitted the claimant to amend his pleadings to include a claim for provisional damages. In *Chewings v Williams* [2009] EWHC 2490, the Court held that a 2% risk of amputation was measurable rather than fanciful. Where the risk is more likely than not to occur, a full and final award (factoring in damages for the risk) rather than a provisional damages award will be appropriate: *Curi v Colina*, Times, 14 October 1998.

In practice, defendants are often reluctant to agree to a settlement on a provisional damages basis as it exposes them to potentially open-ended costs and damages in the future. Some claimants prefer the certainty of achieving a full and final settlement – particularly where a somewhat larger sum is on offer in exchange for abandoning a provisional damages claim, as was the case in *JS v Morey*. This course of action is not without risk. Claimants who accept a full and final damages award in these circumstances should be carefully advised that they will not be able to come back for more money if the risk of serious disease/serious deterioration eventuates, and that in this situation they are likely to be undercompensated.

On the facts in *JS v Morey*, the claimant had already developed post-thrombotic syndrome and was in considerable pain which left her unable to maintain full-time employment, and had also suffered a serious psychiatric injury. It is understandable that in these circumstances, both parties regarded it as appropriate to settle the case by way of a full and final award rather than on a provisional damages basis, as the onset of ulceration may not have transformed the value of the matter. Similar pragmatic settlements are reached in many cases in which a claim for provisional damages has been pleaded.

Joanne Lloyd v Liverpool Women's NHS Foundation Trust (17 May 2019, Unreported)

This interesting judgement dealt with an allegation that a consultant gynaecologist had failed to remove the claimant's complete right ovary in the course of a right salpingo-oophorectomy. The claimant also alleged that the gynaecologist had failed to recognise that her post-operative symptoms had been caused by the incomplete removal of the ovary. The defendant's case was that if pelvic adhesions were present, it would not be negligent to have inadvertently missed a remnant of ovarian tissue.

The expert instructed by the defendant argued that there were dense pelvic adhesions due to previous surgery and recurrent ovarian cysts. The expert for the claimant argued that the adhesions were on the opposite side and were unrelated to the right ovary, and that any adhesions which involved the ovary should have been recorded in the operation note. On the facts, the Court found that the reason why the treating gynaecologist had abandoned the laparoscopy in favour of a laparotomy was the presence of adhesions. The Court accepted the treating gynaecologist's evidence that there were adhesions in the pelvic region.

In finding for the defendant, the Court placed considerable weight upon the expert evidence. The defendant's expert evidence was strongly preferred. The following criticisms were made of the claimant's expert evidence:

> The expert *"jumped to conclusions, e.g. the absence of histology and the ramifications and how he had improperly concluded the mechanics of the operation namely the peeling away of the cyst,*

coupled with an approach that at times was quite argumentative when presented with assertions that there were shortcomings in his report, namely the absence of reference to notes which were perhaps unlikely to be material in any event" [para 82].

The expert's first report *"was seemingly prepared as an 'opening report' and he seemed relatively unconcerned that he had apparently prepared a final version of this report which had not found itself into the trial bundle and on the face of it had not brought a copy of that up-to-date report to court, but which in any event was never disclosed during the trial. This was in my judgment a lack of rigour that one would have expected of an expert giving evidence"* [para 83–84].

These findings can be compared with the criticisms of experts by Turner J in the case of *MC and another v Birmingham Women's NHS Foundation Trust* [2016] EWHC 1334 (QB), which are discussed in the legal commentary at Chapter 11. It can readily be seen that it is crucial for experts to familiarise themselves with all documentation in the case, to take an objective rather than an argumentative stance and to ensure that they are aware of the contents of the final trial bundle. The duties of experts are considered in more detail at Chapter 3.

Clinical Commentary

Peter J O'Donovan and Charles P O'Donovan

Management of Suspected Ovarian Masses in Pre-menopausal Women: Good Practice Guidance

Background and Introduction

These guidelines are to assist clinicians with the assessment and appropriate management of suspected ovarian masses in pre-menopausal women [1].

Up to 10% of women have some form of surgery during their lifetime for the presence of an ovarian mass. In pre-menopausal women, almost all ovarian masses and cysts are benign. The differentiation between a benign and malignant ovarian mass in pre-menopausal women can be problematic, with no test being clearly superior in terms of accuracy. The underlying management rationale is to minimise patient morbidity by:

a) Conservative management where possible.
b) Use of laparoscopic techniques where appropriate, thus avoiding laparotomy where possible.
c) Referral to a gynaecological oncologist where appropriate.

Preoperative Assessment of Women with Ovarian Masses

A thorough medical history should be taken from the woman with specific attention given to risk factors or protective factors for ovarian malignancy and a family history of ovarian or breast cancer. Symptoms suggesting possible ovarian malignancy, such as persistent abdominal distension; appetite change, including increased satiety; pelvic or abdominal pain; increased urinary urgency and/or frequency, should be specifically considered.

A careful physical examination is essential and should include an abdominal and vaginal examination and the presence or absence of local lymphadenopathy.

Although clinical examination has poor sensitivity in the detection of ovarian masses (15–51%) its importance lies in the evaluation of mass tenderness, mobility, nodularity and ascites.

Further Investigations

A serum CA-125 assay does not need to be undertaken in all premenopausal women when an ultrasonographic diagnosis of a simple ovarian cyst has been made.

Lactate dehydrogenase (LDH) α-feta protein and hCG should be measured in all women under age 40 with a complex ovarian mass because of the possibility of germ cell tumours.

Pelvic ultrasound scan is the single most effective way of evaluating an ovarian mass, with transvaginal ultrasonography being preferable due to its increased sensitivity over transabdominal ultrasound.

At the present time, the use of computerised tomography and MRI for assessment of ovarian masses does not improve the sensitivity or specificity obtained by transvaginal ultrasonography in the detection of ovarian malignancy.

Management

Women with small (less than 50 mm diameter) simple ovarian cysts generally do not require follow-up as these cysts are very likely to be physiological and almost always resolve within three menstrual cycles.

Women with simple ovarian cysts of 50–70 mm in diameter should have yearly ultrasound follow-up and those with larger simple cysts should be considered for either further imaging (MRI) or surgical intervention.

Ovarian cysts that persist or increase in size are unlikely to be functional and may warrant surgical management.

Surgical Treatment

The laparoscopic approach for elective surgical management of ovarian masses presumed to be benign is associated with lower post-operative morbidity and shorter recovery time and is preferred to laparotomy in suitable patients.

Laparoscopic management is cost-effective because of the associated earlier discharge and return to work.

In the presence of large masses with solid components, (for example large dermoid cysts) laparotomy may be appropriate.

Laparoscopic management of presumed benign ovarian cysts should be undertaken by a surgeon with suitable experience and appropriate equipment, whenever local facilities permit.

Aspiration of ovarian cysts, either vaginally or laparoscopically, is less effective and is associated with a high rate of recurrence.

Spillage of cyst contents should be avoided where possible as pre-operative and intra-operative assessment cannot absolutely preclude malignancy.

Consideration should be given to the use of a tissue bag to avoid peritoneal spill of cystic contents, bearing in mind the likely pre-operative diagnosis.

The possibility of removing an ovary should be discussed with the woman pre-operatively.

Management of Ovarian Cysts in Post-menopausal Women: Good Practice Guidance

Background and Introduction

Clinicians should be aware of the guidelines published by the RCOG on ovarian cysts in post-menopausal women [2].

Clinicians should be aware of the different presentations and significance of ovarian cysts in post-menopausal women.

In post-menopausal women presenting with acute abdominal pain, the diagnosis of an ovarian cyst accident should be considered (e.g. torsion, rupture, haemorrhage).

It is recommended that ovarian cysts in post-menopausal women should be initially assessed by measuring CA-125 level and transvaginal ultrasound scan.

Initial Assessment

A thorough medical history should be taken, with specific attention to risk factors and symptoms suggestive of ovarian malignancy, and a family history of ovarian, bowel or breast cancer.

Where family history is significant, referral to the Regional Cancer Genetics Service should be considered.

Appropriate tests should be carried out in any post-menopausal woman who has developed symptoms within the last 12 months that suggest irritable bowel syndrome, particularly in women over 50 years of age or those with a significant family history of ovarian, bowel or breast cancer.

A full physical examination is essential and should include body mass index, abdominal examination to detect ascites and characterise any palpable mass, and a vaginal examination.

Further Investigations

CA-125 should be the only serum tumour marker used for primary evaluation as it allows the Risk of Malignancy Index (RMI) of ovarian cysts in post-menopausal women to be calculated [3].

CA-125 should not be used in isolation to determine if a cyst is malignant. While a very high value may assist in reaching a diagnosis, normal value does not exclude ovarian cancer due to the non-specific nature of the test. There is currently not enough evidence to support the routine use of a tumour marker such as CA-19.9, LDH and HCG to assess the risk of malignancy in post-menopausal women's cysts.

A transvaginal ultrasound scan is the single most effective way of evaluating ovarian cysts in post-menopausal women. Transabdominal ultrasound should not be used in isolation. It should be used to provide supplementary information to the transvaginal ultrasound, particularly when the ovarian cyst is large or beyond the field of view of the transvaginal ultrasound.

On transvaginal scanning, the morphological description and subjective assessment of the ultrasound features should be clearly documented to allow calculation of risk of malignancy.

Transvaginal ultrasound scans should be performed by trained clinicians with expertise in gynaecological imaging.

Colour flow Doppler studies are not essential for the routine initial assessment of ovarian cysts in post-menopausal women.

CT, MRI and PET-CT scans are not recommended for the initial evaluation of ovarian cysts in post-menopausal women. MRI scans should be used as a second-line imaging modality for the characterisation of indeterminate ovarian cysts where ultrasound is inconclusive.

Management

Asymptomatic, simple, unilateral, unilocular ovarian cysts, less than 5 cm in diameter, have a low risk of malignancy. In the presence of normal CA-125 levels these cysts can be managed conservatively, with a repeat evaluation in four to six months. It is reasonable to discharge these women from follow-up after one year if the cyst remains unchanged or reduces in size, with normal CA-125, taking into consideration the women's wishes and surgical fitness.

If a woman is symptomatic, further surgical evaluation is necessary.

A woman with a suspicious or persistent complex adnexal mass needs surgical evaluation.

Aspiration is not recommended for the management of ovarian cysts in post-menopausal women except for the purposes of symptom control in women with advanced malignancy who are unfit to undergo surgery or further intervention.

Surgical Treatment

Laparoscopic management of ovarian cysts in post-menopausal women should be undertaken by surgeons with suitable experience and should comprise bilateral salpingo-oophorectomy rather than cystectomy.

Women undergoing laparoscopic salpingo-oophorectomy should be counselled pre-operatively that a full staging laparotomy will be required if evidence of malignancy is revealed.

Where possible, the surgical specimen should be removed without intraperitoneal spillage in a laparoscopic retrieval bag via the umbilical port. This results in less post-operative pain and a quicker retrieval time than when using lateral ports of the same size. Transvaginal extraction of the specimen is also acceptable, if the surgeon has the available expertise.

All ovarian cysts that are suspicious of malignancy in a post-menopausal woman, as indicated by a RMI I greater than or equal to 200, CT findings, clinical assessment or findings at laparoscopy require a full laparotomy and staging procedure.

If a malignancy is revealed during laparoscopy or from subsequent histology, it is recommended that the woman be referred to a cancer centre for further management.

The appropriate location for the management should reflect the structure of cancer care in the United Kingdom. All such cases should be formally discussed at a gynaecological cancer MDT.

While a general gynaecologist might manage women with a low risk of malignancy (RMI I less than 200) in a general gynaecology or cancer unit, women who are at higher risk should be managed in a cancer centre by a trained gynaecological oncologist, unless the MDT review is not supportive of a high probability of ovarian malignancy.

Risks of Hormone Replacement Therapy

Breast Cancer

Breast cancer is the most common cancer in women and today there are estimated to be 550,000 women in the United Kingdom living with breast cancer. Female sex and age are the most important risk factors, but family history, particularly in association with the BRCA1 and BRCA2 gene mutations, is associated with a higher risk of developing breast cancer. Personal factors must be considered; alcohol intake and obesity are considered to be risk factors, while physical activity and breast feeding may be protective. Hormone therapy has been implicated as potential risk factor in randomised and observational studies.

Currently, the question of linkage between breast cancer and hormone replacement therapy used in women over the age of 50 is complex. NICE suggests that we explain to women that HRT with oestrogen alone is associated with little or no change in risk of breast cancer but hormone replacement therapy with oestrogen and progesterone can be associated with an increase in risk [4].

The risk of breast cancer attributable to hormone therapy is small, is duration-dependent and decreases after stopping.

Venous Thromboembolism

Venous thromboembolism is a condition comprising of deep venous thrombosis and pulmonary embolism precipitated by conditions such as immobility, compression of the blood vessel, or increased blood viscosity which causes blood flow to slow.

Hormone replacement therapy is associated with a two-fold increased risk of VTE, which appears to be greatest in the first year of use and in those with increased body mass index.

Oral HRT must undergo first-pass metabolism in the liver, and as such affects the blood clotting cascade by increasing resistance to protein C and protein S (anticoagulants) and increasing fibrinogen, and as a result increasing the clotting risk. Transdermal preparations are absorbed directly into the blood stream through the skin, bypassing this metabolism, and at standard doses are associated with VTE risk no greater than baseline.

Transdermal preparations should be considered in those women with a BMI greater than 30 kg/m^2, but those women at high risk of VTE (e.g. inherited thrombophilias) should be referred to a specialist before considering HRT.

Risks Associated with the Combined Oral Contraceptive Pill

Minor Side Effects

Some women using the combined oral contraceptive (COC) pill may report undesirable side effects resulting from hormone exposure. Fortunately, these symptoms occur significantly less with currently available low-dose COC compared with older preparations. Whilst side effects can be intense in the first few months of use, they frequently resolve with time. Commonly reported side effects such as headache, nausea, dizziness and breast tenderness have actually been reported at the same rate in both treatment groups of placebo and controlled clinical trials [5].

Irregular, unpredictable bleeding can be troublesome. Differences in patterns of bleeding and spotting can vary by COC but generally breakthrough bleeding most frequently occurs after initiation ranging from 10–30% in the first month, decreasing to about 10% by the third [6].

Weight gain has often been perceived to be associated with COC use and is frequently cited as a reason for discontinuation, even though no causal association has been found [7].

The experience of minor side effects, in addition to consideration of more serious complications, can influence both a woman's desire to initiate COC as well as her willingness to continue. Each woman should be provided with appropriate information and offered counselling on the full range of contraceptive options available to her, to ensure an informed choice.

Pregnancy

Perfect use of COC is associated with a failure rate as low as 0.3%, while typical-use failure rates, which better describe COC performance, in practice are as high as 9% [8].

While oral contraception is very effective, the experience of unintended pregnancy as a result of incorrect or inconsistent COC use or from a rare method failure carries significant public health consequences. Women should be advised of the real risks of unintended pregnancy when choosing COC, particularly where other reversible contraceptive methods offering greater protection are available. It should be highlighted, however, that lack of compliance can result in significant risk of unintended pregnancy among COC users [9].

Thromboembolism

The incidence of VTE (8–10/10,000 women-years exposure) and arterial thrombotic events, including both myocardial infarction and stroke (1–4/10,000) are very rare among healthy, reproductive-age users of modern COC. In addition, these incidences are significantly lower than those reported with pregnancy. While the relative risk of VTE is increased approximately three-fold and the relative risk for thrombotic stroke is increased two-fold compared to non-users, the absolute risk for these serious adverse effects among women using COC remains low. Risk of VTE appears to be highest in the first year of COC exposure and decreases with greater duration of use. No differences in the relative risk of myocardial infarction or haemorrhagic stroke have been reported in COC use versus non-use [10,11].

Evidence-based guidelines regarding the safety of COC for use by women with various characteristics and physiological or medical conditions are available to ensure that women's options for effective contraception are not unnecessarily limited due to overestimations of risk [12].

Causes of Litigation

The reasons for litigation arising from both ovarian surgery and also risks of HRT and contraception are as follows:

a) Failure to adhere to national guidelines issued by NICE or the RCOG.

Areas of failure are:

a) Inadequate pre-operative counselling and choices provided.

b) Pre-operative investigations, specifically misinterpretation of investigations. These are more common if cases are not discussed at MDT meetings in the case of ovarian or adnexal masses.

c) Consent and discussion of complications. A full range of consent, including discussing alternatives such as conservative management and conservative surgery to more radical surgical options have to be discussed with the patient, ensuring this includes the full range of options. Also, sufficient information has to be given regarding complications relating to various forms of surgery along with known outcomes if available [13,14,15].

d) Lack of adequate training of surgeons, specifically in various forms of endoscopic surgery, both laparoscopic and hysteroscopic along with specialist areas of training to do with gynaecological cancer management.

e) Specific complications arising from certain types of surgery, such as bladder, bowel or vascular injuries along with failure to adequately follow-up with patients to provide assurance regarding outcomes of surgery..

Avoidance of Litigation

The basic principles of avoiding litigation whilst managing women with ovarian pathology or prescribing HRT/contraception include:

a) Good communication, specifically information regarding therapies provided and also adherence to both national and local guidelines and protocols.

b) Consent. All patients undergoing treatment should be given appropriate information on the nature and purpose of the treatment, benefits, alternatives and risks, and the consent process must comply with the hospital's consent policy. Good practice in consent is more than merely obtaining a patient's signature on the consent form. The consent form is a useful prompt for ensuring that benefits and risks are discussed. On the other hand, a signed consent form is of no value if the patient does not understand what is written on it. Good risk management ensures that staff are aware of good practice in consent.

c) Staff training and development. Appropriate risk management in gynaecology also puts systems in place to ensure the competence and appropriate training of all professional staff and it is important to follow both hospital and national guidelines. It should include, specifically in outpatient clinics, the use of chaperones, obtaining consent, ensuring positive patient identification, logging of specimens dispatched to the laboratory and protecting confidentiality. Women specifically attending for contraception should be advised of alternative methods of contraception, including information regarding failure rates and compliance.

d) Pregnancy tests. These should be readily available in the outpatient or inpatient setting to make sure that this reduces the risk of a women undergoing surgical or medical treatments while having an undiagnosed pregnancy.

e) Operating theatres. Approximately 30% of all litigation relates to intraoperative problems. Gynaecology departments should actively seek to minimise harm to patients during the surgeon's learning process by facilitating supervision, mentorship, peer review and peer support. There should also be a very active system of patient safety incident reporting, including breach of consent, accidental injuries including perforation of viscus, medical errors, wrong patient/wrong procedure, equipment failure and surgical site infections. These should be actively audited and monitored, with regular meetings to learn how these events occurred and how they can be further reduced. A system of audit should feedback patient satisfaction scores to assess the competency of gynaecological surgeons.

f) When things go wrong. When things go wrong, the gynaecologist should be open with the patient. The gynaecologist should lead the way in sharing and learning from patient safety incidents [16, 17].

References

1. Royal College of Obstetricians and Gynaecologists (RCOG). Management of ovarian masses in premenopausal women. Green-top Guideline No. 62. London: RCOG; 2011.

2. Royal College of Obstetricians and Gynaecologists (RCOG). Management of ovarian cysts in postmenopausal women. Green-top Guideline No. 34. London: RCOG; 2016.

3. Tingulstad, S, Hagen, B, Skjeldestad, FE, Onsrud, M, Kiserud, T, Halvorsen, T, et al. Evaluation of a risk of malignancy index based on serum CA125, ultrasound findings and menopausal status in the preoperative diagnosis of pelvic masses. *Br J Obstet Gynaecol* 1996; 103: 826–31.

4. National Institute for Health and Care Excellence (NICE). Menopause: diagnosis and management of menopause. NICE guideline [NG23]. London: NICE; 2015. Available at: www.nice.org.uk/guidance/ng23

5. Coney, P, Washenik, K, Langley, RG, Di Giovanna, J, Harrison, D. Weight change and adverse event incidence with a low dose oral contraceptive: two randomised placebo controlled trials. *Contraception* 2001: 63(6) 297–302.

6. Endrikat, J, Muller, U, Dusterberg, B. A twelve-month comparative clinical investigation of two low dose oral contraceptives containing 30 micrograms ethinyl estradiol/75 micrograms gestodene and 4 micrograms ethinyl estradiol/75 micrograms gestodene with

respect to efficacy, cycle control and tolerance. *Contraception* 1997; 55(3): 131–7.

7. Gallo, M, Lopez, L, Grime, D, Carayon, F, Schulz, K, Helmerhorst, F. Combination contraceptives: effects on weight. *Cochrane Database Syst Rev* 2014; (1): CD 003987.

8. Trussell, J. Contraceptive failure in the United States. *Contraception* 2011; 83(5): 397–404.

9. Osterberg, L, Blaschke, T. Adherence to medication. *N Engl J Med* 2005; 353(5): 487–97.

10. Dinger, J, Bardenheuer, K, Heinemann, K. Cardiovascular and general safety of a 24-day regime of drospirenone containing oral contraceptive: final results from the international active surveillance study of women taking oral contraceptives. *Contraception* 2014; 89(4): 253–63.

11. Peregallo Urrutia, R, Coeytaux, R, McBroom, A, Gierisch, J, Haurilesky, L, Moorman, P, et al. Risk of acute thromboembolic events with oral contraceptive use: a systemic review and met analysis: *Obstet Gynaecol* 2013; 122(2 part 1): 380–9.

12. World Health Organization (WHO). Medical eligibility criteria for contraception use. Geneva: WHO; 2010.

13. Lalchandini, S, Phillips, K. Laparoscopy entry techniques. In: *Complications in Gynaecological Surgery*, edited by Peter O'Donovan. London: Springer; 2008, 3, 20–33.

14. Ogah, J. Laparoscopic surgery. In: *Complications in Gynaecological Surgery*, edited by Peter O'Donovan. London: Springer; 2008, 8, 67–74.

15. Royal College of Obstetricians and Gynaecologists (RCOG). Obtaining valid consent. Clinical governance advice No. 6. London: RCOG; 2004.

16. Hammond, I, Kathigasu, K. Training assessment and competency in gynaecological surgery. *Best Pract Res Clin Obstet Gynaecol* 2006; 20: 173–87.

17. Gray, T, Jha, S, Bolton, H. 'Duty of candour' – The obstetrics and gynaecology perspective. *Obstet Gynaecol* 2019; 21: 165–8.

Incontinence Surgery and Bladder Care

Swati Jha

CASE COMMENTARY

Swati Jha

Successful Claim

Greenhorn v South Glasgow University Hospitals NHS Trust

The Claim

The claimant was 35 years old at the time of referral for stress urinary incontinence and the index surgery (in 1999). She had previously undergone a hysterectomy five years prior to the index event. Urodynamic studies confirmed mixed urinary incontinence and conservative treatment in the form of pelvic floor muscle training had failed to alleviate her symptoms. The patient was overweight with a BMI of 34. She was offered an open colposuspension which she agreed to. This case predates the synthetic midurethral slings when colposuspension was the standard surgical procedure offered for stress urinary incontinence. At the time of surgery, she suffered serious blood loss requiring embolisation of the internal iliac artery.

Damages were claimed on the grounds the supervising surgeon (staff grade) had been negligent in the supervision of an operation and had not established the experience of the lead surgeon (specialist registrar) for the procedure. It was also claimed that the injury occurring was a consequence of substandard care and due to the serious blood loss, she suffered neurological injury.

The Summary

The patient claimed that the blood loss was caused due to the specialist registrar taking stitches out with the usual operating field resulting in uncontrollable haemorrhage whilst performing the operation. It was also claimed that the trainee lacked the necessary experience to carry out the operation as the lead surgeon, given the case was deemed to be technically difficult in view of the patient's BMI. As a consequence of this excessive bleeding, the patient sustained neurological damage.

The defence claimed that the cause of the major haemorrhage was a suture needle injuring an artery in the pelvic floor which could be caused by any surgeon during a colposuspension and did not amount to negligence. Lack of experience of the lead surgeon was also denied as the trainee was sufficiently experienced to undertake the operation under supervision and it was denied that the bleeding was caused by inexperience or inadequate supervision. The senior surgeon could not have predicted that arterial injury leading to massive haemorrhage would occur.

The Judgement

Arterial bleeding requiring management with internal artery ligation was not a recognised risk of colposuspension as it was not mentioned or emphasised in the medical literature. This raised a prima facie case of negligence. Given this was not a known complication of this operation, it was no longer relevant how the injury occurred. This led to the conclusion that the trainee had been inadequately supervised. Had reasonable care and supervision been exercised the trainee would not have performed the manoeuvre which caused the arterial damage. It was also decreed that the senior surgeon had failed to appropriately establish that the trainee had the required expertise and adequate recent experience to carry out the procedure as the lead surgeon.

The judgement was in favour of the claimant and damages paid out.

Unsuccessful Claim

Haughey v Newry and Mourne Health and Social Care Trust

The Claim

The claimant underwent an open colposuspension in 1998. They complained of severe backpain following the procedure and an ultrasound scan the next day found hydronephrosis of the right kidney which was due to ureteric kinking. Further surgery was therefore undertaken following the diagnosis of this complication, the day after the initial surgery to remove some sutures and free the obstruction to the kidney. Removal of the sutures was carried out uneventfully and the claimant made a good recovery. At the time of removal, it was noted that the stitches were not through the bladder or the ureter. The claimant alleged that the ureteric obstruction was a consequence of the sutures being inserted too high and the surgeon undertaking the procedure did not have the adequate experience to perform the surgery.

The Summary

The claimant's expert argued that the obstruction could not occur unless the stitches had been incorrectly placed. However, the surgeon who removed the stitches stated that the stitches were correctly placed at the time of the initial surgery. The defendant's case was that the elevation of the bladder may have caused tethering and immobilisation through lack of elasticity due to previous scarring pre-disposing the ureter to kinking. Following a review of all the evidence, the Judge ruled that this was a known complication of the surgery and the surgery had not been carried out negligently. This judgement was appealed on the grounds that the Trial Judge took into account the evidence of the factual witnesses.

The claimant presented an expert witness whereas the defendants witnesses were the two surgeons involved in the original surgery and the surgeon involved in removal of the stitches in addition to another independent expert. It was suggested by the claimant that the evidence of the expert witness in a clinical negligence case should be preferred to the evidence of factual medical witnesses.

The Judgement

The court held that in contested clinical negligence cases the Court must consider independent expert evidence in conjunction with the evidence of the doctors involved in treatment. The evidence of an independent medical expert was not necessarily to be preferred over the factual evidence submitted in a particular case. Judgement in favour of the defendant was held which stated that, despite normal techniques, kinking can happen in rare instances.

The appeal was also dismissed.

Legal Commentary

Eloise Power

Greenhorn v South Glasgow University Hospitals NHS Trust [2008] CSOH 128

As a preliminary point, this case was determined under Scottish law. The Scottish legal system is separate and distinct from the legal system of England and Wales. Northern Ireland also has a separate legal system, and the Northern Irish case of *Haughey* is considered below. In relation to medical law, the key underlying principles are in general common across the United Kingdom (indeed, the landmark case of Montgomery is a Scottish matter but applies across the country), but the Court system and procedure are different. Medical practitioners should be aware that solicitors and barristers with English and Welsh practising certificates are not licensed to practise in Scotland or Northern Ireland.

Having said all of that, there is no reason to think that the Court of Session's judgement in Greenhorn would have been decided any differently in other areas of the United Kingdom. An important issue of principle in the judgement relates to the circumstances in which the Courts will draw a prima facie inference of negligence from the facts.

Prima Facie Inference of Negligence

This is a concept which often causes concern to medical practitioners. The Latin phrase "prima facie" literally means "at first face" or "at first appearance". When used in the legal context, it refers to evidence which is sufficient to prove a particular point unless it is rebutted.

On the facts in *Greenhorn*, the Court found that once serious arterial damage had been proved by the pursuer, that raised a prima facie inference of negligence. The defenders had failed to provide evidence to rebut this inference and the pursuer succeeded.

Although this argument succeeded in *Greenhorn* on the very extreme facts (there were no reported cases of serious arterial damage during colposuspension reported in the medical literature), there are many examples in the case law where similar arguments have failed on the facts. The *Greenhorn* judgement should be read in conjunction with *Hooper v Young* [1998] Lloyd's Rep Med 61, a Court of Appeal judgement which considered a case involving ureteric damage sustained in the course of a hysterectomy.

In *Hooper v Young*, the plaintiff relied upon another, similar, Latin concept: res ipsa loquitur, which means "the thing speaks for itself". On the facts, the Court of Appeal held that the injury (kinking by a suture) could have occurred with or without negligence. The concept of res ipsa loquitur had no place in the analysis, and there was no reason to infer that the plaintiff's injury had been caused by negligence.

How should we resolve these judgements? As barristers, we are all too well aware of the reality that Courts are unwilling to make assumptions and are generally slow to invoke concepts such as *res ipsa loquitur* or to hold that a particular injury amounts to *prima facie* evidence of negligence. The key lies in the evidence. In *Greenhorn*, the pursuer had suffered an exceptionally rare injury which was not described in any medical literature before the Court. In *Hooper*, the plaintiff had suffered a ureteric injury by a well-known mechanism, and there was no reason for the Court to draw the inference that it was caused by negligence. In short, physicians and medico-legal experts would be well advised to undertake research in the medical literature before arguing that a particular injury speaks for itself.

The concept of a *prima facie* case is also important when considering a different area, namely the approach which the Courts have taken to authoritative guidance (such as NICE guidance). Will a failure to follow NICE guidance amount to a prima facie case in negligence?

Haughey v Newry and Mourne Health and Social Care Trust [2013] NICA 78

This is a judgement of the Court of Appeal of Northern Ireland. The Northern Irish legal system is separate from the English and Welsh legal system and from the Scottish legal system, but (as with the case of *Greenhorn* above) there is no reason to think that the case would have been resolved differently in other United Kingdom jurisdictions. Indeed, the approach taken in the *Haughey* judgement is consistent with the approach taken by the Court of Appeal of England and Wales in *Hooper v Young*, which is considered above.

The case of *Haughey* raises similar issues to the case of *Greenhorn*, but it arguably delves deeper into the relevant legal principles (perhaps because the factual background was less extreme than in *Greenhorn)*. We will consider four principles arising from the *Haughey* judgement.

Principle 1: Approach to *res ipsa loquitur*

On the facts in *Haughey*, the plaintiff did not attempt to argue *res ipsa loquitur* in respect of the obstruction of the ureter. The Court of Appeal approved the following observation of the trial judge: *"he was doubtful whether it* [res ipsa loquitur] *could ever apply in a complex contested medical negligence case."*

The plaintiff's argument was more sophisticated: their case was that the trial judge should have considered whether obstruction of the ureter in the absence of misplacement of the sutures was *"a remote or theoretical possibility"* or due to a *"highly unlikely combination of circumstances."* Higgins LJ, giving judgement for the Court of Appeal, held that this was essentially an issue of fact and evidence for the trial judge, finding: *"Whether that was only a remote or theoretical possibility or due to a highly unlikely set of circumstances would depend on the nature of the evidence given on that issue."*

The effect of this approach is to limit the practical usefulness of *res ipsa loquitur* and analogous arguments: while it remains open to claimants to argue *res ipsa loquitur* and/ or to argue that there is only a remote or theoretical possibility that a particular injury could occur in the absence of negligence, care must be taken to ensure that such arguments are properly supported by the evidence.

Principle 2: Approach to Medical Literature

On the facts of this case, the Court of Appeal upheld the trial judge's finding that the medical literature was inconclusive upon the question of whether ureteric obstruction could occur in the absence of negligence – even though the Court accepted that *"the thrust of the literature was in favour of surgical error as the cause of ureteric obstruction"*. Particular consideration was given to literature which indicated that fibrosis from previous pelvic surgery could cause kinking of the ureter (this would amount to a non-negligent explanation for the complication).

Importantly, the Court of Appeal found that the trial judge *"was quite entitled to consider the literature in the context of the other evidence in the case namely the factual experiences of the medical witnesses, whom he believed, about cases that had not been reported and commented upon in the literature. To have rejected their honest testimony in favour of non-conclusive literature would not have been a satisfactory outcome."*

This finding lends support for a holistic approach in relation to the evidence in clinical negligence cases: it is ultimately for the Court to determine the weight which should be given to the factual evidence, expert evidence and scientific and medical literature in each case. We will consider this issue in more detail in Chapter 7 in relation to the important judgement in *Schembri v Marshall*, a case which concerns the approach which the Court should take to statistical evidence.

The finding also provides support for witnesses who wish to rely upon professional experience which goes beyond the published literature. On the facts of this case at least, the trial judge was prepared to accept the witnesses' professional experience and to give their experience considerable weight in arriving at his judgement.

Principle 3: Approach to Expert Evidence

The Court of Appeal held that *"In the field of clinical negligence expert evidence is relative. In some cases it can be conclusive but in other instances it may require to be considered in the context of the other evidence in the case."* The expert evidence *"has to be considered in the context of all the evidence"* and cannot be considered and acted upon *"in isolation from the other evidence in the case."*

This approach provides further support for the holistic role of the Court in weighing and considering all of the evidence in the case – not merely the expert evidence.

Principle 4: Finding an Expert in a Small World

Counsel for the plaintiff in the *Haughey* case made much of the fact that the defendant's lay witnesses and expert witness were known to one another due to the small numbers of urogynaecologists in practice in Northern Ireland at that time (according to the material presented to the Court, there were only six practising urogynaecologists within the jurisdiction). The Court rejected this approach:

> The fact that Northern Ireland is a small jurisdiction, that there are limited numbers of specialists, that they may be known to one another or members of the same specialist medical society are not of themselves reasons to deprive the parties of their expert advice or evidence. In the case of expert witnesses the declaration above cannot be taken lightly.

This issue has resonance beyond the Northern Irish jurisdiction. Given the highly specialised nature of clinical negligence practice, it is frequently the case in practice that the pool of available experts is tiny and that experts may be known to the lay witnesses. While this is not an ideal situation by any means, the approach taken in *Haughey* indicates that the mere fact that an expert knows a lay witness through work will not necessarily amount to a conflict of interest.

As a caveat to this, any relationship (including an ordinary working relationship) between an expert and a lay witness must be disclosed at the very earliest opportunity. In *EXP v Barker* [2017] EWCA Civ 63, the Court of Appeal of England and Wales upheld the trial judge's finding that the independence and objectivity of the defendant's expert witness (a consultant neuroradiologist) had been undermined by his failure to disclose that he had previously worked with the defendant and had co-authored papers with him.

Clinical Commentary

Swati Jha

Good Practice Guidance

Initial Assessment

When a patient presents with urinary incontinence, a detailed history and physical examination should be undertaken. The aim is to categorise the incontinence as stress, urgency or mixed urinary incontinence. Bladder diaries should be used in this initial assessment of women. Preliminary treatment is started on the basis of the predominant symptom presentation. Predisposing factors such as obesity, chronic cough, constipation should be identified, as these may need addressing before other treatments are commenced. An abdominal examination is an important component of this examination as occasionally an abdominal cause for the urinary leakage will be found, such as a mass arising either from the ovary or the uterus. At the initial assessment, digital examination to assess pelvic floor muscles should be undertaken. This allows judgement of whether pelvic floor muscle training will be beneficial. This is done on the Oxford scoring, where pelvic floor muscles are graded from 1 to 5 based on strength of contraction [1]. The urine should be tested with a dipstick to rule out infection. Where an infection is present or suspected, a course of antibiotics should be prescribed. Enquiry about voiding patterns and problems may identify high residual urine. Where women present symptoms of voiding problems, a post void bladder scan should be undertaken. If facilities to manage patients with voiding dysfunction do not exist locally, they should be referred. A symptom scoring and quality of life questionnaire should be used to assess the impact of urinary incontinence on activities of daily living. This is particularly helpful in women who have both urinary incontinence in conjunction with prolapse, to establish which is more bothersome. This also allows assessment of whether the treatments being offered are effective.

Concurrent Prolapse and Incontinence

Where patients present with concurrent urinary incontinence and prolapse, conservative treatment for urinary incontinence should be initiated. If the patient is more bothered by urinary incontinence than by a prolapse that is at or beyond the introitus, treatment for the prolapse should be considered prior to invasive treatments of the urinary incontinence. This is because prolapse is known to cause overactive bladder and obstructive voiding which needs to be addressed prior to any continence surgery. In addition, treatment of prolapse treats the urinary incontinence approximately one third of the time [2]. Therefore, a potential cause of dissatisfaction following concurrent incontinence and prolapse surgery is the argument that if the procedures had been done in two stages, the incontinence surgery may not have been required in the first place.

Best practice would always be to treat the most bothersome complaint first, but where both are present, and the prolapse is significant, i.e. at or beyond the introitus, most clinicians would treat the prolapse in preference to the incontinence for the reasons stated.

Further Investigations

Though most clinicians do perform urodynamic tests prior to invasive treatments for urinary incontinence, testing is not a mandatory requirement prior to surgical intervention for stress urinary incontinence. However, if this is not performed, assessment of bladder function through alternative means such as bladder diaries, voiding cystometry, symptom assessment questionnaires and demonstrable leakage on examination must be documented to explain the rationale for not performing these tests. Occasionally, patients will decline the urodynamic tests, and this too should be documented in the records.

In all cases where the patient describes stress urinary incontinence (SUI) in conjunction with urge-predominant mixed urinary incontinence, anterior compartment prolapse, voiding dysfunction or a history of past incontinence surgery, urodynamics should be performed routinely prior to surgical interventions.

Non-imaging urodynamics is routine, but in cases of recurrent SUI, consideration should be given to video urodynamics, particularly as it is useful to know whether patients have intrinsic sphincter deficiency or a hypermobile bladder neck.

Referral to Subspecialist

Referral to specialist services should be considered in the following situations:
- double incontinence (faecal and urinary incontinence)
- suspected neurological disease
- urogenital fistula
- persistent bladder pain syndrome not responding to initial therapy
- previous continence surgery
- previous cancer surgery/pelvic irradiation.

Management

Conservative Management

All patients should be given lifestyle advice as part of their physiotherapy or bladder retraining regime. This includes reduction of caffeine, modification of total fluid intake and losing weight where this is over a BMI of 30. They should also be offered a trial of supervised physiotherapy, with pelvic floor muscle training (PFMT) for at least three months as a first-line treatment. It is also important to emphasise at this point that the NICE recommendations are for supervised physiotherapy, though in someone with good pelvic floor muscles it could be argued that supervision would not provide added value. It is therefore essential to make a note of the pelvic floor tone in women who are not referred for supervised physiotherapy. In women who decline supervised physiotherapy, this should be clearly documented in the medical records. Bladder retraining should be for a minimum of six weeks.

In women who suffer complications from surgery, it is not uncommon for claimants to argue that if they had been offered conservative therapies they would have accepted and could therefore have avoided surgery, as success rates of up to 60% are quoted for PFMT alone [3,4].

NICE have issued guidance for women choosing to manage their problem through the use of absorbent containment products for long-term management [5].

Medical Management

Women with urgency symptoms should be offered medical treatment including anticholinergics or beta 2 agonists (Betmiga) and should be screened for contraindications and cautions before commencing. Women with genitourinary syndrome of the menopause (atrophy) should be offered intravaginal oestrogen.

When commenced on medications, these should be reviewed four to six weeks after commencing therapy, to assess satisfaction to treatment.

Multidisciplinary Team Discussion

All patients in whom invasive therapies for stress or urge incontinence is contemplated should be discussed at the MDT.

Invasive Treatment for Detrusor Overactivity and Overactive Bladder

Women not responding to conservative management of their overactive bladder symptoms should be offered urodynamic studies to see if they have underlying detrusor overactivity. Once confirmed, treatment in the form of bladder wall injection of Botulinum toxin A may be considered. If not confirmed, an MDT review should take place if intravesical Botox is being offered. Patients should be warned of the risk of voiding problems and the need for intermittent self-catheterisation. The initial starting dose recommended is 100 iu. Other treatments for detrusor overactivity include sacral nerve stimulation and percutaneous tibial nerve stimulation (PTNS), which is usually offered in specialised units. Augmentation cystoplasty and urinary diversion are both highly invasive operations that are reserved for patients where all other options have been exhausted.

Surgical Management of Stress Urinary Incontinence

In women with stress urinary incontinence who have exhausted conservative treatments and are considering surgery, the NICE patient decision aids should be utilised to promote shared decision-making. These should be used in conjunction with patient information leaflets to allow patients to reach a decision based on their personal values and choices. A detailed discussion of the pros and cons of each of the procedures, as well as the option of not operating and continuing to use continence pads, should be discussed with the patient.

It should be borne in mind that the guidelines being adhered to are the most up to date ones. For the treatment of stress urinary incontinence, in the recent NICE guidelines from 2019, there is an emphasis on offering patients all options for stress urinary incontinence. This poses the problems that not all surgeons can perform all procedures, but there needs to be clear documentation that this process ensued and where the procedure of choice was not available locally, a referral to alternative hospitals where the procedure the patient wishes is available.

Where women wish for a definitive cure, options include:

- colposuspension
- autologous fascial sling
- mid-urethral synthetic sling (MUSS)

Table 22.1. Complications of incontinence surgery

Infection

Bleeding and need for blood transfusion

Clots in legs and lungs (thrombosis)

Injury to bladder, bowels and ureters

Need for laparotomy

Voiding problems;, need for self-catheterisation

Overactive bladder symptoms

Failure

Recurrence

Failure to achieve the desired result

Chronic pain

Sexual problems

Hernia formation (*this risk is greater with autologous fascial sling procedures*)

Problems arising from synthetic mesh where a mid-urethral synthetic sling was used (*mesh exposure and extrusion into adjacent organs and the need for further surgery to deal with these complications should be discussed*)

Problems arising from non-dissolvable sutures if used for colposuspension (*suture migration and need for further surgery*)

Success and failure of each of these, as well as complications associated with continence surgery, should be discussed in detail. The complications that should be mentioned are shown in Table 22.1. The difference between the operations in terms of anaesthesia used, expected length of hospital stay, recovery post-surgery, the type and location of surgical incisions should be discussed.

If a MUSS is performed, a device made of type 1 polypropylene mesh should be used with high visibility for ease of insertion and revision. A retropubic device should be used in preference to an obturator device unless there are very specific clinical circumstances. An obturator device should not be routinely offered. The additional risks of mesh exposure into the vagina and extrusion into the bladder should be discussed and the implication of this, i.e. the need for further surgery, sometimes major to correct this problem. Patients should also be informed that it is a permanent implant and complete removal may not be possible.

Where a colposuspension is performed, a minimum of two stitches should be used to anchor the paravaginal tissue to the ileopectineal ligament. When a laparoscopic procedure is performed, this should be by a clinician who has adequate caseload of performing these procedures. In patients undergoing a colposuspension, where non-dissolvable stitch is used, patients should be informed of this and given the option of having a dissolvable stitch. Success rates quoted in literature of laparoscopic colposuspension is with the use of non-dissolvable suture. If dissolvable suture is used when performing a laparoscopic colposuspension, patients should also be informed of this, as this may impact on success rates.

Once given these choices, patients should be given ample opportunity to consider these before proceeding to surgery (cooling off period). Where surgery is not available locally, patients should be referred to the nearest specialist unit offering the procedure of choice for the patient.

With continence surgery, the consent should be viewed as a multi-stage process, with the first consultations aimed at educating patients about their options and encouraging them to complete decision aids and read the information leaflets before proceeding to decisions about surgical intervention.

Where patients are not willing to accept risks and complications associated with the aforementioned procedures, they may also be offered urethral bulking agents. The reduced effectiveness compared to the other surgical procedures should be made clear.

Recommendations are that patients are given documented information if they have any synthetic mesh or non-dissolvable suture used during surgery or if a urethral bulking agent is injected, so they know what has been implanted during the course of the procedure. This includes the following information:

- which mesh has been used (brand and unique identifiers of the device)
- which sutures were used
- which urethral bulking agent was used

All cases of continence surgery should be entered into a national registry/database.

Postoperatively and prior to discharge after major surgery, post-void residuals should be checked to ensure voiding has returned to normal or appropriate precautions for bladder emptying with either an indwelling catheter or self-catheterisation have been made.

All patients should be offered a follow-up appointment within six months. For women who have a MUSS, a vaginal examination should also be performed to rule out mesh exposure. Women should be advised to seek assistance in case of problems, recurrence of symptoms or complications arising in future. Women who report new onset symptoms after mesh surgery should be investigated for mesh-related complications. These symptoms include any of the following:

- pain provoked, such as with sexual intercourse and movement, or unprovoked occurring in the vagina
- urinary problems including recurrent infections, incontinence, retention or difficulty during voiding
- vaginal problems such as bleeding, discharge, dyspareunia or hispareunia
- symptoms of infection

Where it is confirmed that symptoms are related to mesh complications, patients should be referred to a specialist centre to manage the mesh complication.

Where incontinence surgery fails, they should be referred to a specialist centre for further management, particularly if they require recurrent incontinence surgery. If the patient does not wish further surgery, advice about further conservative management should be offered.

Post-operative Bladder Care

Post-operative assessment of voiding is important after continence surgery. Prolonged bladder overdistention in excess of 120% of normal bladder capacity can result in primary, temporary neurogenic detrusor dysfunction causing retention [6]. The use of an indwelling catheter should be for the shortest length of time to prevent a UTI. Protocols for a trial without catheter should be in place. This will typically involve removing the catheter at the optimal time (based on type of surgery undertaken), followed by instructions to the patient to void when they have a strong desire to pass urine or when four hours have passed (whichever occurs first). The volume of urine passed should be measured and the bladder scanned or catheterised to check the residual volume of urine within 15 minutes of voiding. The definitions of high residual volume vary, and some protocols will use a volume (usually of 100 ml) whereas others will use a residual greater than one third of the voided volume as abnormal. This measurement of the post-void residual will usually be carried out twice before assuming that voiding is normal. In women with high residuals, an indwelling catheter will usually be left in situ, or alternatively the patient will be taught clean intermittent self-catheterisation. The objective is to avoid overdistention and subsequent injury to the bladder.

Post-operative bladder care is relevant not just after incontinence surgery, but after any gynaecological surgery, regional anaesthesia and childbirth. There are currently no national guidelines for post-operative bladder care after gynaecological surgery and therefore local guidance should be developed and adhered to. These should be in keeping with the NICE guidelines on intrapartum and postpartum bladder care [7,8].

Failing to consider urinary retention following surgery, inadequate early monitoring of bladder emptying, failing to insert an indwelling catheter following prolonged over-distention and inadequate assessment of voiding dysfunction after prolonged catheterisation are all considered substandard care and can result in litigation.

Concurrent Incontinence and Prolapse Surgery

Urodynamic tests should be performed prior to concurrent incontinence and prolapse surgery and voiding problems ruled out.

When performing concurrent incontinence and prolapse surgery, there should be clear documentation of the reasons why incontinence and prolapse surgery were undertaken together. Patients should always be offered a two-stage procedure. Patients should be informed that if prolapse is treated first there is a possibility that the urinary incontinence may improve [2], though there is also a possibility that this may actually deteriorate or get worse as well. As surgical procedures for both conditions can cause voiding problems, it is also important to make them aware that it is difficult to know post-operatively whether the problems with voiding are caused by the prolapse or the incontinence surgery.

Patients should be warned of the increased risk of complication [9], as the patient is having two surgical procedures rather than one.

Training of Clinicians Undertaking Incontinence Work

Clinicians looking after women with urinary incontinence should be urogynaecologists or gynaecologists with a special interest in urogynaecology. If undertaking surgery for SUI, they should be able to demonstrate that they have had adequate training either as a trainee doctor or gained competence through the mentorship scheme as a consultant. In the United Kingdom, the various training programmes for doctors in training performing continence surgery are as follows:

- Advanced training skill modules (ATSM) in vaginal surgery
- Subspecialty training in urogynaecology

For consultants already in post, there is a training programme established by the British Society of Urogynaecology which allows them to acquire this training through a process of formal mentorship by another consultant [10].

They should also be able to demonstrate they maintain their skills through an adequate caseload which is evidenced through the appraisal process. They should be able to demonstrate they audit their outcomes for surgery and adhere to national recommendations for incontinence surgery, including the use of patient decision aids to promote shared decision-making and data entry into a national registry/database.

Going forwards, increasingly clinicians will be asked to demonstrate they are adequately trained to perform the incontinence surgeries they are undertaking. They may also be required to demonstrate they can perform the tests for incontinence as well, i.e. urodynamics.

Causes of Litigation

The reasons for litigation arising from continence surgery include the following:

- Failure to adhere to national guidance issued by NICE: given the emphasis on following guidelines, this continues to be a common cause of litigation, particularly if it is demonstrated that guidelines have not been adhered to.
- Pre-operative counselling/choices provided
- Pre-operative investigation/misinterpretation of investigations
- Consent and discussion of complications
- Lack of adequate training of surgeon
- Complications during/arising from the procedure and failure to advise of these complications (bladder, urethral, ureteric, nerve, rectal or blood vessel injury, fistula formation, voiding dysfunction and self-catheterisation, retropubic haematoma, prolapse problems following colposuspension, groin pain for trans-obturator tapes, need for a laparotomy, sexual dysfunction, failure, recurrence)
- Failure to follow-up
- Longer-term problems
- Inadequate assessment of voiding and failing to identify retention post-operatively
- In women undergoing concurrent prolapse and incontinence surgery: failing to offer a two-stage procedure, failing to adequately investigate before surgery, failing to advise of increased risk of complications, particularly voiding, and failing to advise that sometimes incontinence improves after prolapse surgery thereby mitigating the need for continence surgery altogether, can all result in litigation.

Avoidance of Litigation

To avoid litigation when performing continence surgery, ensure the following have been taken into account:

- Offer conservative treatment in the form of supervised PFMT.
- Ensure medical treatments are considered where appropriate.
- Ensure appropriate investigations, including but not exclusively urodynamic studies, are carried out prior to any surgical intervention.

- If offering surgery, shared decision-making tools such as patient decision aids (PDA) should be used.
- Patients should be given adequate time to consider their options.
- All risks and complications of the various options should be discussed, as well as the option of no treatment.
- Patients should be informed when they have synthetic mesh, non-dissolvable sutures or urethral bulking injected, as these are permanent materials that stay in a patient's body (they should be given written information on this where feasible).
- Patient information leaflets should be provided for all procedures in conjunction with the PDA.
- Ensure protocols are in place for the assessment of voiding post-operatively and clear guidelines for nursing staff for the management of high residuals as well as trial without catheter (TWOC).
- Post-operative bladder function should be documented in the medical records.
- Post-operative follow-up should be performed, and this should be face to face where a synthetic tape is used.
- Patients undergoing synthetic mid-urethral mesh procedures presenting with unusual symptoms should be reviewed promptly to rule out mesh complications.
- Where mesh complications arise, referral to specialist centres where this can be managed should be promptly expedited.
- Clinicians undertaking these procedures should be able to demonstrate they have had the training and maintain their caseload. Data for this surgery should be entered on a registry/database.
- Where concurrent incontinence and prolapse surgery is undertaken, ensure adequate precautions, as listed previously, have been taken.

References

1. Laycock, J. Pelvic muscle exercises: physiotherapy for the pelvic floor. *Urol Nurs* 1994; 14(3): 136–40.

2. Borstad, E, Abdelnoor, M, Staff, AC, Kulseng-Hanssen, S. Surgical strategies for women with pelvic organ prolapse and urinary stress incontinence. *Int Urogynecol J* 2010; 21(2): 179–86.

3. Dumoulin, C, Hay-Smith, J. Pelvic floor muscle training versus no treatment, or inactive control treatments, for urinary incontinence in women. *Cochrane Database Syst Rev* 2010; (1): CD005654.

4. Dumoulin, C, Hay-Smith, J, Habee-Seguin, GM, Mercier, J. Pelvic floor muscle training versus no treatment, or inactive control treatments, for urinary incontinence in women: a short version Cochrane systematic review with meta-analysis. *Neurourol Urodyn* 2015; 34(4): 300–8.

5. National Institute for Health and Care Excellence (NICE). Urinary incontinence and pelvic organ prolapse in women: management. Nice guideline [NG123]. London: NICE; 2019.

6. Madersbacher, H, Cardozo, L, Chapple, C, Abrams, P, Toozs-Hobson, P, Young, JS, et al. What are the causes and consequences of bladder overdistension? ICI-RS 2011. *Neurourol Urodyn* 2012; 31 (3): 317–21.

7. National Institute for Health and Care Excellence (NICE). Postnatal care up to 8 weeks after birth. Clinical guideline [CG37]. London: NICE; 2015.

8. National Institute for Health and Care Excellence (NICE). Intrapartum care for healthy women and babies. Clinical guideline [CG190]. London: NICE; 2017.

9. van der Ploeg, JM, van der Steen, A, Oude, RK, van der Vaart, CH, Roovers, JP. Prolapse surgery with or without stress incontinence surgery for pelvic organ prolapse: a systematic review and meta-analysis of randomised trials. *BJOG* 2014; 121(5): 537–47.

10. British Society of Urogynaecology. BSUG Mentorship Scheme. 2020. Available at: https://bsug.org.uk/pages/information/ nonmesh-continence-surgery-mentorship-scheme/123

Vaginal Prolapse

Ian Currie

CASE COMMENTARY

Swati Jha

Successful Claim

Jane Duffett v Worcestershire Acute Hospitals NHS Trust (2007) Out of Court Settlement

The Claim

The claimant attended hospital with menorrhagia while at the same time trying to get pregnant. She had a second-degree uterine descent and underwent a vaginal hysterectomy even though she wished to try for a pregnancy. She claimed that all options for her menorrhagia had not been tried and she was not given alternative options to a hysterectomy, being informed this was her only option.

The Summary

The claimant had an elongate cervix coming down to the introitus and a cystocele. When she initially presented to her GP, she was managed conservatively with progesterone and ring pessaries. The pessary failed to control her symptoms, so she was referred to hospital. The defendant made the case it was reasonable to offer her a hysterectomy and she was fully aware of the implications on her fertility. The defendant denied that alternative treatments would have worked for the menorrhagia and therefore the hysterectomy was not causative of the other postoperative problems. Following the hysterectomy, she developed urinary and bowel incontinence, an adjustment disorder and also went on to develop vault granulation requiring further treatment under general anaesthetic, and subsequently a vault prolapse. She underwent a repair of the rectocele.

The Judgement

The urinary incontinence was not related to the hysterectomy and was due to previous childbirth. The claimant was unable to run her business following the procedure and was also unable to continue with her hobbies. The case was settled out of court with no breakdown of damages at £45,000.

In the case of M v Barking Havering & Redbridge University Hospital NHS Trust (2013), the claimant underwent a vaginal hysterectomy which was complicated by a postoperative bleed requiring a laparotomy. Four litres of blood were evacuated from the abdomen. She was subsequently found to have a right-sided ureteric obstruction which required further treatment. Her recovery was significantly delayed and she developed severe anxiety, panic depression and agoraphobia. It was claimed that the claimant had sustained injury to the bladder and kinking of the ureter and though she recovered from the physical issues, had been left with severe psychiatric problems resulting in an out-of-court settlement for £220,000.

Unsuccessful Claim

Sem v The Mid Yorkshire Hospitals NHS Trust [2005] EWHC 3469 (QB)

The Claim

The claimant, Mrs M, presented with uterine prolapse aged 41 years, for which she underwent a vaginal hysterectomy, McCall culdoplasty and an anterior with posterior vaginal wall repair. It was claimed that the defendant did not give any alternative options to the surgery, either surgical or non-surgical. The secondary allegations were that a non-absorbable suture (Ethibond) was used for the McCall culdoplasty without informing the claimant of this and a posterior repair was performed where it was not necessary.

The Summary

The claimant was diagnosed to be suffering from a somatoform disorder based on her past medical history. This is the presence of physical symptoms that suggest a general medical condition but are not fully explained by the condition or other mental health disorders or the use of substances. In this condition there is no medical condition to account for the physical symptoms. When she presented with vaginal prolapse, she was referred to see a urogynaecologist. She also had problems with urinary incontinence and some faecal incontinence. An ultrasound scan and urodynamic investigations were performed, but were essentially normal, and at the fourth consultation with the defendant, the claimant was offered surgery. The defendant did not offer any alternatives to the said procedure or any non-surgical options. The claimant describes the onset of pain in the postoperative period which has been ongoing since then. She was referred to the bowel surgeons, urologists and other gynaecologists for a second opinion. She underwent a diagnostic laparoscopy, and laparotomy for adhesiolysis, though adhesions were minimal. She underwent further laparoscopic adhesiolysis but was no better following this surgery. This left her in a state of permanent disability where her husband had to care for her and she had to give up her business.

The Judgement

Though it was admitted that the defendant failed to give Mrs M the different options for her prolapse, it was felt that she was too young to use pessaries long term and it was unlikely they would have addressed her problems. Alternative surgeries such as the Manchester repair would also not have been suitable. It was ruled that even if given all the options, the claimant would still have chosen to have this operation, even though it was more invasive. This was evident by the fact that when given the option of the less invasive laparoscopic adhesiolysis versus open, she opted for the more invasive option. In light of the opinion of the experts, surgical intervention would have been required in any event, this would have triggered Mrs M's illness and she would have been in a similar situation, requiring the same treatment. The decision on causation in this case was therefore not established. The claim was dismissed.

Legal Commentary

Eloise Power

Duffett v Worcestershire Acute Hospitals NHS Trust (Unreported, Lawtel 30 June 2008)

The issues raised in the case of *Duffett* are typical of many cases involving elective gynaecological surgery, prolapse and urinary incontinence which are encountered in practice. The claimant suffered from menorrhagia, urinary stress incontinence and urgency and a cystocele. She alleged that she was advised that there was no treatment option other than a hysterectomy, and that she consented to treatment on that basis. Following the hysterectomy, she developed a vault prolapse and enterocele and underwent a trans-anal repair of a rectocele. The issues in dispute were (a) consent and (b) causation. The matter settled out of court; the claimant's solicitors estimated that litigation risk was in the region of 35%.

In practice, lawyers frequently encounter consent issues in cases relating to prolapse surgery. Unlike some other areas of gynaecological practice (for example, the treatment of malignancy), prolapse in itself is not a fatal condition or an emergency, and patients have a meaningful choice to make as to when and whether to undergo surgery at all. In many cases encountered in practice, such as *Duffett*, claimants allege that they were not meaningfully counselled about risks, benefits and (in particular) alternative options.

In the light of *Montgomery* (which is considered in detail at Chapter 4), the relevant legal principles are clear:

> The doctor is therefore under a duty to take reasonable care to ensure that the patient is aware of any material risks involved in any recommended treatment, and of any reasonable alternative or variant treatments [para 87].
>
> The significance of a given risk is likely to reflect a variety of factors besides its magnitude: for example, the nature of the risk, the effect which its occurrence would have upon the life of the patient, the importance to the patient of the benefits sought to be achieved by the treatment, the alternatives available, and the risks involved in those alternatives [para 89].

In the particular factual context of treatment for prolapse, alternative treatment options are likely to include conservative management with a review, pelvic floor physiotherapy and pessaries, as well as alternative forms of surgery. Montgomery postdates the settlement in Duffett, but similar factual issues seem to have been considered.

The case of *Duffett* is also typical due to the relatively complicated causation issues which it raised: it appears that the claimant initially advanced the case on the basis that her urinary problems had resulted from the negligent treatment, but by the time of settlement, the experts instructed by the claimant seem to have acknowledged that the majority of her urinary problems were as a result of childbirth rather than the negligent treatment.

SEM v Mid Yorkshire Hospitals NHS Trust [2005] EWHC 3469 (QB); [2005] 9 WLUK 164, also Reported as M v Mid Yorkshire Hospitals NHS Trust

This case, which predates the *Montgomery* judgement, turned upon the causation which flowed from a number of admitted failings in the consenting process. The claimant underwent a vaginal hysterectomy, McCall culdoplasty and an anterior with posterior vaginal wall repair. It was common ground that she should have been informed of alternative procedures, including: (1) doing nothing apart from reassurance and physiotherapy; (2) the use of medical devices such as ring or Hodge pessaries; (3) alternative surgical procedures, which included anterior repair alone, the Manchester-Fothergill operation, or vaginal hysterectomy and anterior repair.

Despite the acknowledged deficiencies in the consenting process, the claimant's case failed on causation. The Court took the following approach to causation in the hypothetical scenario:

> Assuming that Miss F had properly advised Mrs M, giving due weight to her own views and experience, she would have provided a menu of approaches but would have recommended a vaginal hysterectomy with McCall's procedure. In my judgment Mrs M, acting as a reasonable patient and even if one leaves out of the equation her particular psychiatric condition, would have been likely to follow the surgeon's advice. Patients do normally follow the advice of a consultant, and I cannot see in this case any factors which lead me to suppose that Mrs M would have done otherwise.

If the case of *SEM* had been decided after *Montgomery*, it is likely that causation in the hypothetical scenario would have been approached differently. Lords Kerr and Reed held that *"the question of causation must also be considered on the hypothesis of a discussion which is being conducted without the patient's being pressurised to accept her doctor's recommendation"* [para 103, underlining added]. Further, the discussion of risks should be *"sensitive also to the characteristics of the patient"* [para 89]. However, even if the court in *SEM* had approached causation in the manner set out in *Montgomery*, it seems unlikely that this would have led to a different result. On the facts, the claimant's pre-existing somatoform disorder was taken into account: the expert psychiatrists agreed that the claimant would have been *"highly dissatisfied with any treatment intervention other than surgery"*. The Court observed that this *"shipwrecked"* the claimant's case on causation [para 55].

Counsel for the claimant in *SEM* advanced a number of creative arguments based upon *Chester v Afshar* [2004] UKHL 41 in support of his position that the claimant should succeed even if she could not demonstrate that she would have acted differently if properly consented. These arguments failed. The legal commentary to Chapter 18 contains a summary of various cases in which claimants have unsuccessfully sought to raise similar arguments after *Montgomery*. By way of a general observation, those acting for claimants in consent cases would be well-advised to think through the implications of their case on causation in detail at the earliest opportunity.

Mesh Repairs for Prolapse

In recent years, cases arising out of mesh repairs for pelvic organ prolapse are becoming increasingly prominent. A comprehensive review of the rise and fall of trans-vaginal mesh for pelvic organ prolapse, and the suffering which many patients have experienced, can be found in the report of the Independent Medicines and Medical Devices Safety Review of July 2020, commonly known as the "Cumberlege Report".[1]

From a medico-legal viewpoint, claims arising out of mesh repairs for pelvic organ prolapse tend to fall into two categories: (1) clinical negligence cases against Trusts or individual doctors alleging the failure to obtain properly informed consent for the use of trans-vaginal mesh and (2) product liability cases against device manufacturers alleging that the trans-vaginal mesh was "defective" under the Consumer Protection Act 1987. Some claimants bring multi-party actions which fall into both of these categories.

The first category of cases is governed by the principles set out in *Montgomery*. By way of a caveat, the *Montgomery* principles have not as yet been considered in detail by the higher courts in the particular factual context of the selection of medical devices.[2] Permission to appeal was granted by the Court of Appeal in the case of *Grimstone v Epsom and St Helier University Hospitals NHS Trust* [2015] EWHC 3756 (QB). The issues which would have fallen for consideration by the Court of Appeal included: (a) the information with which patients should be provided where a doctor proposes to use a novel product with no or limited published follow-up data; (b) the extent of detail about alternatives which should be provided in this situation; (c) whether doctors have a duty to inform patients of commercial links with manufacturers of medical devices which they propose to use in a patient. Unfortunately, the case did not reach a full hearing before the Court of Appeal.[3] An important issue relating to consent in mesh cases is the interplay between product information provided by manufacturers and the consenting process between doctors and patients: in a nutshell, if the manufacturers have produced misleading product information in relation to the risks posed by vaginal mesh, to what extent will this be a defence to doctors who have passed on the same information to patients? It remains to be seen how these issues will be approached in practice by the Courts.

The second category of cases is governed by the principles under the Consumer Protection Act 1987 and the law of negligence. Under the Consumer Protection Act 1987, manufacturers are liable for personal injury and property damage caused by "defective" products. There is a defect in a product if *"the safety of the product is not such as persons generally are entitled to expect."*[4] *"All the circumstances"* are taken into account when assessing defect, including:

> *(a) the manner in which, and purposes for which, the product has been marketed, its get-up, the use of any mark in relation to the product and any instructions for, or warnings with respect to, doing or refraining from doing anything with or in relation to the product;*

> *(b) what might reasonably be expected to be done with or in relation to the product; and*

> *(c) the time when the product was supplied by its producer to another.*[5]

---

[1] www.immdsreview.org.uk/. The section on pelvic mesh is from p138–79 of the report; it covers TVT as well as mesh for POP.

[2] The case of *Shaw v Kovac* [2017] EWCA Civ 1028 concerned a trans-aortic valve implant, but the judgement of the Court of Appeal turns on issues which are not specific to medical device cases (in particular, whether free-standing damages are available for the loss of autonomy as a result of the failure to obtain informed consent).

[3] Eloise Power acted for the claimant at the appellate stage in Grimstone (though not at first instance).

[4] Section 3 (1).

[5] Section 3 (2).

Defect is not inferred simply by the fact that a product which is supplied at a later date is safer than the product in question. There are a number of defences available to manufacturers, including (but not limited to) the "development risks defence": *"that the state of scientific and technical knowledge at the relevant time was not such that a producer of products of the same description as the product in question might be expected to have discovered the defect if it had existed in his products while they were under his control."*[6]

As things stand, there is ongoing High Court litigation against Johnson and Johnson Medical Limited known as the "Pelvic Organ Prolapse Products Litigation."[7] The litigation concerns a number of trans-vaginal mesh products, including Prolift, a pre-cut mesh kit which was inserted into the lead claimant in the litigation. The claimants' case is that trans-vaginal mesh conferred no additional benefits on patients over and above the benefits of the main alternative procedure (native tissue repair), whereas it exposed them to significant additional risks such as the risk of mesh erosion/exposure. Further, the product information provided to doctors downplayed the risks and over-emphasised the perceived benefits. At the time of writing, the matter has not been listed for trial. A case brought in Australia,[8] which raised similar issues, succeeded at trial: *Gill v Ethicon Sàrl (No 5)* [2019] FCA 1905. The judgement was upheld on appeal: *Ethicon Sàrl v Gill* [2021] FCAFC 29. The Court upheld the trial judge's finding that the manufacturer had misled surgeons and patients by exaggerating the benefits of the mesh products and minimising the risks, and observed that *"no matter how learned the intermediary may be, it is highly unlikely, if not inconceivable, that the intermediary would know as much about the product as the manufacturer itself"* (para 404 (7)).

Clinical Commentary

Ian Currie

Introduction

Within this chapter, the author aims to focus on the clinical issues surrounding the management of vaginal and uterine prolapse with specific reference to litigation issues, rather than reproduce guidelines which are already in the public domain. Guidelines for clinical practice however do form the basis of clinical management, and it is encouraged that all clinicians performing prolapse surgery maintain not only their surgical skills, volume of workload but also their knowledge base around guidelines from relevant institutions (e.g. NICE, BSUG, IUGA).

It is also recognised that prolapse surgery is often carried out in conjunction with surgery for stress urinary incontinence. For the purpose of this chapter, the author will focus solely on prolapse surgery.

---

[6] Section 4 (1) (e).
[7] Eloise Power acts for the lead claimant in the Pelvic Organ Prolapse Products Litigation, and Swati Jha is an expert instructed in the litigation. The information provided in this paragraph is in the public domain.
[8] Australian product liability law has marked similarities with the law in our jurisdiction.

Classification

In clinical practice, prolapse surgery can be divided into different subsets. Division into primary and secondary (repeat/ revision) surgery is an important distinction to make.

Primary surgery has historically not required the use of mesh, the controversies of which are beyond the remit of this chapter. Suffice to say, the success of each repeat repair operation decreases with each operation and the lack of longevity and success of repeat surgery should be clearly explained to patients when contemplating repeated fascial repair. Quite often this simple fact is implied in the medical records but rarely documented accurately.

The use of a multidisciplinary team (MDT) is invaluable and now a necessary part of clinical management and governance, but it must be remembered that the MDT team decision should be advisory and should not disregard less favourable options but merely explain the reasons why one procedure may be more suitable than another. The MDT team can also advise when further surgery may be inappropriate. Emphasis in dealing with difficult clinical issues is usually not documented well in the medical records in the author's opinion, other than saying it was the MDT opinion. MDT discussion documentation that is comprehensive and advisory along with good clinical records that support the decision-making process for surgery are invaluable when faced with a clinical negligence claim.

Repeated surgery also causes further scarring and may cause narrowing of the vagina above and beyond what is required for a satisfactory repair. This can cause symptoms to occur which were not present before, for example dyspareunia. There are many examples of patients being unable to achieve penetration at intercourse after prolapse surgery.

Fibrosis from either repeated surgery or insertion of mesh will be discussed later in the chapter. Rarely are surgeons criticised for not performing surgery but moreover many legal cases have focussed on the hourglass narrowing of a combined anterior and posterior repair. Explanation regarding the potential mismatch in healing when repairing more than one vaginal wall, leading to fibrotic narrowing, is even more important with the younger patients.

Surgery can be subdivided by surgical site and the apparent defect may be more prominent under anaesthetic than what was first noted at clinical examination. Discrepancies in clinical findings are often looked at by medical experts, particularly when procedures have been performed that were not consented for. Explanation in the notes is essential when discrepancies occur, particularly if hysterectomy is contemplated and especially if a surgeon changes the proposed procedure from that which was previously consented for. The surgeon may have the patient's best interest in mind, but a surgeon needs to be aware that all patients may not see it in that way and may consider the action as inappropriate, particularly if the outcome was not as desired.

Surgery Types
- Primary
- Secondary (revision)

Site Specific
- Cystocele
- Rectocele

(**FAILURE**)Poor fibrosis◄----(**CURE**)----► Excessive fibrosis (**PAIN**)

Figure 23.1 Example diagram of the effects of fibrosis.

- Enterocele
- Uterine

Specialist Areas
- Use of mesh
- Post-hysterectomy (abdominal mesh v vaginal mesh v sacrospinous ligament fixation)
- Uterine preserving surgery

Any operation for prolapse requires an element of scar/fibrosis formation in order to prevent protrusion of tissues (cystocele, rectocele, enterocele) or support structures such as the uterus. This concept will be discussed later in relation to vaginal mesh issues.

Explanation to patients by the clinician that the "new" tissue created is not the original tissue is a useful start in the counselling process. The explanation that scarring/fibrosis can fail to form resulting in surgical failure, or indeed can form in excess giving pain, tethering and nerve entrapment should form part of good counselling. Documentation, either written or in a dictated letter, is best practice.

The author uses this model (see Figure 23.1) at the outset, highlighting that the majority of patients lie between these two extremes of healing and therefore get a desired result. Lifetime reoperation rates/failure are quoted at approximately 30% and so setting expectations for patients at the outset is desirable when reflecting when results have not lived up to expectations. A simple diagram in the records will add weight to the discussion that has taken place

Some issues regarding surgery are common to most operative surgery and so the chapter will focus on the specific issues surrounding prolapse surgery which the author feels are most relevant for the clinician to be aware of with respect to litigation.

Decision-Making for Surgery

It is important to document all forms of conservative treatment and whether they have been tried, offered and accepted (e.g. self -directed pelvic floor exercises (PFE), formal physiotherapy or vaginal pessary management).

Regarding PFE/physiotherapy – the clinician should be aware that many patients believe that the pelvic exercises they performed many years previously are what the clinician is referring to when asked, and so documentation of when and who provided the treatment is important. Many patients seeking litigation frequently feel they were "railroaded" into surgery and that non-surgical options were not explored, particularly if the surgery was not successful. This is a particular factor for patients with mild prolapse as they are more likely to respond to conservative measures.

Any management starts with a concise history. Concerning prolapse, there are certain aspects in the history that take on more prominence.

Particular documentation around pre-existing pain, particularly vaginal pain, dyspareunia is important. Pain and sexual function issues are frequent issues that patients seek to redress. It is not just the presence or absence of discomfort but moreover the type and description of the pain if present. A patient may admit that pain was present previously but state that it has changed in character, is more severe and having a greater impact on quality of life. This is equally important in the immediate postoperative phase. Pressures on the NHS have made follow-up of postoperative patients more difficult to carry out but the author is of the opinion that a remote consultation should be the bare minimum following surgery and that if there are concerns, a face-to-face appointment should be arranged.

Treatments offered to try and alleviate dyspareunia/vaginal atrophy should be considered routine. The discomfort should not be presumed to be related to the prolapse itself. The use of vaginal pessary may obviate the need for surgery.

Reference should be made to any other pre-existing conditions such as fibromyalgia and other musculoskeletal disorders. This aspect of history-taking is frequently overlooked. If a patient already has significant widespread pain then greater detail is needed when documenting preoperative symptoms. The mere recording of these conditions and an acceptance that they are present is not sufficient.

Information should not, however, be solely given in written format (patient information leaflet), without reviewing the patient back later and crucially checking understanding of the decisions that have been arrived at. Reflection and understanding is now mandatory.

The clinician should also check whether the patient has understood the information they have been given, and whether or not they would like more information before making a decision. Ideally, they should make it clear that they can change their mind about a decision at any time.

Above all, the clinician should not "choose" the operation but guide the patient in her decision-making and show evidence that this has happened.

A clinician should avoid the use of such terms as "I've discussed all the options in detail" or "I have fully counselled the patient regarding her options". These terms retrospectively are open to many interpretations and are not helpful. Diagrams however are helpful, particularly in explaining anatomy and quickly bulleting complications. Review of medical records with an annotated diagram shows there has been interactive discussion and an attempt by the clinician to give the information in a clear and concise way.

Interactive prolapse software is available and if used should be documented by merely stating that it was used to aid discussion.

Procedure-specific consent forms are available and avoid the common issue of junior doctors consenting and missing major complication issues on the consent form. In the author's opinion, however, it is quite often the consultant who misses major complications and the risks documented by junior staff are invariably thorough. The consent form should ideally be filled in by the person who is carrying out the procedure, but documentation as to what consent form was given, and direction to websites should be recorded (BSUG). The decision-making aid from NICE [1] is helpful in showing retrospectively what influenced the patient's decision-making process.

A follow-up visit should be organised. Frequently the tick box confirmation area on the consent form is not filled in. Additional information at the time of consent could be "shown video" or specific reference made to state that it was received, read and understood in an attempt to align information/decision-making with *Montgomery*.

In accordance with *Montgomery v Lanarkshire Health Board and GMC* (2015) UKSC 11, a clinician is under a duty to take reasonable care to ensure that the patient is aware of **any** material risks involved in any recommended treatment, and of any **reasonable** alternative or variant treatments.

Consent Process

General Medical Council Good Practice

Frequently, clinicians ignore guidance published by the General Medical Council (GMC) relating to consent. This guidance specifically highlights the following in relation to informed consent:

1. The clinician must give patients the information they want or need about the diagnosis and prognosis.
2. They should also highlight any uncertainties about the diagnosis or prognosis, including possible options for further investigations.
3. They should discuss reasonable alternative options for treating or managing the condition, including the option not to treat.
4. They should explain carefully the purpose of any proposed investigation or treatment and what it will involve.

Risks that Should Be Mentioned on the Consent Form

1. Exposure where mesh protrudes from the vagina
2. Erosion if mesh used
3. Organ perforation
4. Infection – vaginal discharge, odour, erosion, bladder infection, cystitis
5. Bleeding
6. Dyspareunia
7. Vascular injury
8. Bladder or rectal injury
9. Voiding difficulty
10. Significant chronic pain
11. Psychiatric injury if at risk
12. Avoidable remedial surgery to extract mesh
13. Original symptoms not treated, continued, recurrence of prolapse and/or incontinence
14. Worsening of their present condition
15. Urge and urgency may start or get worse
16. Permanence of the mesh implant
17. The need for self-catheterisation and the long-term recurrence of infection

Operative Recording

Accurate assessment of the extent of prolapse is essential when recording operative details. Correlating with the outpatient examination and explaining differences is important, particularly if traction on the cervix is employed. Recording the technique of dissection (sharp or blunt) as well as any concern regarding previous scarring. Recording of careful dissection and not using the term "routine repair" also helps when postoperative issues subsequently arise. Similar recording of the calibre of the vagina at the end of the procedure is helpful, particularly if there has been postoperative infection which may increase scarring and narrowing.

Recognition and Management of Postoperative Complications

A frequent concern is often a delay in the management of complications rather than the complication itself. It is always good practice that the recording of urinary incontinence before any prolapse operation is accurate as well as the discussion about risk of latent stress incontinence. However, sudden onset of urinary incontinence after the procedure should raise concerns about trauma to the urinary tract. There are many cases whereby persistent profound incontinence is treated as a urinary tract infection or detrusor overactivity when later it is revealed that there is a fistulous tract. Any incontinence occurring postoperatively should be investigated thoroughly. Whilst tampon tests/methylene blue investigations may be helpful, it must be recognised that these tests do not rule out a fistula. Imaging with a CT urogram or retrograde cystogram are the initial investigations of choice.

A similar management strategy should be adopted for potential damage to the rectum. Investigation of a persistent malodorous smell should alert the clinician to the potential for harm, especially if the discharge is unresponsive to antibiotics. Early opinion with colorectal surgeons is essential in such cases and a proactive approach regarding what has happened may avoid litigation. Patients who perceive their doctor has been caring, compassionate and has listened to their concerns are much less likely to seek redress through the legal system.

Early Failure

When prolapse symptoms return within weeks or months after a procedure, the question that is most asked is whether the operation failed or whether the wrong operation was performed. There are three main circumstances in which this occurs:

Firstly, a decision made at the time of surgery to not perform a hysterectomy and then to later find out that the cervix and uterus are part of the recurrent prolapse. This may be explained by progressive deterioration of the prolapse with time but it is much more difficult to explain if the time interval to recurrence is short.

Secondly, the failure to correct a vault prolapse and not support the vault adequately. This may occur by not performing a concomitant vault prolapse procedure when carrying out a vaginal hysterectomy. Current guidance states that a vault supportive procedure should be employed if there is descent of the cervix/uterus to the introitus (stage 2 prolapse). It is recognised there are some instances whereby the uterine body is well supported but the component of the prolapse is an elongated cervix. Clear documentation over the decision to not perform hysterectomy or vault procedure is important. Describing the "uterine body – well supported" or "very high Pouch of Douglas" are always useful in relaying the decision-making process.

Thirdly, there are situations when a high enterocele/vault descent is present but the surgeon elects to perform a double repair. In the author's experience this does not correct the high prolapse issue and only narrows the vagina excessively.

Postoperative Clinic Visits

Whether a postoperative visit is performed remotely or face to face, it is an opportunity for the clinician to again explain the procedure that was undertaken and accurately record any concerns made by the patient. The visit is usually set at the time of discharge from hospital, but the clinician must be responsive to postoperative concerns and be adaptive if necessary. They should try and avoid breakdown in communication, particularly if it is evident that a patient is concerned by symptoms. Taking personal ownership of any concerns, rather than just passing the issue on to the GP, is essential in avoiding litigation.

Mesh Issues

The incidence of vaginal mesh for surgery is decreasing and it may be that in future mesh is used primarily in abdominal/laparoscopic sacrocolpopexy or sacrohysteropexy only.

Mesh use in the United Kingdom has for a large part been used solely in revision surgery after repeated attempts at fascial surgery has failed, but there are many examples of mesh being used in primary surgery. It is the author's opinion that these patients should be the exception to the rule and require even more meticulous documentation through the governance process of an MDT team. However, if a clinician decides to use mesh for primary surgery, they need to highlight specific indications as to why it has been offered, e.g. inherited collagen disorder

A young age with prolapse has often been used as an argument for intervention with mesh, with the idea that one needs a more robust repair as it has to last longer. However, the excessive fibrosis associated with vaginal mesh in particular can cause significant dyspareunia.

Fibrosis/pain syndrome issues surround mesh are discussed at length in litigation. Subsequent pain from surgery may be from the following:

1. Direct nerve injury from trocars (mesh kits)
2. Excessive scarring with contraction of the mesh
3. Repeated surgery to remove exposed mesh

Fibrosis

One of the key factors in the development of granulation tissue is the migration, activation and proliferation of fibroblasts. This mechanism is controlled by many growth factors that are released by platelets, inflammatory cells, injured epithelial cells and endothelial cells.

Some of these factors switch on fibroblast formation to produce a matrix of proteins.

It is these fibroblasts that are involved in the formation of granulation tissue (scar tissue). Some fibroblasts may contain myofibrils and therefore express skeletal protein smooth muscle. These so called "myofibroblasts" have contractile properties and are thought to play a role in contraction of wounds and scarring.

The simplest form of wound healing occurs when uninfected skin incisions are closed promptly by suturing as in the context of closure of the vaginal epithelium. This is referred to as healing by **first intention** (or primary union) and it is characterised by the formation of only minimal amounts of granulation tissue. It is a rapid process and contrasts with healing by **secondary intention**, which may occur in open wounds or when there is infection or a foreign body present such as vaginal mesh.

When an incision is made in the skin, blood escapes from cut blood vessels and the blood clots on the wound surface, filling the gap between the wound edges. In a sutured wound the gap is narrow. Fibre in the clot then acts as a glue, which holds the cut surfaces together. The dehydrated blood clot on the surface forms a scab, which seals the wound.

After 24 hours there is a mild inflammatory reaction at the wound edges with exudation of fluid and migration of polymorphs (white blood cells).

Within 24–48 hours there is enlargement of cells within the epidermis and cells in the deeper part of the epithelium begin to proliferate and slide over each other, creating a healing process. These new cells however will migrate only over viable tissue.

This is an important factor when considering healing by secondary intention. This type of healing is where there is an open, gaping wound that leads to the formation of more substantial amounts of granulation tissue, which grow on the base of the wound to fill the defect. Angiogenesis (growth of blood vessels) and fibroblast proliferation are much more abundant and healing takes longer than that following healing by primary intention. There is a massive emigration of neutrophils and macrophages.

Healing by secondary intention is a more prolonged process, and if a wound does not heal because of a foreign body such as vaginal mesh, then the inflammatory process continues to occur, constantly laying down more fibroblasts and excessive scar tissue. The healing of an open wound is helped by the movement of the edges towards the centre of the wound, brought about by so-called myofibroblasts. This leads to the term "contracture" and this word is used when the repair process ultimately leads to distortion or limitation of movement of the tissues. This may result either from contraction of the wound itself or from scarring of the deeper muscles and soft tissues. Fibrosis around terminal sensory nerve endings can lead to neuralgic discomfort and pain in the affected area and the subsequent fibrosis will lead to reduced mobility in the tissues.

The mechanism of excessive fibrosis and scarring is frequently enquired about during litigation. A knowledge of the principles of what is forming the success or complication of prolapse surgery is important both for the surgeon, medical expert and legal team.

Causes of Litigation

- Failure to offer conservative treatment
- MDT not giving options to the patient and being unidirectional
- Not documenting previous sexual history (pain) accurately and whether patient is sexually active
- Failing to explain risk factors increasing complications/recurrence rates above what would be considered acceptable
- Failure to document risks of procedure until the day of operation
- Description in operation notes of "routine"
- Dismissive of postoperative incontinence

Avoidance of Litigation

- MDT should give conservative and surgical options (plural if possible) and give reasons as to why it may favour one option over another. It should not present the patient with a fait accompli. Where options are firmly discounted then clear reasons should be articulated.

- Destruction of sex life is often a route for litigation. Clear documentation of pre-existing sexual difficulties (if any) clearly allows one to make comparison before and after the event.
- Clearly noting pre-existing conditions which have symptoms that may overlap with complications of prolapse surgery with clear categorisation of pain (groin, suprapubic, vaginal)
- Avoid using overarching terms such as "counselled extensively"
- Ensure verbal and ideally written information is provided to the patient in a timely fashion, allowing for reflection. Document how the signposting has occurred
- Clear written operative records describing dissection technique, particularly with revision surgery
- Prompt recognition of urological trauma (e.g. fistula
- Investigate postoperative urinary leakage promptly and thoroughly

References

1. www.nice.org.uk/guidance/ng123/resources/surgery-for-stress-urinary-incontinence-patient-decision-aid-pdf-6725286110

Subfertility and Assisted Conception

Raj Mathur

CASE COMMENTARY

Swati Jha

Successful Claim

Richard Holdich v Lothian Health Board [2013] CSOH 197, 2013 WL 7117501

The Claim

The claimant was diagnosed with testicular cancer and prior to receiving treatment, as this would render him infertile, deposited three samples of semen in the defender's facility. The sperm was deposited to preserve his ability to become a father following the treatment through IVF. However, due to a mishap with the storage vessel and resultant inability to safely use the semen provided, he claimed for the loss of the chance of fatherhood and compensation for the distress and depressions arising from this.

The Summary

Storage of semen is in a cryogenic storage facility. There was a malfunction which involved a leak of the cooling medium which was liquid nitrogen. As a consequence, the temperature of the storage vessel rose from minus 190 degrees to minus 53 degrees. All the sperm was stored in the same vessel, hence deteriorated following this event. The claimant was advised that using these sperms carried a reduced chance of conception and increased risk of chromosomal abnormalities, miscarriage and birth defects. He therefore opted not to use this sperm due to these risks and the loss of the chance of fatherhood is characterised as "loss of autonomy". The case in question was whether there was mental injury consequent on bodily injury, whether this was pure mental injury or whether semen could be classed as moveable property and mental injury was a consequence of damage to moveable property. The defendant sought to have the claim "struck out" on the basis that the law in Scotland does not compensate for mental injury in such circumstances or for "mere distress", and does not recognise "loss of autonomy" as a compensable category.

The Judgement

Though the defendants claimed that because the breach of contract case was likely to fail, it should follow on that psychiatric injury based on negligence must therefore fail. It was observed by the Judge that the claimant's property and breach of contract case did face difficulties, it was not bound to fail, and was therefore allowed to go to proof. As a consequence, the whole of the pursuer's claim was permitted to go to trial. It was ruled that an infringement of the ability to father children could result in mental injury, and loss of autonomy was not rejected as an independent damage in its own right. The judgement did not go so far as to recognise autonomy as a right, suggesting that such cases may be better subsumed within general claims for mental distress.

Unsuccessful Claim

ARB v IVF Hammersmith and R [2018] EWCA

The Claim

ARB and R opted for IVF at a clinic and several embryos were created. Following the birth of their son, the couple separated. R went on to have another child using one of the frozen embryos and ARB claimed that the clinic failed to obtain his consent for use of the embryo. ARB sought damages for the losses incurred due to shared parental responsibility and shared residence in respect of both children.

The Summary

When the couple were still together and attended the clinic at the start of the IVF treatment, they signed a form which required that they both sign and give written consent before any embryos could be thawed and replaced in future. This was also the case in the event of separation or divorce. Following the birth of their first child through IVF treatment, R wished to have another child. They attended clinic together just before their separation, but when they separated a few months later, failed to inform the clinic of this. The clinic therefore continued treatment on the assumption they were still together. R attended subsequent clinic appointments alone. According to the standard operating procedure (SOP), if both partners attended the frozen embryo replacement clinic, the clinic's employee confirmed the understanding of each of them to the consequences of the procedure and then witnessed their consents and each of their signatures. Where one of their partners failed to attend, the SOP permitted the employee to delegate the responsibility for obtaining consent to the attending partner. It provided for no witnessing of the non-attending partner's signature, still less any effective check that the consent had been validly obtained from the non-attending partner. The result was that in precisely those circumstances where forgery was most likely, the safeguards for obtaining written consent were significantly reduced. In this case, the consent to thaw frozen embryos which required a signature from both partners was forged on behalf of ARB by R.

The Judgement

ARB succeeded in the primary case against the clinic for breach of contract but it was ruled that ARB was not entitled to recover damages for the cost of upbringing of the second child. This subsequently went to the Court of Appeal and it was reaffirmed that the damages claimed for the upbringing of a healthy child were too remote and not recoverable under the contract which ARB had with the clinic. This was not a loss for which the defendant assumed responsibility hence the appeal too was dismissed.

Legal Commentary

Eloise Power

Richard Holdich v Lothian Health Board [2013] CSOH 197, 2013 WL 7117501

The Scottish case of *Holdich v Lothian Health Board* considered a preliminary issue, namely whether the pursuer's pleadings disclosed a cause of action relevant in law.

The pursuer was allowed to proceed with his case both in contract and in delict (the Scottish equivalent to tort). Lord Stewart held that the trial judge should determine the issue of whether an award for "loss of autonomy" (in relation to the pursuer's ability to father children) should be made as a stand-alone head of loss or whether it should be taken into account under other heads of loss. The concept of a free-standing award for "loss of autonomy" or the loss of a claimant's opportunity to live the life which s/he wanted to live derives from the case of *Rees v Darlington Memorial Hospital NHS Trust* [2003] UKHL 52, which is considered in the legal commentary to Chapter 5.

Lord Stewart also held that the issue of whether damages were recoverable for the pursuer's distress, and the question of where the line is to be drawn between distress and mental illness, were matters for trial; he observed, *obiter*, that *"I think it is reasonably clear that the judicial outlook is now sufficiently flexible to recognise that distress can be the precursor of more serious mental symptoms"* [para 98]. This accords with the approach taken in certain English and Welsh cases: see, for example, the judgement of Martin Spencer J in Zeromska-Smith v United Lincolnshire Hospitals NHS Trust [2019] EWHC 980 (QB), which is considered in the legal commentary to Chapter 8.

Similar issues to those considered in *Holdich* were given substantive consideration by the Court of Appeal in *Yearworth and others v North Bristol NHS Trust* [2009] EWCA Civ 37. In *Yearworth*, the claimants were cancer patients who had banked sperm samples at the defendant's fertility unit. The sperm was banked free of charge, and was damaged due to an equipment failure. In a unanimous judgement, the Court held as follows:

(a) The damage to the sperm did not constitute "personal injury". The Court rejected the argument (based upon a German court decision) that a woman's eggs which had been extracted from the body with a view to future reimplantation retained a functional unity with the body, and that it would be illogical for the law to treat damage to sperm differently from damage to eggs.[1] The Court found as follows: *"We must deal in realities. To do otherwise would generate paradoxes, and yield ramifications, productive of substantial uncertainty, expensive debate and nice distinctions in an area of law which should be simple, and the parameters clear."*

(b) Notwithstanding that various limitations were placed upon the use of the sperm under the Human Fertilisation and Embryology Act 1990, the claimants had ownership of the sperm. The Court placed considerable weight upon the requirement for consent under the HFEA: *"their negative control over their use remains absolute"* [para 45 (b)(ii)].

(c) The claimants had a distinct cause of action against the defendant under the law of bailment.[2] A bailment arises where a bailee (here, the defendant) acquires exclusive possession of a chattel (here, the sperm) or a right in relation to it. If a bailee chooses to take possession of a chattel, they assume duties over it. The Court found that the defendant had extended and had broken a particular promise to the men, namely that the sperm would be stored at minus 196 degrees centigrade.

---

[1] I am not aware of any case in our jurisdiction which has considered the issue of whether damage to frozen eggs or embryos would amount to a personal injury to the mother/birthing parent. It would be interesting to see whether Yearworth could be successfully distinguished. In practical terms, the same/a better result is likely to be achievable in contract or bailment, which would discourage claimants from attempting to distinguish Yearworth.

[2] The claims were not argued under the law of contract: it is unlikely that any contract would have arisen on the facts, as the claimants had not provided any consideration in exchange for the storage of the sperm.

(d) The law of bailment provided the claimants with a remedy under which the claimants were entitled to compensation for psychiatric injury or mental distress; the issue of damages was remitted for determination by a lower court.

Some doubt was cast upon aspects of the *Yearworth* judgement by Lord Stewart in the Scottish case of *Holdich v Lothian Health Board*: in particular, Lord Stewart observed, *obiter*, that he did not have "*the same difficulty with the idea of functional unity as the Court of Appeal did in* Yearworth" [para 9], and appeared open in principle to the idea of revisiting the concept of whether damage to sperm could amount to personal injury. However, this issue did not fall for consideration before the Court of Session, as the pursuers had chosen not to advance this argument. *Yearworth* remains good law and binding in England and Wales.

ARB v IVF Hammersmith and R [2018] EWCA Civ 2803

In *ARB v IVF Hammersmith and R* [2018] EWCA Civ 2803, a heterosexual couple underwent fertility treatment and froze five embryos. They subsequently separated. The female ex-partner attended the clinic alone for fertility treatment, claiming that the couple had agreed to have another child. She was allowed to take away the consent form to obtain a signature from her partner. She forged the male ex-partner's signature on the consent documents, underwent embryo implantation and gave birth to a healthy child. The male ex-partner brought an action in contract against the clinic and the female ex-partner.

The Court of Appeal found that – regardless of the significant failings on the part of the clinic – the legal policy barring damages for the pure economic loss of raising a child should apply in breach of contract as much as in tort. Accordingly, the father was not entitled to damages. The law relating to wrongful birth, and to the losses attributable to raising a child, is considered in more detail in Chapter 5.

Recoverability of Damages for Surrogacy

In the landmark judgement of the Supreme Court in *Whittington Hospital NHS Trust v XX* [2020] UKSC 14, the legal principles relating to recoverability of damages for surrogacy were considered in detail. The claimant had suffered a loss of fertility due to the defendant's admitted negligence, which arose from a delay in diagnosing cervical cancer. Prior to undergoing treatment for cervical cancer, she underwent egg freezing and had eight mature eggs collected and frozen in storage. Following treatment by way of surgery and chemo-radiotherapy, she was left completely infertile and unable to bear children in her own uterus. The three issues which fell for consideration by the Supreme Court were as follows [para 8]:

(1) Are damages to fund surrogacy arrangements using the claimant's own eggs recoverable?

(2) If so, are damages to fund surrogacy arrangements using donor eggs recoverable?

(3) In either event, are damages to fund the cost of commercial surrogacy arrangements in a country where this is not unlawful recoverable?[3]

---

[3] Commercial surrogacy is unlawful in the United Kingdom as the law presently stands, and contracts for surrogacy are unenforceable.

In answering these questions, extensive consideration was given to the legal framework around surrogacy in the United Kingdom, previous case law and policy documents. Lady Hale, with whom the majority of the Supreme Court agreed, answered the questions as follows:

(1) On general principle, where the prospects of success were reasonable, if not good, damages should be recoverable for surrogacy arrangements using the claimant's own eggs [para 44].

(2) Subject to reasonable prospects of success, damages should be recoverable for surrogacy arrangements using donor eggs: *"a woman can hope for four things from having a child: the experience of carrying and giving birth to a child; the perpetuation of one's own genes; the perpetuation of one's partner's genes; and the pleasure of bringing up a child as one's own... Donor egg surrogacy using a partner's sperm gives her two of those... If this is the best that can be achieved to make good what she has lost, why should she be denied it?"* [para 47–48].

(3) The question of the costs of foreign surrogacy was regarded as more difficult, but the Court concluded that it was *"no longer contrary to public policy to award damages for the costs of a foreign commercial surrogacy"*. Certain limiting factors were put in place: the proposed programme of treatment must be reasonable; it must be reasonable for the claimant to seek the foreign commercial arrangements proposed rather than to make arrangements within the United Kingdom; foreign surrogacy was unlikely to be reasonable unless the foreign country has *"a well-established system in which the interests of all involved, the surrogate, the commissioning parents and any resulting child, are properly safeguarded"*; the costs involved must be reasonable [para 53].

The Court observed that it is *"scarcely surprising that the claimant's clear preference is for a commercial surrogacy arrangement in California"* [para 22] given that in California, surrogacy arrangements are binding, and the mother chooses the intended surrogate rather than vice versa. The Court also recognised the reality that social and legal attitudes towards surrogacy and towards family life in general had changed since the issue of damages for surrogacy was previously considered in 2001[4]: *"More dramatic still have been the developments in the law's ideas of what constitutes a family. Traditionally, families were limited to those related by consanguinity (blood) or affinity (marriage). Hence at first only opposite sex married couples could apply for parental orders. Now they have been joined by same sex married couples, by same sex and opposite sex civil partners, and by couples, whether the same or opposite sexes, who are neither married nor civil partners, but are living together in an enduring family relationship. They have also been joined by single applicants"* [para 30].

The judgement in *Whittington Hospital NHS Trust v XX* accordingly represents a significant milestone, not only in relation to the issue of recoverability of damages for surrogacy, but also in relation to the wider issue of the recognition of the increased diversity of family life in the United Kingdom.

---

[4] By an earlier Court of Appeal judgement in *Briody v St Helen's and Knowsley Area Health Authority* [2001] EWCA Civ 1010.

Clinical Commentary

Raj Mathur

Background

Subfertility is defined by the National Institute for Health and Care excellence (NICE) as "inability to conceive after one year of unprotected vaginal sexual intercourse, in the absence of any known cause of infertility" [1], and is estimated to affect one in six couples. It is important to bear in mind that the desire for a child is not restricted to heterosexual couples, or indeed restricted to couples. In addition, patients facing a loss of potential fertility due to a medical condition or its treatment constitute a group requiring care from fertility specialists.

The investigation and management of subfertility encompasses primary, secondary and tertiary levels. Most patients commence their care with a visit to their GP. However, the major part of fertility treatment occurs after referral from primary care. Ovulation induction and surgery for conditions such as endometriosis and fibroids are usually carried out in secondary care, with tertiary centres used for complex cases and assisted conception. Uniquely for healthcare in the United Kingdom, the major proportion of assisted conception cycles are performed in private clinics, usually stand-alone and not linked to a hospital or acute trust. This raises specific challenges in delivering continuity of care as well as in adherence to the evidence base.

Professionals looking after patients presenting with concerns about their fertility are required to exercise adequate levels of clinical knowledge and skill, but beyond that to facilitate shared decision-making, taking into account the specific circumstances and values of the patients. Communication skills and empathy are useful in arriving at a shared understanding of issues and potential solutions.

Good Practice Guidance

Relevant sources of guidance include NICE, the Human Fertilisation and Embryology Authority (HFEA), Royal College of Obstetricians and Gynaecologists (RCOG) and professional bodies such as the British Fertility Society (BFS) and the Association of Reproductive Clinical Scientists (ARCS). In order to implement these diverse sources of guidance effectively, clinicians should develop evidence-based local protocols reflecting local resources and pathways. NICE guidance covers the whole range of fertility investigations and treatment, although continuous technological innovation means that the guidance is not exhaustive. Awareness of professional body guidance and the literature is therefore useful in ensuring care is based on up-to-date evidence.

Initial Management

Failure to conceive after 12 months is a valid starting point for investigations relating to fertility. However, in cases where there is a known condition affecting fertility (e.g. endometriosis) or factors in the history point to an obvious potential cause (e.g. irregular menstrual cycles, previous testicular surgery), investigation should commence without delay. For same-sex female couples and single women trying to conceive with the use of donor sperm, investigation is recommended after six unsuccessful insemination cycles.

The aims of initial investigation are to arrive at a diagnosis and prognosis for the likelihood of a healthy baby, through spontaneous conception or treatment. Any medical or social factors that may impact on pregnancy should be identified and managed, seeking multi-disciplinary input where needed. Examples are diabetes, epilepsy, thyroid disorders, anxiety and depression, where treatment and control should be optimized prior to conception.

A thorough history is the first essential step in evaluating patients of subfertility. This should include the duration of subfertility, previous conceptions and outcomes, menstrual pattern, presence or absence of significant pelvic pain, coital frequency and timing, smoking and medications (a proforma is likely to be helpful). Menstrual irregularity points to ovulatory disorder, while dyspareunia and congestive dysmenorrhea should prompt consideration of endometriosis. In this way, investigations can be targeted to the likely underlying problem.

It is recognized that in approximately 30% of couples, no clear cause is identified for the lack of conception. This proportion will vary depending on how extensively patients are investigated and what causation is attributed to conditions such as minor endometriosis and reduced ovarian reserve. It should be recognized that this can be an unsatisfactory position for many patients, and requires sympathetic and careful explanation. Not every patient would benefit from, or should have, every test available. For instance, in couples with a long history of subfertility and a significant male factor, tubal patency testing is unlikely to add value in terms of altering management. In such situations, it is important to explain why a test, otherwise perceived as routine, is not being advised (Table 24.1).

A proper evaluation of male factor infertility and involvement of the male partner in treatment decisions is a crucial part of delivering good care. Since the major part of initial fertility care is carried out in clinics within gynaecology departments, this is an important element to recognise. NICE guidance states that *"A specific male factor should be identified and corrected where possible to try to initiate natural pregnancy. The diagnosis of 'mild' male factor infertility is an example of a situation where natural conception remains a possibility and is equivalent to unexplained infertility".* Men with azoospermia and severe oligozoospermia require further evaluation, including testicular ultrasound scan, chromosomal analysis and cystic fibrosis carrier screening. Endocrine evaluation of azoospermia may reveal a correctable cause such as hypogonadotropic hypogonadism, which can be treated with gonadotropins leading to a high chance of successful conception. Hence, due attention must be paid to male partners.

Gynaecological Co-morbidities

Examples of gynecological conditions that are relevant to fertility include endometriosis, fibroids and pelvic inflammatory disease. Women with endometriosis should be offered a documented discussion of the risks and benefits of laparoscopic surgery versus assisted conception, taking into account other fertility factors, female age, ovarian reserve and patient preference. Surgery for endometrioma carries a risk of reduction in ovarian reserve, but may improve access to follicles at oocyte retrieval. NICE Quality Standards recommend that women with suspected or confirmed deep endometriosis involving the bowel, bladder or ureter are referred to a specialist endometriosis service [2]. Submucous fibroids are likely to reduce the likelihood of implantation and removal is advised. For intramural fibroids, the evidence remains poor and an individualized discussion is

Table 24.1. The salient features of investigation of subfertility at primary and secondary level

Male

• Semen analysis (SA) – WHO reference values

Semen volume: $\geq$1.5 ml

pH: $\geq$7.2

Sperm concentration: $\geq$15 million spermatozoa per ml

Total sperm number: $\geq$39 million spermatozoa per ejaculate

Total motility (percentage of progressive motility and non-progressive motility): $\geq$40% motile or $\geq$32% with progressive motility

Vitality: $\geq$58% live spermatozoa

Sperm morphology (percentage of normal forms): $\geq$4%

• Sperm antibody screening not recommended

• Repeat SA if first test is abnormal (three-month gap between tests recommended)

Female

• Post-coital test not recommended

• Ovarian reserve testing

Use age as an initial indicator

Total antral follicle (AFC) $\leq$4 = low response; >16 = high response

Anti-Müllerian hormone (AMH) $\leq$5.4 pmol/l = low response; $\geq$25.0 = pmol/l high response

Follicle-stimulating hormone (FSH) >8.9 IU/l = low response; <4 IU/l = a high response

• Luteal phase progesterone for ovulation status

• Prolactin, thyroid function test, endometrial biopsy should not be routinely performed

• Women without history of fertility-related comorbidities should be offered tubal assessment, with the remainder being offered a laparoscopy and dye test

• Rubella status

• Chlamydia test

needed [3]. IVF success rates are reduced by 40% in the presence of hydrosalpinges [4], hence removal or obstruction is recommended prior to starting IVF treatment [5]. This can be counter-intuitive to a fertility patient, particularly if a "see-and-treat" approach is taken to laparoscopy.

Assisted Conception

Assisted conception techniques involve manipulation of gametes (eggs or sperm) and/or embryos outside the body. Techniques include intra-uterine insemination (IUI), *in-vitro* fertilization (IVF) and intra-cytoplasmic sperm injection (ICSI). Additional measures may include the use of donor gametes or embryos. Over 60,000 cycles of assisted conception are performed annually in the United Kingdom.

Assisted conception is the only field of medical practice in the United Kingdom with its own act of parliament (Human Fertilisation and Embryology Act 1990, amended in 2008). The Human Fertilisation and Embryology Authority (HFEA) is an arms-length government body that licenses and inspects clinics, sets standards for clinical practice and research and provides authoritative information to patients and public. Every clinic is mandated to have a Person Responsible (PR), who should have enough understanding of the scientific, medical, legal, social, ethical and other aspects of the centre's work to be able to supervise its activities properly, besides possessing integrity, managerial authority and capability. The PR does not have to be a clinician, but must possesses a diploma, certificate or other evidence of formal qualifications in the field of medical or biological sciences. The PR has overall responsibility for ensuring the clinic and its staff comply with the law [6]. Broadly speaking, the PR must ensure that the functioning of the clinic is compliant at all times with the regulations of the HFEA.

The HFEA publishes a Code of Practice [7], which is an essential resource for professionals working in assisted conception. The Code of Practice lays out standards for investigation and information to be provided to patients and donors prior to assisted conception. It also covers procuring, processing, storage, import and export of gametes, screening and compensation for donors, egg sharing arrangements, surrogacy, traceability and premises and facilities. Clinics are inspected against these standards at regular intervals, including unannounced visits. A breach of standards may result in serious consequences for the clinic, and professional consequences for the PR. Sanctions against clinics are proportional to the gravity of breach of standards. In severe cases, a clinic may lose its license to provide treatment, or have restrictions imposed on its ability to provide certain treatments.

Structural Risk Factors in United Kingdom Fertility Care

Certain features of fertility practice in the United Kingdom are relevant to understanding medicolegal risk in this field. Patients commonly begin their care at primary level and progress through their local gynaecology service before accessing assisted conception. Referral processes need to be robust in order to avoid duplication of tests, and also to ensure that relevant test results are available to the professional looking after the patient. Where a gynaecological pathology such as hydrosalpinx is identified prior to referral for assisted conception, management of this may not have been discussed with the patient at the point of diagnosis. In such a situation, the onus falls on the tertiary clinic to ensure that the patient has adequate information and is given the chance to have the pathology corrected if appropriate. Since many United Kingdom clinics are stand-alone structures, this can be difficult to arrange and is often associated with patient dissatisfaction. If a patient develops a complication of assisted conception, such as ovarian hyperstimulation syndrome (OHSS), she may require further management in a location other than the clinic that carried out her fertility treatment. Clinics should have arrangements for the care of their patients seen in local acute units.

The predominance of private clinics in the United Kingdom has led to a competitive market, with clinics using advertising and social media to attract patients. An important factor in patient choice is the "success rate" of a clinic. The HFEA providers validated results on its website, but these are often out of date by two or more years due to the length of time from treatment to live birth, and the time needed for processing submitted data. In this situation, clinics display their own unvalidated data, which can leave them open to accusations of misinforming patients about their true likelihood of success. A further consequence of the marketisation of assisted conception is the prevalence of "add-on" treatments, which are not essential parts of treatment but may be promoted by clinics or demanded by patients in the hope of increasing the likelihood of successful treatment. When the patient is considering paying for treatment that has a scant evidence base, the clinician must ensure and document that the patient has been fully informed.

Causes of Litigation

- Missed or misinterpreted results of investigations
- Delay in investigations and diagnosis, leading to futile treatment or a reduced likelihood of success due to female age
- Miscommunication of investigation results and diagnosis
- Providing assisted conception with inadequate preliminary investigation, missing a potentially significant finding such as hydrosalpinx, uterine septum or submucous fibroid.
- Advising assisted conception when a less invasive option is available with a reasonable prospect of success (e.g. ovulation induction).
- Inadequate counselling prior to treatment about the risks and implications of treatment.
- Failure to complete valid consent forms for legal parenthood prior to start of donor sperm treatment, leading to uncertainty in legal parenthood of a child born from treatment.
- Complications of treatment – OHSS, pelvic infection following egg collection.
- Complications relating to adjuvant treatment for which the evidence base is poor, e.g. immunosuppressive treatment for recurrent implantation failure.
- Laboratory errors, for instance use of mis-identified "wrong" gametes or embryos, errors in performing or reporting genetic tests on embryo biopsy.

Avoidance of Litigation

- Establishment of local pathways and criteria based on NICE guidance for referral and investigation of subfertility.
- Clinicians must ensure that the results of investigations ordered are acted upon and explained to patients.
- With pre-existing conditions, if advice is required from another specialty (e.g. genetics, haematology or neurology) the clinician must ensure that this advice has been obtained and acted upon prior to treatment designed to achieve pregnancy.
- Open communication, an empathetic approach and clear documentation are helpful in preventing medicolegal challenges.
- The PR must be able to perform their role in accordance with the HFEA Code of Practice. This requires the PR to have adequate time to carry out their role, as well as the confidence of senior management.
- Clinic success rates should be advertised according to HFEA guidelines, ensuring accuracy and completeness. The Competitions and Marketing Authority (CMA) is in

the process of developing guidance to help assisted conception units that treat patients who pay for their treatment meet their obligations under consumer law.

- Clinical practice that is in keeping with the Code of Practice is likely to be sufficient to avoid regulatory sanction and certain types of litigation, for instance relating to legal parenthood.

- Specific clinical guidance from the RCOG, BFS and other professional bodies covers most aspects of clinical practice in fertility and assisted conception. United Kingdom clinicians who base their practice on such guidance may legitimately claim to deliver care at a reasonable level of competence.

- Where practice diverges from guidelines, patients should be clearly informed that this is the case and be made aware of the risks and potential benefits of treatment. For instance, professional guidance is clear that tests and treatments based on uterine or blood "natural killer" cells are not supported by the evidence base. Nonetheless, several clinics and competent clinicians prescribe these in their practice.

- Guidelines exist for the prevention and management of OHSS [8,9]. In order to reduce the risk of litigation, it is important to document adequate patient counseling and the use of applicable preventative measures such as GnRH antagonist protocol, agonist trigger or embryo cryopreservation ("freeze-all").

- Care should be taken to prevent both under- and over-diagnosis of OHSS, including local training and protocols. Clinicians are sometimes quick to label women presenting with any abdominal pain after fertility treatment as suffering from OHSS. This carries the risk of missing serious pathology. It should be kept in mind that severe abdominal pain, pyrexia and peritonism are not features of OHSS and an alternative diagnosis should be sought if these are noted, or if features of severe OHSS such as ascites and haemoconcentration are absent. Diagnoses that have been wrongly attributed to OHSS include Group B Strep pelvic sepsis following IUI, ovarian torsion and appendicitis.

- Serious infection following egg retrieval is uncommon, but can occur, especially in women with endometriosis or pelvic inflammatory disease. It may be a reasonable defence to say that an endometrioma had to be traversed at egg collection, in order to access follicles that were otherwise inaccessible. Provision of prophylactic antibiotics in such cases would constitute a reasonable precaution, even though this has not been subject to randomized trials.

- A patient reporting significant abdominal pain at embryo transfer should be assessed clinically to rule out pelvic infection or another complication, and it may not be appropriate to proceed to embryo transfer in such cases.

References

1. National Institute for Health and Care Excellence (NICE). Fertility problems: assessment and treatment. Clinical guideline [CG156]. London: NICE; 2013.

2. National Institute for Health and Care Excellence (NICE). Endometriosis quality standard. 2018. Available at: www.nice .org.uk/guidance/qs172

3. Pritts, EA, Parker, WH, Olive, DL. Fibroids and infertility: an updated systematic review of the evidence. *Fertil Steril* 2009; 91(4): 1215–23.

4. Camus, E, Poncelet, C, Goffinet, F, Wainer, B, Merlet, F, Nisand, I, Philippe, HJ. Pregnancy rates after in-vitro fertilization in cases of tubal infertility with and without hydrosalpinx: a meta-

analysis of published comparative studies. *Hum Reprod* 1999; 14(5): 1243–9.

5. Tsiami, A, Chaimani, A, Mavridis, D, Siskou, M, Assimakopoulos, E, Sotiriadis, A. Surgical treatment for hydrosalpinx prior to in-vitro fertilization embryo transfer: a network meta-analysis. *Ultrasound Obstet Gynecol* 2016; 48: 434–45.

6. Human Fertilisation and Embryology Authority (HFEA). www.hfea.gov.uk/media/2993/person-responsible-role-description-and-key-behaviours.pdf

7. Human Fertilisation and Embryology Authority (HFEA). Code of Practice, 9th edition. Published 2018.

8. Royal College of Obstetricians and Gynaecologists (RCOG). The management of ovarian hyperstimulation syndrome. RCOG Green-top Guideline No. 5. Published 2016.

9. Gebril, A, Hamoda, H, Mathur, R. Outpatient management of severe ovarian hyperstimulation syndrome: a systematic review and a review of existing guidelines. *Hum Fertil* 2018; 21(2). http://dx.doi.org/10.1080/14647273.2017.1331048

Gynaecological Precancer

John Murdoch

CASE COMMENTARY
Swati Jha

Successful Claim

Morrissey v Health Service Executive [2020] IESC 6

The Claim

Ms Morrissey was diagnosed with terminal cervical cancer in 2018. In 2009 and 2012 she had received two cervical smear results reported as normal, however, following an audit it was disclosed that both results were incorrect. It was claimed that if the 2009 and 2012 smears had been accurately reported, then the pre-cancerous condition would have been diagnosed and she would have been successfully treated.

The Summary

In Ireland, the Health Service Executive (HSE) is responsible for running the cervical screening programme. It contracts out to labs to assess the samples taken. The claimant had smears tests as per the National Cervical Screening Programme (CervicalCheck) in 2009 and again in August 2012 and her smear test was reported as negative for abnormalities and she was given a clear result. In May 2014, following symptomatic bleeding, a biopsy and an MRI scan, she was diagnosed with cervical cancer and underwent surgery which appeared to be successful. However, following a recurrence in 2018 she was given a terminal diagnosis. Following her initial diagnosis, the earlier tests were audited in 2015. It was found that the 2009 sample had borderline abnormalities, and the 2012 sample was found to be "scanty", which required that the test be repeated. Neither abnormal results were communicated to the claimant until 2018, who was informed that both results were normal.

The Judgement

The high court judged in favour of the claimant. The HSE was found to be vicariously liable for the actions of the laboratories and reporting had to be by standards of "absolute confidence" in determining breach of duty in this case. It was noted that in cases of screening, there was no role in imposing a standard of approach on a professional but the standards of the profession itself. The case went to appeal to the Supreme Court of Ireland on several grounds, both for liability and for quantum. The appeal for issues of liability were turned down, but on the issue of award of damages for losses attributable to having to replace services which would have been provided to the family by Ms. Morrissey, had it not tragically transpired that she would have a significantly reduced life expectancy, the appeal was upheld.

Other successful cases include *Whittington Hospital NHS Trust v XX* [2020] UKSC 14, in which the Supreme Court considered whether the claimant was entitled to recover as damages the costs of surrogacy arrangements using her own eggs, the costs of surrogacy arrangements using donor eggs, and the costs of commercial surrogacy arrangements in the United States, and found for the claimant. This case will be discussed in further detail in the "Legal Commentary" for Chapter 24.

Similar to the *Morrissey* case, in *McGlone v Greater Glasgow Health Board* [2012] CSOH 190, an award totalling approximately £2,000,000 was proposed for loss, injury and damages caused by the misinterpretation and misreporting of two cervical smear tests, resulting in a subsequent diagnosis of invasive adenocarcinoma. In the case *of XX v Whittington*, the claimant recovered as damages the costs of surrogacy arrangements using her own eggs, the costs of surrogacy arrangements using donor eggs, and the costs of commercial surrogacy arrangements in the United States.

Unsuccessful Claim (Partially)

Beverley Pidgeon v Doncaster Health Authority [2001] 10 WLUK 238

The Claim

A smear taken when Mrs Pidgeon was 35 was sent to the defendants and reported as negative. On a subsequent smear nine years later there was severe dyskaryosis and this was subsequently confirmed to be a stage 2A or 3B cervical cancer requiring extensive treatment. It was claimed that the first smear had been reported incorrectly and this led to the development of a cervical cancer.

The Summary

Ms Pidgeon underwent a cervical smear which was reported as normal and she was noted to be pregnant soon after. Following this, she was invited repeatedly for her routine smear tests approximately seven times but failed to attend. Approximately nine years after the first smear reported as normal, she presented with abnormal bleeding and when a smear was repeated it showed evidence of severe dyskaryosis. Following further tests and investigations she was diagnosed to have cervical cancer stage 2B, for which she received radiotherapy and required resection of her bowel. This led to the initial smear being reanalysed and it was confirmed that there were several severely dyskaryotic cells in the initial smear that had been reported as normal. It was claimed that if this initial smear had been accurately reported, the treatment would have been an excision of the abnormal area of the cervix and would have prevented progression to a cervical cancer.

It was contended that if she had responded to these calls the gradually progressive abnormality of the smears missed on the initial smear would have been identified and treated before becoming an advanced cancer. Her failure to attend therefore broke the chain of causation and was contributory negligence to the harm suffered. The defendant also made the case that their duty to take reasonable care extended just to the three years till the next routine smear was due under the screening programme. Also, the development of full-blown cancer from severe dyskaryosis takes from seven to ten years, so had the claimant attended for her subsequent routine smears, the abnormality would have been detected and treated.

The Judgement

The health authority was liable for the negligent evaluation of a cervical smear test which failed to reveal a pre-cancerous condition. However, the claimant was held two thirds responsible for the development of cervical cancer as she had failed to attend screenings in the following nine years. The patient was therefore only entitled to one third of the payment (£18,500 instead of £55,500). While failing to attend for subsequent smears did not break the chain of causation, it did mean the patient was contributorily negligent. It was also ruled that GPs should continue to encourage attendance at smears.

Legal Commentary

Eloise Power

Morrissey v Health Service Executive and Others [2020] IESC 6

This case was determined by the Supreme Court of Ireland, who held that the principles set out in the case of *Dunne v National Maternity Hospital* [1989] IR 91 continued to apply to clinical negligence cases in Ireland. As discussed at Chapter 20, the Irish principles in *Dunne* are broadly equivalent to the English/Welsh principles in *Bolam*.

The key issue in the case was whether the trial judge had been correct in holding that the cytology screeners needed to have *"absolute confidence"* that the slide was negative before classifying the smear as normal. This finding had caused concern among commentators about the correct legal principles governing clinical negligence in Irish law. This concern was misconceived, as the Supreme Court of Ireland recognised,

> imposing such a standard of approach does not derive from the Court but rather from an assessment of the evidence given on all sides concerning the standard actually applied by professionals in the area in question. It is those experts, not the Court, who identified the standard expected of a normally competent screener as being one which precludes giving a clear result in a case of doubt [6.30].

In other words, in the particular context of the standard expected of a reasonably competent cytology screener, a reasonable standard of care requires that the screener should not give a negative result in a doubtful case. The legal principles are unchanged.

In the course of giving judgement in *Morrissey*, the Supreme Court of Ireland spent time analysing the principles established by the English case of *Penney and others v East Kent Health Authority* [2000] Lloyd's Rep Med 41. These principles, and their application in subsequent cases, are worthy of particular consideration in relation to cases involving the misreporting of cervical smears, and in the wider context of cases involving other types of misreporting of test results.

Approach to "Pure Diagnosis" Cases

In the case of *Penney* (supra), the Court of Appeal considered four cases of misreporting of cervical smears and addressed in particular the applicability of *Bolam/Bolitho* principles in relation to such cases. The Master of the Rolls held as follows [para 27]:

In addition, the Bolam test has no application where what the judge is required to do is to make findings of fact. This is so, even where those findings of fact are the subject of conflicting expert evidence.

He approved the following three questions [para 27]:

What was to be seen in the slides?

At the relevant time could a screener exercising reasonable care fail to see what was on the slide?

Could a reasonably competent screener, aware of what a screener exercising reasonable care would observe on the slide, treat the slide as negative?

The first question is a question of fact to which *Bolam/Bolitho* principles would not apply, whereas *Bolam/Bolitho* principles govern the approach to be taken to the second and third questions.

As we have seen in the Irish case of *Morrissey*, the concept of "absolute confidence" obfuscated the analysis of the issues to a certain extent until the situation was clarified by the higher courts. In a similar manner to that seen in *Morrissey*, the Court of Appeal explained that "absolute confidence" merely derived from the expert evidence on these particular facts, rather than being a legal test: *"The phrase 'absolute confidence' was no more than shorthand for the approach which on examination of the transcripts it seems to us all the experts endorsed"* [para 40]. Although the trial judge had questioned the relevance of *Bolam* in this factual context, the Court of Appeal made clear that *Bolam/Bolitho* was applicable to the questions which involved an examination of the screeners' skill and judgement, i.e. the second and third questions identified above.

In the case of *Muller v King's College Hospital NHS Foundation Trust* [2017] EWHC 128, Kerr J considered the applicability of the *Penney* principles in a case involving a pathologist who missed a malignant melanoma. The Court made some interesting observations on the relevance of the *Bolam/Bolitho* principles in the context of "pure diagnosis" cases [para 48–50]:

> In my judgment, the difficulty has arisen because, unfortunately, the authorities applying the conventional Bolam approach to negligence in this field do not sufficiently differentiate between two types of case. The first type is a case such as the present, where the patient's condition is unknown, and what is alleged to be negligent is a doctor's diagnosis of the condition, in the form of a report, with no decision made or advice given about treatment or further diagnostic procedures. The diagnosis is either right or wrong and, if wrong, either negligently so or not. Such a case could be called a "pure diagnosis" case. At the other end of the spectrum is the second type of case: a "pure treatment" case, where the nature of the patient's condition is known, and the alleged negligence consists in a decision to treat (or advise treatment of) a condition in a particular manner. The second type of case is the paradigm for application of the Bolam principle...

Despite these observations, which were *obiter dicta*,[1] Kerr J came to the conclusion that the *Bolam/Bolitho* principles applied to "pure diagnosis" cases, and that the Court of Appeal's approach in *Penney* was binding:

---

[1] In other words, they were not essential to the rationale of the judgement and hence not legally binding.

the case most closely analogous to the present case is Penney v. East Kent Health Authority; and I regard Penney as authority permitting the court to choose between competing expert opinion on the issue the court has to decide: whether the act or omission of the defendant's employee fell below the standard reasonably to be expected of her. However, I am bound by the law as it currently stands, to approach that issue by reference to a possible invocation of the Bolitho exception [para 78–79].

The approach to be taken to "pure diagnosis" cases fell for further consideration by Irwin LJ in *Brady v Southend University Hospital NHS Foundation Trust* [2020] EWHC 158, which concerned allegations of negligence on the part of a radiologist. Following a review of *Penney* and of *Muller*, the Court held as follows:

> It follows that determining what the CT scans show (e.g. (i) omental infarction or infection, (ii) whether the mass involved the lesser omentum, (iii) whether the mass was infiltrating the transverse colon), are essentially questions of fact for the Court to determine on the balance of probabilities, with the assistance of the witness and expert evidence provided. It is a separate question as to whether Dr Tam's or Dr Jain's assessments, even if conflicting with the Court's findings of fact, were negligent or not negligent. In that respect, I judge their work in accordance with Penny [sic] by invocation of the Bolitho exception. Insofar as I am required to assess their views on advancing differential diagnoses or recommending further investigation or treatment, as well assessing Mr Wright's conduct, there can be no question but that the Bolam test, with the Bolitho qualification, applies.

As the law stands, the principles which can be derived from this line of cases are as follows: (a) The *Bolam/Bolitho* test has no application to pure questions of fact such as what was objectively present on a cytology slide or a CT scan; (b) Bolam/Bolitho continues to govern the Court's approach to questions of professional skill and judgment, such as the second and third questions in *Penney*; (c) the concept of "absolute confidence" is not a legal test, but was merely a way of summarising the expert evidence heard in relation to a particular factual context, namely the approach which a reasonably competent cytology screener should take to an ambiguous slide. In the light of Kerr J's comments in *Muller*, various commentators have recommended that *Bolam/Bolitho* should not apply to "pure diagnosis" cases,[2] and it is possible that these issues will be revisited by the higher courts in the future.

As a point of good practice, when analysing a "pure diagnosis" case, it is generally relevant to explore whether the particular discipline involved has any form of audit system or grading system for discrepancies/misdiagnoses. The Royal College of Pathologists has a system of categorisation for discrepancies which postdates the events in *Muller*.[3] Such a system would not bind a Court, but would be likely to be regarded as evidentially valuable.

Beverley Pidgeon v Doncaster Health Authority [2001] 10 WLUK 238

The case of *Pidgeon*, which was determined by HHJ Bullimore sitting in the County Court in 2001, is of interest for a different reason: it is one of a relatively small number of

---

[2] See Paul Sankey. The test of breach of duty. *Personal Injury Law Journal* 2020; 184: 19–21.

[3] Royal College of Pathologists, Guide to Conducting an Investigative Audit of Cellular Pathology Practice, August 2017. Available at: www.rcpath.org/uploads/assets/5549a110-285a-4bb6-b9eba8d5b8192cb9/GuideInvestAuditCP.pdf

clinical negligence cases in which the Court has been prepared to make a finding of contributory negligence on the part of the claimant.

As background, the claimant had undergone a cervical smear test in 1988 which was wrongly reported as negative. The defendant accepted breach of duty in relation to the 1988 smear. The issue before the Court was whether the claimant's subsequent actions in failing to attend for repeat smears on multiple occasions broke the chain of causation, or alternatively amounted to contributory negligence.

On the facts, the Court found that the claimant was spoken to on *"not less than seven occasions by one of her panel doctors about the need for her to have a smear, and in 1991 and again in 1994 she received two letters from the screening programme urging her to do so"* [para 15]. The defendant argued (a) that their duty of care did not extend significantly beyond the recall date of three years for a repeat smear, (b) that the claimant's failure to attend for repeat smears on multiple occasions amounted to a *novus actus interveniens*,[4] breaking the chain of causation, and (c) that the claimant's actions amounted to contributory negligence.

The Court rejected the first argument: the claimant had never made an agreement with the defendant that she would participate in the screening programme, and the Court observed that *"The effects of the Defendants' admitted negligent failure would have been the same, if there had been no screening programme at all"*. The Court also rejected the second argument: the claimant's conduct was not regarded as *"so unreasonable as to eclipse the Defendant's wrongdoing"*, and did not suffice to break the chain of causation altogether.[5]

The defendant's third argument succeeded: the claimant was found to have been contributorily negligent. In the course of giving evidence, the claimant accepted that her doctors would have explained the importance of having a smear test, and she also accepted that she had *"probably been warned that pre-invasive cancer would not be picked up"* if no smear test was performed. The Court was unimpressed with the claimant's reasons for non-attendance:

A temporary discomfort or pain would have to be borne at 3 yearly intervals... She was plainly used to attending her GP and had been seen by other doctors while pregnant or after having given birth, and must have undergone a number of intimate examinations. Such may be embarrassing, but the level of embarrassment must lessen" [para 32].

There is nothing in the judgement to suggest that any weightier barrier to cervical screening was applicable in the claimant's particular case.

In the premises, the Court found that the claimant's own conduct was culpable: *"To fail to attend once in 1991 was blameworthy and showed some unreasonable care for her own health and welfare; to fail to respond again in 1994 was doubly so, against a background of increasingly strong warnings from her GP"* [para 33]. The Court held that the claimant was two thirds responsible for her own misfortune, and she only recovered one third of the damages and interest which had been agreed.

---

[4] Literally "a new intervening act", used in law to refer to an action which breaks the chain of causation.

[5] Para 22, citing *Emeh v Kensington and Chelsea and Westminster Area Health Authority* [1984] 3 All ER 1044.

The *Pidgeon* judgement serves as a salient reminder to claimants and defendants that in appropriate cases, contributory negligence can be a relevant and important issue. Where a claimant has failed to attend for important diagnostic tests, it is essential to explore the reasons in detail and provide a salient explanation to the Court.

Clinical Commentary

John Murdoch

Good Practice Guidance

Introduction

Cervical disease is the dominant issue here and the other sites will be dealt with briefly. The lower genital tract is dominated by human papilloma virus (HPV) and the upper tract dominated either by hormones or the aetiology is obscure.

Vulval and Vaginal Precancer

Vulval intraepithelial neoplasia (VIN) is one of the vulval dermatoses and is associated with cancer progression in 30% to 90% of cases, depending on the series referenced, all of which are small and of short duration hence the wide range of incidence. Lichen sclerosis et atrophicus (LSA) is statistically associated but the aetiological association is obscure.

The dermatoses are protean in their manifestation and timely biopsy is key. One exception is classic LSA which can be managed by a short sharp course of steroids with review. If there is no rapid response, then reconsideration and biopsy is essential. Otherwise, the key is to beware of any uncertain skin change, any complex lesion and any lesion with developing or changing symptoms which must be assessed in a vulval clinic and biopsied. Steroid treatment is good for symptom relief but if VIN is present then antivirals may help and if appropriate excision should be contemplated. Destruction of VIN is often unsatisfactory. Follow-up is unfortunately long-term given the long latency of VIN and careful explanation, management of expectations and repeat treatment is often the case.

Vaginal intraepithelial neoplasia (VaIN) is usually an extension of cervical disease and careful inspection of the vagina in large cervical lesions is important, with care required to diagnose it. Thereafter antivirals and local destruction may help. Care is required when there is disease involving the vaginal vault scar after hysterectomy, as disease progression can occur in the scar out of sight. Upper vaginectomy is a tricky and potentially traumatic procedure to be undertaken by experienced surgeons with caution.

Cervical Precancer

Colposcopy was first described in 1927 by the German Hans Hinselmann but it did not find its place in Western medicine until the late 1960s onwards. This was probably because of the difficult polysyllabic German words used, the political turmoil of the first half of the twentieth century and the absence a clear role in gynaecology. The situation was transformed by the increasing use of cervical cytology in the 1960s and the development of comprehensive cervical screening programmes. The only alternative response to an abnormal smear was hysterectomy and colposcopy found its role which

I would define as: the maintenance of a woman's cervical health while protecting as far as possible her psychological, sexual and reproductive well-being.

In clinical practice, colposcopy is inextricably linked with cervical screening and this feeds through to medico-legal issues. Colposcopy can be viewed as the motor arm of a reflex arc where cytology is the sensory arm. In the United Kingdom, the NHS has been key to the development of one of the best examples of a population screening programme which has seen cervical cancer rates and deaths plummet. This has created its own problems, with the risk of over-medicalisation and over-treatment of minor cervical problems. Alternatively, the rarity of overt cancer has led to missed diagnoses in General Practice where current GPs will be unlucky to see more than one cervical cancer in their professional lives and even gynaecologists in other subspecialties will seldom see a case. While cervical cytology is not my area of expertise, I will touch on the issue of screening misdiagnoses and the considerations for an expert in addressing the needs of her patient when an audit reveals an apparent error years before a cancer diagnosis and those of the expert asked to comment on causation in such cases.

The explosion in colposcopy coincided with the evidence-based revolution in medicine. Medicine based on expert opinions of a few doyens and viewed as largely an art has given way to the application of well worked high quality evidence, large observational studies and collated expert opinion. Molecular biology has shown us the clear causal role of human papilloma virus (HPV) high risk subtypes. This has resulted in widely accepted comprehensive clear guidelines [1]. This guidance is so well written, so well accepted and backed up by a robust quality assurance programme that it has evolved the status of Mandate rather than simple guidance. This means that there is limited scope for deviation and any deviation must be fully justified in writing to ensure high quality care and protection from litigation. Good clinical practice and avoidance of litigation is almost always co-terminal. Ultimately successful litigation is seldom unjust; no matter how aggrieved a clinician may feel during the process.

Cervical Cytology

Cervical screening is imprecise, diagnostically relying on repeat testing in the average 10 years latency from exposure to HPV and cancer. Colposcopists base their actions on the cytology report. Expert cytopathologists have reached a fair degree of consensus about the numbers of abnormal cells and their degree of abnormal morphology beyond which no reasonable cytoscreener should have missed the diagnosis. Errors are found at audit of the last 10 years of available cytology after a cancer diagnosis, backed by external review. The expert colposcopist contributes by:

1) Counselling a patient with cancer about her audit result, often some time after diagnosis and treatment. The information can be an overwhelming burden on top of the strain of dealing with the fear, anxiety and pressure of life changes imposed by the cancer and its treatment for many patients. The colposcopist or treating gynaecological oncologist most well-known to the patient must fully engage in the sensitive open and honest disclosure of the facts to ensure that the patient has a balanced understanding. Patient reactions vary dramatically and the doctor has to listen as intensely as she gives information. The aim for the colposcopist is to maintain trust with the patient that she has been open and balanced, acting as the patient's advocate and friend. This helps with their present and future relationship

through treatment. The involvement of a clinical nurse specialist (CNS) can be very helpful.

2) At litigation, the expert colposcopist, who is usually a gynaecological oncologist, provides an opinion on causation. Usually, there are no clinical issues at the time of a false negative test as the patient has no symptoms. The expert gives an opinion, on the balance of probability, on the stage at presentation and treatment compared to what would have happened if the sample had been reported appropriately. This aids quantification of the excess harm or risk the patient suffered by the alleged error. To reach an opinion about the state of the cervical epithelium at the time of the incident test, the expert relies on her knowledge of the natural history of HPV/CIN, her understanding of symptoms and signs of abnormalities of the cervix, and a realistic understanding of the concept of cervical doubling times.

Tumour doubling times are based on poor science and are fraught with error. A precise numeric volume by back-calculation from an estimated tumour volume at presentation risks inadvertently misleading the Court with pseudo-accuracy. My practice is to use the simplest calculation of volumes (volume = 1/2 (product of the three principle diameters of the tumour)), calculated from MRI and/or histology; with an average doubling time of three months (range two to four months). This provides a framework against which the known symptoms and the natural history of the disease can be compared. Most experts can agree with this, thereby assisting the Court. Usually, it is possible to define the likely stage of the disease, treatment and outcomes. Occasionally, a calculation places a patient on a border such as that where a radical trachelectomy would be considered reasonable, with its impact on future fertility. Here the expert is required to be explicit about the uncertainties so the Court can make its judgement.

Colposcopy

Litigation in colposcopy is unusual in my experience because widespread adherence to the guidelines ensures quality assurance. This can be subdivided:

The Symptomatic Patient Under the Age of Twenty-five -- The correct management for a GP when presented with a young patient with symptoms of discharge, post-coital bleeding and irregular vaginal loss is to take a menstrual, contraceptive and sexual history, to examine the cervix and take appropriate swabs for treatment of infection. Many patients cannot understand the sound statistical reasons why screening is potentially counterproductive in this age group. It is sensible to emphasise the need for review if the symptoms do not settle. Overt cervical cancer is rare in general practice and GPs are naturally cautious when they see unusual appearances. This generates urgent suspected cancer referrals for benign ectopy or Nabothian follicles. The referral route is to an urgent referral suspected cancer clinic or a colposcopy clinic. The advantage of the former is a speedy satisfactory service for most patients with benign problems. The drawbacks are that these clinics can be staffed by gynaecologists inexperienced in the diagnosis of cancer and that an apparent benign ectopy can be accompanied by a surrounding but invisible halo of CIN. Alternatively, colposcopy offers the advantages of a speedy, highly accurate diagnosis of clinical normality resulting in removal of anxiety and clarity when cancer is the likely diagnosis and involvement of the cancer CNS and the oncology service if required. It allows the identification of invisible CIN which can be treated if necessary or observed to allow regression if appropriate. I favour colposcopy.

Delays in Assessment once Referral Has Been Made -- All services are under considerable pressure to achieve the two-week target for 93% of patients with moderate or severe dyskaryosis and 18 weeks for lesser results [1]. The direct referral system from cytology lab into the colposcopy service has hugely reduced administrative delay. While some services fail to achieve the standard, it is rare, apart from a patient failing to attend or engage in the programme, for a delay to impact on care or outcome, with consequent absence of causation. I have never been instructed under these terms.

Errors in Assessment and Diagnosis -- Individual smears are diagnostically imprecise, with accuracy of 50% to 90% against histopathology. An abnormal result is saying that there is probably a lesion with some indication of the severity of the lesion. Similarly, colposcopic assessment is not accurate [2]. Colposcopists are heavily influenced by the severity of the referral cytology. Colposcopy defines where a lesion is and if the whole lesion is visible. An experienced colposcopist should be able to identify true invasion on the one hand and normality on the other. Diagnosis of minor CIN lesions and indeed differentiation of high activity CIN3 and microinvasion can be problematic [3].

The colposcopist should exclude overt invasion and define the upper limit of the lesion then take a directed punch biopsy of the maximum abnormality. Alternatively, if the patient gives her informed consent, the visible lesion is compatible with a high-grade smear and the patient's age and fertility requirements are clear, then, tailored loop diathermy on a "see and treat" basis is appropriate.

A common failure is to take an inadequate loop biopsy. Loop diathermy is almost universally used in colposcopy compared to other treatment modalities. Its simplicity, cheapness and versatility are attractive but careless use of the term large loop excision of the transformation zone (LLETZ) which should be confined to treatment of type1 transformation zones and the use of loop cone [4] for a cone biopsy for type 2 and 3 lesions results in loose thinking and intent. The key is the position of the squamo-columnar junction in the endocervical canal. Type 1 lesions require excision to a depth of 7–10 mm. Type 2 lesions require excision to 10–15 mm and type 3 lesions require excision to 15–25 mm. Treatment should be performed under local anaesthesia, with 80% of specimens removed in one piece. This requires a compliant consenting patient, a good colposcopy assistant administering "verbal anaesthesia", an accessible lesion and a skilful colposcopist. Sometimes, it is entirely appropriate to resort to a short general anaesthetic or to take a sample in sections.

The depth of excision is a major determinant of subsequent pregnancy performance. This is relevant in young women with fertility plans. Excessive conservatism to preserve cervical tissue in older women with no fertility aspirations is pointless and risky.

Failure of Adequate Counselling and Consent -- Clear information sheets and online information are valuable. Time taken outlining likely options prior to examination is well spent. A relaxed patient, confident in the colposcopist's skill is essential. A clear understanding of the patient's comprehension and wishes is central. Consent is seldom an issue with regards to immediate and early complications of bleeding and infection. The relatively small risk of future pregnancy difficulties set against the importance of ongoing cervical health does need specific mention to avoid the risk of a late complaint.

I well remember two cases where careful discussion was necessary between doctor and patient. One was a young woman who had persisting abnormal endocervical cells on cytology after deep conisation against a fierce desire to have children. An anxious three years followed until, after two rapid pregnancies, a hysterectomy revealed focal high grade cervical glandular neoplasia (HGCGIN). The other case was a patient being worked up for infertility who had a double cervix with fluctuating mild cytological abnormalities in both cervixes and unsatisfactory colposcopy. At the time of my retirement, she was still trying for pregnancy with no progression in the cytological abnormalities.

Treatment Complications –– Failure to counsel for, or adequately manage immediate complications of bleeding and infection is rare.

Minimising problems is a matter of learned technique comprising:

- Carefully sited subcutaneous local anaesthetic and a suitable vasopressor to achieve a blanching oedema peripheral to the lesion.
- Diathermy blended settings which allow a snag free steady passage of the loop to an appropriate depth without too much power causing collateral tissue damage and uncontrolled passage through the tissues.
- Rapid conversion to ball diathermy coagulation of the excision edges and any active bleeding vessels before the cavity fills with blood resulting in simply boiling blood without coagulation.
- Avoiding time-wasting dabbing before haemostasis is achieved.
- Targeted packing of the diathermy cavity with a tampon or ribbon gauze soaked in Monsels solution, rather than uncomfortable ineffective vague vaginal packing.
- Simple effective cryotherapy for secondary haemorrhage rather than ineffective vague packing of the vagina or traumatic ineffective suturing.

Alternatively, damage to the vagina or worse, bladder or bowel, is never defensible and can be avoided by:

- Patient selection within the experience of the colposcopist.
- Reversion to general anaesthesia when the risks from access or patient compliance are high.
- Inducing subcutaneous oedema with the local anaesthetic where the lesion is close to the vagina, thereby creating tissue separation.
- Selecting the correct size loop to achieve the ideal single specimen but being willing to use a smaller loop with more than one pass if access is challenging.
- Use a q-tip pressed against the fornix diagonally opposite the area of most risk to make the cervix nod towards the q-tip away from the risk while resecting away from the maximum risk to safety.
- Stabilising the insulated shaft of the loop against the outer edge of the speculum and use as a fulcrum to stop "operator shake".

The risk of preterm delivery in a subsequent pregnancy from cervical incompetence caused by cervical excision appears to be dependent on the volume of excised tissue relative to the volume of the available cervix [5]. LLETZ for type 1 lesions needs no special preparation. For type 2 and type 3 lesions, women with pregnancy aspirations require specific counselling about the limited additional risk a cone biopsy poses contrasted with the need for a healthy cervix and the avoidance of cancer for future health. Careful follow-up without treatment of minor cytological problems looking for cytological or colposcopic progression, may be appropriate in women planning pregnancy. It is worth remembering that such conservatism is not relevant in older women whose child-bearing is complete and whose primary concern is a rapid return to cervical health.

Failure of Follow-up and Communication –– Current advice on follow-up after treatment for CIN is clearly via community-based cytology for most patients [1]. This builds on early advice that involvement of excision margins is not a good indicatory of residual disease [6]. The follow-up of selected patients with treated HGCGIN and some patients with treated CIN where there is anticipated difficulty getting a good cervical sample is best accomplished via colposcopy. There is no point in a GP smear-taker struggling and failing to get a useful result to the disillusion and discomfort of a patient when it is critical to get a good sample. This is most easily achieved with a colposcopically directed endocervical sample offering a good quality sample to the relief of patient and attendant alike.

Good communication following assessment with or without treatment is central to GMC guidance on good medical practice. I was an early adopter of the practice of writing to the patient copy to the GP with reports couched in lay terms on the grounds that:

1) The patient is the most important participant.
2) Effective understanding by the patient of the diagnosis maximises compliance in ongoing surveillance which is a central component of failsafe mechanisms to find persistent disease in a process where cytology and colposcopy carry inherent weaknesses and even gold standard histology can be wrong.
3) The GP is better able to interpret lay language into medical understanding than the other way around as occurs when the GP is written to with a copy to the patient.
4) Failure to effectively communicate the need for follow-up can result in the tragedy of a patient assuming all is well having been discharged from the clinic only to ignore developing important symptoms in subsequent years.

In summary, colposcopy is a highly researched, tightly controlled, relatively simple clinical process with simple core rules. These are clearly enshrined in well accepted national guidance backed up by well organised quality assurance and multidisciplinary team (MDT) working. Adherence to guidelines will result in good clinical practice which will result in security from litigation. Colposcopists working within the limits of their experience with reference to experienced clinical leaders as required will seldom have problems. Individual variations from established clinical pathways should be clearly reasoned and documented. Patient involvement in their care is paramount for their current care and future compliance in follow-up.

Endometrial Hyperplasia

Divided into two subgroups, hyperplasia is either cytologically simple and hormonally driven or atypical with a less clear association, probably reflecting the two broad malignant categories of type 1 and 2 cancer. Both can be managed with progestogens but the malignant potential from already co-existing invasive disease or subsequent progression in atypical hyperplasia can occur in up to 60% of cases in reported series. Atypical hyperplasia is therefore best treated by hysterectomy unless there are contra-indications or patient dissent. Non-surgical management with intrauterine hormonal treatment or high dose oral treatment in patients unsuitable for surgery is helpful but requires clear and careful explanation of risks and failure rates.

Ovarian Precancer

More correctly termed fallopian tube precancer, this is a histological diagnosis which confirms the tubal origin of serous cancers and is not usually detectable prior to surgery. Borderline tumours of the ovary of uncertain malignant potential are just what the name suggests. The diagnosis is uncertain without full histological assessment and the only time I have seen this condition appear in a medico-legal context is when a surgeon fails to completely remove a complex ovarian mass for examination by a specialist pathologist.

Causes of Litigation

- Failure to reassess the presumed diagnosis if a vulval lesion does not respond to treatment as expected
- Failure to biopsy an atypical or changing vulval lesion
- Collateral damage in treating VaIN
- Failure of adequate counselling
- Deviation from cervical treatment guidelines without specific written justification
- Failure of adequate treatment
- Inadequate follow-up
- Taking on cases outside a clinician's ability

Avoidance of Litigation

- Adhere to guidelines
- Fully justify variation from guidelines
- Keep your patient on board with clear information
- Ensure treatment is appropriate to the patient and her circumstances
- Stay within your skill and experience

References

1. www.gov.uk/government/publications/cervical-screening-programme-and-colposcopy-management

2. Ruan, Y, Liu, M, Guo, J, Zhao, J, Niu, S, Li, F. Evaluation of the accuracy of colposcopy in detecting high-grade squamous intraepithelial lesion and cervical cancer. *Arch Gynecol Obstet* 2020; 302: 1529–38.

3. Murdoch, JB, Grimshaw, RN, Morgan, PR, Monaghan, JM. The impact of loop diathermy on management of early invasive cervical cancer. *Int J Gynaecol Cancer* 1991; 2: 129–133.

4. Mor Yosef, SAD, Lopes, D, Pearson SE, Monaghan, JM. Loop diathermy cone biopsy. *Obstet Gynecol* 1990; 75(5): 884–6.

5. Sasieni, P, , A, Landy, R, Kyrgiou, M, Kitchener, H, Quigley, M, Poon, LCY,

Shennan, A, Hollingworth, A, Soutter, WP, Freeman-Wang, T, Peebles, D, Prendiville, W, Patnick, J. Risk of preterm birth following surgical treatment for cervical disease: executive summary of a recent symposium. *BJOG* 2016; 123(9): 1426–9.

6. Murdoch, JB, Morgan, PR, Lopes, A, Monaghan, JM. Histological incomplete excision of CIN after large loop excision of the transformation zone (LLETZ) merits careful follow-up, not retreatment. *Br J Obstet Gynaecol* 1992; 99: 990–3.

Gynaecological Malignancy

Helen Bolton, Anastasia Georgiou

CASE COMMENTARY

Swati Jha

Successful Claim

Loretta Oliver v Gary Williams [2013] EWHC 600 (QB)
The Claim

The claimant saw her GP (defendant) with symptoms of stomach cramps, bloating and diarrhoea. Following a normal stool result the GP referred her to the hospital but failed to tell the patient that an urgent referral to rule out other pathology had been made. It was claimed that the GP, by failing to alert her to the urgent referral, resulted in the patient not following up the referral and as a consequence there was a delay in the diagnosis by five to six months. It was initially alleged that her life expectancy had been reduced as a result of the delayed diagnosis and due to the psychological effect she was less able to deal with chemotherapy or resume work as she would have wished.

The Summary

The initial referral made by the GP to the hospital was misplaced. There was no arrangement in place to ensure the patient received a referral. Because the patient had not been informed to expect an appointment from the hospital, she was not aware of the need to follow this up and when her symptoms persisted, she returned to see the GP again. The defendant stated he had made the patient aware of the referral but this was denied by the claimant who only had recollection of attending for a review of moles she was worried about. There is a documentation in the notes that a referral was being made but the defendant failed to tell the patient. Her symptoms persisted and she was seen by another GP six months later when it was identified that the initial referral had not been actioned. On referral to the hospital, she was found to have widespread and disseminated malignancy with deposits throughout the abdomen. She was debulked and received multiple courses of chemotherapy.

The Judgement

The delay in referral meant that her surgery was delayed by 5.5 months. However, the experts agreed that this delay did not make a difference to the disease staging or the treatment options as the cancer was already advanced. The objectives of surgery, had this been performed earlier, would have been the same i.e. to debulk the patient and provide chemotherapy. Therefore, it was not admitted that a delay in diagnosis made a material difference to the life expectancy, however it did mean she went through considerable discomfort and worsening symptoms on account of it. In the judgement it was also denied that the inability to work or the psychological problems were a cause of the delay in diagnosis and would have occurred anyway due to the advanced stage of disease.

Though successful, the pay-out was for £7,500 (£2,500 for suffering during the period of delayed diagnosis and £5,000 for the psychiatric injury attributable to the breach)

In the case of JD v (1) Wye Valley NHS Trust, (2) Gloucestershire Hospitals NHS Foundation Trust, (3) Worcestershire Acute Hospitals NHS Trust (2017), an out-of-court settlement was reached when the cervical biopsy had been insufficient to test for CIN and the histopathologist had advised a repeat biopsy. This led to a delay in diagnosis resulting in more extensive surgery with an early onset of menopause and loss of fertility. The change in the stage of diagnosis meant the pay-out was for a greater sum of £87,500.

Unsuccessful Claim

Devonport v Gateshead Health NHS Foundation Trust [2016] EWHC 1729 (QB)

The Claim

Mrs Devonport (claimant) was diagnosed with stage 2A cervical cancer and underwent a Wertheim's hysterectomy. She developed multiple complications subsequently following this surgery, including a psoas abscess, stricture of the ureter and an ovarian mass, and required multiple further interventions to manage these complications. It was claimed that the injury to her bowel during surgery caused the psoas abscess and the formation of the ovarian mass, which resulted in the pressure and stricture of the ureter. It was also alleged that the gynaecologist failed to involve the urologists in performing the salpingo-oophorectomy, resulting in further surgery for the ureter at a later date.

The Summary

The claimant was fit and well prior to the diagnosis of cervical cancer. When consenting to the hysterectomy she was informed of its complications, including infection and injury to internal viscera. The contemporaneous records for the surgery were uneventful and the claimant given antibiotics as per hospital protocol. She made an uneventful postoperative recovery and was discharged home after eight days with an adequate postoperative plan. Eleven days after discharge she presented to her GP, was treated for infection but when this did not settle was referred to hospital and found to have a psoas abscess. There was evidence of inflammation around the ureter on the affected side resulting in hydronephrosis of the affected kidney. The abscess was drained under radiological guidance. When reviewed three months post-surgery, she was found to have lesion on her ovary with a stricture of the ureter on the same side. The claimant had a stent inserted and 10 months after the index procedure was scheduled for removal of the ovarian mass. The claimant appears to have been told by the consultant gynaecologist that there may have been an inadvertent bowel injury at the time of the index procedure which resulted in the psoas abscess and ovarian mass. However, the possibility of bowel injury was denied during the hearing.

Following the replacement of the stent, the urologists sent correspondence to the gynaecologists stating that if the stricture persisted the claimant would need a reimplantation of the ureter. However, this would not have result in a joint procedure at the time of the removal of the ovary, hence a discussion regarding a joint procedure was not initiated. This meant the claimant required a further operation for ureteric reimplantation at a later date.

The Judgement

Both the allegations were denied. The formation of a psoas abscess was an unusual but significant complication of surgery occuring due to infection rather than negligence. This infection subsequently led to the ovarian mass and fistulated into the bowel. The stricture of the ureter was managed appropriately and the surgery for ovarian mass was also appropriate, with no indication to involve the urologists in this second procedure. The claim was therefore dismissed.

In the case of *Baxter v McCann* [2010] EWHC 1330 (QB), a claim of negligence was dismissed against a GP for failing to identify a rare ovarian cancer during the course of an examination. The GP met the standard of care by performing an abdominal vaginal and bimanual examination.

Legal Commentary

Eloise Power

Legal Framework Relating to Cancer Claims

The judgements of the House of Lords in *Gregg v Scott* [2005] UKHL 2 remain the leading source of authority governing delayed diagnosis of cancer claims (as well as other clinical negligence claims involving reduced prospects of a more favourable outcome). On the facts, the claimant's GP negligently misdiagnosed a lump under the claimant's arm as benign. In fact, the claimant suffered from non-Hodgkin's lymphoma. The negligence led to a nine-month delay in the claimant receiving treatment. During this period, his cancer spread to the left pectoral region. His prospects of 10-year disease-free survival were reduced as a result of the delay from 42% to 25% [para 64].

The key issue which fell for consideration was whether or not the claimant had suffered a recoverable loss. Should damages in clinical negligence be recoverable for the loss of a chance, even a less than likely chance, or should the Court take the view that the claimant had lost nothing given that he was unlikely to survive for 10 years on the balance of probabilities regardless of the negligence?

This has long been a controversial and divisive issue. As Lord Nicholls put it, *"This appeal raises a question which has divided courts and commentators throughout the common law world"* [para 1]. The judgements in *Gregg v Scott* cite various academic authorities and judgements from other jurisdictions as well as historic judgements from this jurisdiction. The House of Lords itself was divided, with two justices (Lord Nicholls and Lord Hope) dissenting from the majority decision.

Ultimately, the majority of the House of Lords (Lord Hoffman, Lord Phillips and Baroness Hale) decided that damages in clinical negligence should not be recoverable for the loss of a chance of survival and that causation had to be approached on the balance of probabilities. The claimant's appeal was dismissed.

To an extent, the harshness of the outcome in *Gregg v Scott* has been mitigated by some observations in their Lordships' judgements which have been developed in the subsequent case law. In the course of her judgement in *Gregg v Scott* Baroness Hale observed (obiter) that the claimant would have been entitled to damages for any adverse outcomes which were caused by the defendant's negligence on the balance of probabilities. She observed that

> The defendant is liable for any extra pain, suffering, loss of amenity, financial loss and loss of expectation of life which may have resulted from the delay. If without the delay, the claimant would have achieved a longer gap before more radical treatment became necessary, then he should be entitled to damages to reflect the acceleration in his suffering. If the pain and suffering he would have suffered anyway was made worse by the anguish of knowing that his disease could have been detected earlier, then he should be compensated for that [para 206].

She proceeded to explore the possibility of a claim arising from a modest reduction in life expectancy based upon a comparison between the non-negligent and the negligent scenarios [para 207]. Unfortunately, there was no material before the House of Lords upon which to consider the case on this basis, as the claimant had chosen to fight upon loss of a chance alone. As Lord Hope put it, "All the appellant's eggs were, so to speak, put in this one basket" [para 97].

The observations of Baroness Hale in *Gregg v Scott* were applied by Bean J in *JD v Mather* [2012] EWHC 3063 (QB). On the facts, the claimant suffered a seven-month delay in diagnosis due to her GP's negligent failure to diagnose a malignant melanoma. The Court found that the claimant's prospects of 10-year survival were already under 50% at the date of the consultation with the GP. His primary claim therefore failed by application of the majority decision in *Gregg v Scott*. His secondary claim, in which he alleged that he had suffered a loss of life expectancy as a result of the delay, succeeded: the Court found that the negligence caused a three-year reduction in life expectancy and awarded damages to be assessed upon this basis.

As a matter of good practice, it is advisable for lawyers and experts working on delayed diagnosis of cancer cases to be aware of the following points:

(a) It is sensible to investigate both the percentage by which a claimant's chance of survival has been reduced by the delay and the overall reduction in life expectancy (expressed in years) as a result of the delay.

(b) Other forms of damage besides reduction in life expectancy should also be explored (e.g. additional painful treatment with associated side effects, symptoms during the delay period, psychiatric damage as a result of the delay).

(c) Most clinical negligence cases take years to come to trial or to settlement. During the period when the case is ongoing, the expert evidence in relation to survival prospects both in the actual scenario and the hypothetical scenario may well change. It is important to ensure that expert evidence remains up to date.

(d) The House of Lords considered the claimant's percentage chance of survival over a 10-year period in *Gregg v Scott*; essentially, 10-year survival was regarded as equivalent to a cure. The use of the 10-year period derived from the expert evidence heard at trial in *Gregg v Scott*. A 10-year time period is unlikely to be appropriate for all forms of cancer; expert evidence should be sought on the appropriate time period in each specific case. It may be possible to distinguish the approach taken in *Gregg v Scott* if the expert evidence establishes that a different time period should apply for a different type of cancer.

"Lost Years" Claims and Fatal Cases[1]

The judgements discussed above, and the approach to cancer cases in general, should be considered in the context of the general legal framework relating to claims involving reduced life expectancy. By way of background:

(a) Under section 1 of the Law Reform (Miscellaneous Provision) Act 1934, the estate of a deceased person can sue (or be sued) in respect of any cause of action which is in existence at the date of their death. There are certain exceptions. In particular, the estate cannot claim any damages for loss of income in respect of any period after the deceased's death under the 1934 Act.

(b) Under section 1 of the Fatal Accidents Act 1976, the dependants[2] of a person whose death has been caused by *"any wrongful act, neglect or default"* can bring an action for damages for the benefit of the dependants. A restricted list of dependants[3] can also claim damages for bereavement. Claims under the 1976 Act can include claims brought by dependents for financial dependency and dependency upon services such as childcare and housework.

(c) A living claimant with a reduced life expectancy can claim damages for the loss of income during the "lost years", i.e. the years by which his or her life has been shortened as a result of the negligence. A "lost years" claim cannot be brought in respect of a deceased claimant[4] as this could amount to double recovery given that the dependants of the deceased may well have a claim under the Fatal Accidents Act 1976.

If a claimant has settled a claim in life, the dependants cannot bring a further action following death: see the judgement of Langstaff J in *Thompson v Arnold* [2007] EWHC 1875. Langstaff J observed that a claim for income dependency brought on behalf of the dependants after death under the Fatal Accidents Act is *"always likely to be higher than a claim for loss of income during the 'lost years'"* [para 22]. There are a number of reasons for this. The main reason is that the conventional deduction for living expenses made in a 'lost years' claim is 50%, whereas the conventional deduction for the amount which the deceased would have spent upon himself/herself in a Fatal Accidents Act claim is 33.3% (or 25% where the deceased left a spouse and children). This is something of a legal anomaly.[5]

---

[1] See chapter 27, *Clerk and Lindsell on Torts*, 23rd edition, sections 4–5, for a more comprehensive discussion of this area of law than it is possible to give here.

[2] Defined at section 1 (3)–1 (5) of the Act.

[3] Husband, wife, civil partner, cohabiting partner as defined by section 2A of the Act, and parents/mother of a deceased minor.

[4] Section 4, Administration of Justice Act 1982.

[5] In *Gregg v Scott*, Lord Phillips suggested that *"It would be much better if the claimant had no right to recover for such loss of earnings and the dependants' right to claim under section 1 (1) of the Fatal Accidents Act 1976 subsisted despite the claimant's recovery of damages for his injury. I am not persuaded that this result could not be achieved by a purposive construction of that section"* [para 182].

As an aside, it is not always the case that the value of a Fatal Accidents Act claim is higher than the value of a "lost years" claim. The present author recently settled a case acting for a lone parent with a terminal cancer diagnosis. The "lost years" claim spanned the lone parent's entire career to retirement age, whereas the dependency claim only covered the period until her youngest child turned 21. Hence the "lost years" claim worked out as higher value than the dependency claim, even though the percentage by which the annual income was reduced was greater. It is important for practitioners to be alert to this possibility, and not to make the assumption that a claim after death will in all cases be higher value than a claim in life.

In the more typical scenario encountered in practice, where a claim brought by dependants after death is likely to be higher in value than a claim brought in life, claimants with reduced life expectancy have various options. In cases where liability has been admitted, an interim payment can be sought in life, with the remainder of the claim being settled after death. An adjournment of the trial can also be sought. In some circumstances, defendants may be amenable to settlement of claims on a Fatal Accidents Act basis even where a claimant is still alive (particularly if death is imminent). In addition, claims for further damages under an existing provisional damages order may be brought by the estate of the deceased after death,[6] although in practice defendants are often reluctant to agree to orders for provisional damages. Obtaining specialist advice is essential; this is a difficult area of law which is often profoundly upsetting for claimants with reduced life expectancy.

Oliver v Williams [2013] EWHC 600 (QB)

In the case of *Oliver v Williams*, Simeon Maskrey QC, sitting as a Deputy Judge of the High Court, found that there had been no reduction in life expectancy due to a 5.5-month delay in diagnosing ovarian cancer on the particular facts of the case. Counsel for the defendant encouraged the Court not to make an assumption that the delay probably translated into a reduction in life expectancy merely because *"the idea that delays in diagnosis and treatment of cancer patients adversely affect survival is deeply ingrained in our psyche."* Rather than making such an assumption, the Court looked closely at the expert evidence. Although the Court accepted that as a matter of general principle, the less the volume of cancerous tissue left after surgery, the better the prognosis for survival, there was no evidence before the Court as to what proportion of residual cancerous tissue would have been left if it had not been for the delay [para 40]. The experts did not give a clear answer beyond stating that *"slightly less tumour"* would have been left. There was no trial data evaluating the impact of different volumes of residual material on life expectancy. Under the circumstances, the Court was not prepared to find that there had been a reduction in life expectancy based on the particular facts.

The Court made an award of £2,500 for the claimant's increased pain and suffering due to her symptoms during the delay period and her poorer health at the onset of chemotherapy (which she would have required in any event). A further award was made for psychiatric injury. The psychiatric evidence before the Court did not clearly differentiate between the psychiatric impact of the cancer (which the claimant would have suffered in any event) and the psychiatric impact of the delay. The Court held that the

---

[6] *Guilfoyle v North Middlesex University Hospital NHS Trust* (2018), unreported, HHJ Roberts.

majority of the psychiatric damage was attributable to the cancer, but awarded £5,000 for the psychiatric injury attributable to the negligence.

In *Kadir v Mistry* [2014] EWCA Civ 1177, the Court of Appeal went one step further: damages were awarded for the deceased claimant's mental anguish occasioned by an apprehension of early death based upon her well-founded fear that her life had been curtailed as a result of a delay in diagnosing cancer. It appears that there was no psychiatric evidence before the Court. In the absence of directly relevant case law, an award of £3,500 was made on account of mental anguish in the final three months of life.

Devonport v Gateshead Health NHS Foundation Trust [2016] EWHC 1729 (QB)

In the case of *Devonport*, Whipple J considered allegations of negligence arising from two surgical procedures which the claimant had undergone for treatment of carcinoma of the cervix, namely a hysterectomy and a salpingo-oophorectomy.

The allegations in relation to the hysterectomy failed on the facts. As the Court observed: *"To dispose of the case, it is enough that I conclude that the negligent explanation for the Claimant's problems is no more likely than the non-negligent explanation. On that basis, the case must fail. . ."* [para 84]. The Court found that infection in the lower pelvis is a known and relatively common complication of radical hysterectomy. Although the precise location of the infection was otherwise unknown after radical hsyterectomy (it formed an abscess in the psoas muscle), the Court found that this *"can best be explained as a particularly unusual feature of an otherwise, sadly, unsurprising case"* [para 82].

The allegations arising out of the salpingo-oophorectomy similarly failed on the facts: the Court found that the claimant's case (to the effect that a urologist should have been present at the time of the salpingo-oophorectomy which would have prevented her from suffering a ureteric stricture leading to a right nephrectomy) *"seems to me to go far beyond identifying the reasonable minimum standard of care which the Claimant was entitled to expect, and to have become a 'counsel of perfection'"* [para 95].

This interesting judgement illustrates (a) the potential for clinical negligence cases to arise out of alleged negligence in the course of cancer treatment, as well as delayed diagnosis and (b) the difference between a particularly poor outcome and an incidence of clinical negligence. Although the claimant suffered serious complications arising from two separate surgical procedures, no breach of duty was found to have occurred.

Clinical Commentary

Helen Bolton and Anastasia Georgiou

Background

Missing a diagnosis of cancer is an understandable fear for clinicians and patients alike, and it is this fear that drives the investigation of many symptoms and subsequent monitoring and follow-up. However, successful litigation for negligence related to gynaecological malignancy is rare, and when it does happen the defendants are more likely to be primary care practitioners such as GPs, radiologists, pathologists or the laboratories that provide services for the NHS cervical screening programme.

Gynaecologists play an important role in the recognition of symptoms and signs of gynaecological cancer. They are responsible for organising appropriate investigations and subsequent referral for management if malignancy is confirmed. A minority of gynaecologists (Unit Leads or Centre Sub-specialists) will also be responsible for the ongoing management and surgical treatment of patients with suspected or confirmed gynaecological cancer. Apart from the fear of a missed or delayed diagnosis of cancer, there are other areas of practice that have the potential to result in litigation if not managed appropriately. Additionally, other medicolegal issues may arise when managing patients with suspected or confirmed gynaecological cancer, particularly in situations where women lack the capacity to consent for investigations or treatment.

Good Practice Guidance: Providing a Quality Service

Delivering good quality healthcare will inevitably reduce the potential for litigation. Providing a quality service requires input and commitment from the healthcare organisation, as well as from the individual clinicians working within that organisation. Both parties need to work collaboratively to make certain that requirements and responsibilities are met. Gynaecologists who have concerns about the organisational aspects of their service have a duty to raise their concerns and work with their organisation to improve the service. Likewise, organisations are responsible for ensuring that the individuals delivering their service are appropriately trained and that their performance is monitored and confirmed to be acceptable. This should be implemented through the organisation's governance processes.

Organisational Aspects of Care

The importance of organisational aspects of cancer care within the NHS was first recognised in 1995 following the publication of the Calman-Hine Report [1] in response to variation in cancer care within the United Kingdom. This set out principles for cancer care and the clinical organisation requirements for effective service delivery. There have since been several government publications [2–5] making further recommendations and requirements to improve the care of patients diagnosed with cancer.

The cancer service provider must have a sufficient number of relevant healthcare professionals to support the caseload of patients referred, in addition to an adequate team of administrative staff. All team members need to be allocated sufficient time to support both their clinical and administrative roles.

It is good practice for all cancer service providers to have published documents setting out their "cancer services structure", with clearly defined pathways, roles and responsibilities. Clinicians working within the service should ask to see a copy of this and familiarise themselves with how their organisation provides the service.

The Multi-Disciplinary Team Meeting

A key element in the national reform of cancer services was the introduction of the multi-disciplinary team (MDT) meeting; team decision-making is now the expected standard of care for patients with cancer. It is essential for the healthcare organisation to provide adequate infrastructure to support the effective functioning of the MDTM.

This includes protected time in job plans to make certain that the relevant members of the team are able to prepare and attend in person, in addition to providing adequate physical space, and information technology (IT) support. All MDTs should have a dedicated MDT co-ordinator whose role is to support the administrative running of the meeting. In addition to their primary role in supporting team decision-making, the organisation and individual members of the MDT should recognise the secondary roles of MDTs in education, governance and research. The organisation should provide support for these secondary roles and regularly review the MDT processes at regular business meetings.

Evidence-Based Practice

The healthcare organisation has additional responsibilities to make sure that agreed processes are followed. This includes following evidence-based guidelines, such as those published by the National Institute for Health and Care Excellence (NICE) and specialist societies such as the Royal College of Obstetricians and Gynaecologists (RCOG), the British Society for Gynaecological Oncology (BGCS) and the British Society for Colposcopy and Cervical Pathology (BSCCP). The organisation must be reactive to publications of new and updated guidance, and support any necessary changes in practice.

National Cancer Waiting Times Standards (NHS England)

These national standards were first introduced following publication of the NHS Cancer Plan [3] and provide operational standards for cancer waiting times. This includes time from referral for suspected cancer, from referral to first treatment, and from diagnosis to first treatment. These standards are monitored and published by NHS England, with all cancer service providers required to submit their data. Guidance is provided by the NHS to help organisations manage capacity and demand, and this guidance encourages engagement and collaboration with clinicians working within the service.

"Cancer Pathways" and Failsafe Administrative Support

As a direct result of the national cancer waiting times standards, cancer service providers developed "Cancer Pathways". Patients with suspected cancer, or having treatment for cancer, are placed on these pathways and their care is formally tracked by administrative staff, often the MDT co-ordinator. Not only does this support timely diagnosis and treatment, the Cancer Pathway also ensures that patients are tracked and not inadvertently "lost" in the system. This is especially important for those patients who do not attend their appointments, or the more complex cases that are referred for an opinion from other specialities.

Responsibilities of Individual Healthcare Professionals

Gynaecologists should be supported by their healthcare organisations to fulfil their duties of a doctor as required by the General Medical Council [6]. This is usually monitored through the annual appraisal process. Individuals must take responsibility for keeping up to date with their practice and should direct their continuing professional development programme appropriately. Clinicians must attend MDT meetings on a regular basis.

Training, Accreditation and Sub-specialisation

In the United Kingdom, gynaecological oncology is recognised as a subspecialty, requiring specific training, accredited by the General Medical Council, or equivalent. There is national agreement on the differing roles and responsibilities of cancer units, which can be delivered by gynaecologists, and of cancer centres, which must be led by subspecialist gynaecologists. The majority of women requiring surgical treatment for gynaecological cancer will be referred to specialist cancer centres for their care. In contrast, the diagnosis of gynaecological malignancy does not require specialist training. However, it is good practice for cancer units to be led by a gynaecologist with a special interest in gynaecological cancers. These clinicians usually have evidence of additional training, such as completion of the Advanced Training Study Module (RCOG ATSM) in gynaecological oncology, and they should undertake continuous professional development within this field. It is essential that all gynaecologists recognise the limitations of their training and experience, and seek advice from their cancer unit lead clinician, or cancer centre sub-specialist colleagues whenever they encounter difficult or unusual cases. Likewise, subspecialists must provide a responsive service, offering support and advice to their colleagues whenever a specialist opinion is requested. Gynaecologists working within cancer units must not undertake work that is recognised to be within the remit of the subspecialist, even if it may seem within their skillset. Clinicians who provide colposcopy services within the United Kingdom should be accredited by the BSCCP. This requires successful completion of a training programme, including an assessment, with reaccreditation occurring on a three-yearly basis.

Recognising Cancer Pathways and Referring Appropriately

Although the majority of cancer service providers now have the necessary infrastructure to support cancer pathways, it is essential that clinicians are familiar with how the system works. It is the responsibility of the individual clinician to recognise when their patient should be upgraded to a formal cancer pathway, and to know how to implement this within their own organisation. Problems may arise when a patient is referred on a non-cancer pathway, or is referred between specialities, and so slips through the net of the more common primary-care referral for suspected cancer. Unnecessary delays and misunderstandings may occur when a clinician inadvertently uses the "Urgent" pathway, rather than "Cancer Pathway".

Communication

To minimise the risks of errors or delays, individual healthcare practitioners must communicate well with their patients, and with any other healthcare professionals involved in delivery of care. It is now considered to be good practice to write letters directly to the patient about their care, and to include copies of correspondence to their GP and other professionals involved. Likewise, recommendations from the MDTM must be clear, unambiguous, and be a true reflection of the professional discussion held at the time of decision-making. Recommended actions should be clearly delegated in the written output so that there is no confusion about who is responsible for implementing the action.

Potential Causes of Litigation in Gynaecological Malignancy

The potential reasons for litigation in gynaecological malignancy can be classified as those that are "generic" to providing a diagnostic and surgical service, and those that are "specific" to gynaecological cancer work.

Generic Causes of Litigation Include

- Failure to adhere to national guidance, unless explicit reason to take alternative action
- Failure to organise or act on appropriate tests for presenting condition
- Inadequate pre-treatment discussion of options, their alternatives and consequences ("consent" and information sharing dialogue)
- Surgical complications and postoperative care
- Failure to organise or communicate appropriate follow-up plans or further management

Litigation Specific to Gynaecological Oncology

- Missed or delayed diagnosis of cancer
- Wrong diagnosis with inappropriate treatment
- "Over treatment" for suspected cancer
- "Under treatment" of condition which subsequently turns out to be cancer
- Wrong site/side surgery on lymph nodes (Never Event)
- Vulval surgery with cosmetic or functional sequelae
- Failure to offer or discuss fertility-sparing treatment
- Premature menopause following treatment

Most litigation can be avoided by working within an organisation that delivers a quality service, adhering to guidelines, and making certain that patients are kept informed of their choices and fully involved in their decision-making. It is acceptable and defendable to differ from guidelines, provided there is a justifiable reason, and that the patient has been involved in this decision wherever possible. High quality, contemporaneous documentation is key to preventing successful litigation.

Specific Considerations in Gynaecological Malignancy

Delayed Diagnosis

Members of the public and many healthcare professionals believe that an earlier cancer diagnosis will result in a better outcome for the patient. Consequently, it is often presumed that if breach of duty is proven, then litigation will be successful. However, these claims are frequently defended by the NHS on the basis of causation; the delay is often successfully argued to have made no difference to the patient. The issue of causation can be particularly complex in these cases.

In most cases of delayed diagnosis there has been a failure to refer. Consequently, the majority of claims are brought against primary healthcare providers. Occasionally gynaecologists and obstetricians may be responsible for a patient with a benign condition who volunteers symptoms suggestive of cancer, or receives an unexpected test result such as an abnormal scan. The clinician then has a duty to investigate or refer further. Delays can be avoided with failsafe pathways that ensure investigation results are received in a timely manner. Findings concerning for cancer that require further action should be subject to an "alert" or "flag", with a pathway that continues even if the responsible clinician is not available, either through planned or unexpected absence. Additionally, patients should be informed that they are being referred, and given a clear timeframe for when to expect to be contacted for the next steps in their management. Keeping the patient involved adds a further layer of safety, as many will contact their clinician if there are unexpected delays.

Diagnostic Uncertainty and the Potential Impact for over- or under-Treatment

In some situations, imaging may show concern for malignancy but the final diagnosis will remain unknown until after the abnormality is removed surgically. This can occur in suspected uterine sarcomas and some complex ovarian masses, especially on the background of endometriosis. For younger patients, treatment recommendations and decisions have the potential to result in irreversible loss of fertility and iatrogenic menopause. If the final pathology confirms malignancy, then the patient may have received the treatment with the greatest chance of "cure", with a good outcome. Conversely, if the final pathology is benign then the patient will have been over-treated and will have to live with the long-term consequences of this treatment.

Some women who no longer require fertility, or are post-menopausal, may also find the loss of their uterus and ovaries difficult to accept, and no assumptions should be made about their views. They may also feel that they were subjected to unnecessary major surgery, especially in the context of subsequently proven benign disease.

These situations highlight the importance of considering the role of supplementary diagnostic tests to help assess the likelihood of malignancy. In cases of possible uterine sarcoma and some complex ovarian masses, magnetic resonance imaging (MRI) may be helpful and should be considered if the information would be expected to help direct the patient's choice for her treatment. Uncertainties must be shared clearly with the woman, and the choice of possible management options and their consequences should be explored together prior to any treatment decisions. The dialogue should include the potential consequences of over-treatment, in the case of benign disease, and the alternative option of more conservative treatment. Although more conservative treatment may result in under-treatment, this will be acceptable and defendable provided it is clearly documented that the patient was fully informed of the potential consequences, with confirmation that this was her own choice, and that she was willing to accept the risks of this approach.

Choices should not be presented to the patient as neutral options if there is a clear steer towards an approach with a better outcome. In difficult cases, or when the clinician senses that the patient is uncertain about her decision, consideration should be given to requesting a further review in the MDTM, as well as offering the patient a second opinion from another specialist.

Impact on Fertility and Ovarian Function

Treatment for gynaecological malignancies frequently requires hysterectomy and bilateral salpingo-oophorectomy. This can result in loss of fertility and iatrogenic menopause. Even if the patient is approaching the menopause, or has completed her family, these effects should be discussed explicitly and the discussion documented in her medical records. Conversations should also explore the potential suitability of HRT after treatment, when relevant.

Surgery for Lymph Nodes

Gynaecological surgery does not usually require pre-operative site marking. Occasionally imaging may show unilaterally enlarged lymph nodes. The MDTM may recommend surgical removal of the enlarged nodes to help with staging and subsequent treatment planning. Site marking must be carried out prior to anaesthesia, cross-checking with imaging, and confirming the site through the WHO Surgical Checklist [7] procedure. The failure to remove nodes on the correct side has the potential to result in suboptimal adjuvant treatment recommendations, which could result in a poor outcome for the patient.

Cervical Cancer

Cervical cancer in the United Kingdom is now very rare, due to the success of the national screening programme. However, negligence cases involving cervical cancer constitute the majority of gynaecological oncology cases that are decided at formal court proceedings. Cervical cancer is almost entirely preventable, and late presentation often results in significant morbidity and potential mortality in younger women. Hence claims for loss of fertility, long-term pain and suffering, in addition to compensation for loss of earning are usually high value and consequently less amenable to out-of-court settlements.

Primary care and cervical screening laboratories are usually the focus for delayed diagnosis negligence cases in cervical cancer. However, gynaecologists must remain vigilant, and remember that a full pelvic examination, including direct attempts to visualise the cervix, should be carried out when a woman presents with abnormal vaginal bleeding. Clinicians must not be falsely reassured by a normal pelvic ultrasound scan as this imaging modality cannot reliably detect tumours. Additionally, it must be remembered that a negative smear test does not exclude cancer; cervical cancer can still develop within the normal screening interval. Women often express that they would rather not undergo pelvic examination whilst they are bleeding. Although the woman's views should be respected, it is important to recommend examination if her bleeding persists, and to explore options to reduce any embarrassment or anxiety.

Cervical screening and colposcopy service providers are required to follow national guidelines that provide standards on organisational and clinical pathways [8]. This includes the requirement to discuss significant discrepancies between cervical screening results, colposcopy and histology results in the colposcopy MDTM.

Ovarian Cancer

Delay in diagnosis, or failure to act on abnormal results, may result in litigation in ovarian cancer. This usually occurs in primary care. However, ovarian abnormalities are common coincidental findings on scans (gynaecological and non-gynaecological imaging) and should be investigated appropriately. Clinicians should be encouraged to seek advice from the MDTM if there are diagnostic uncertainties.

Women with ovarian cancer usually undergo surgery. Those with advanced disease may require extensive surgery, known as ultra-radical cytoreductive or debulking surgery, with associated risks. Litigation can be avoided with careful and well documented pre-operative discussions, particularly covering the material risks of serious complications, including their impact on subsequent treatment, outcome and quality of life.

The woman's views on the extent of surgical effort, including the possible need for bowel resection and stoma, should be explored, and documented clearly.

Endometrial Cancer

All cases of post-menopausal bleeding, or persistent unscheduled bleeding in pre-menopausal women, should be considered as potential endometrial cancer and investigated appropriately. The incidence of endometrial cancer in younger women is increasing, especially in those who are overweight. Fertility and ovary-sparing options should be considered carefully in younger women and discussed at the MDTM. All women who are overweight with bleeding abnormalities should be counselled about the importance of weight loss, as this is a significant risk factor for endometrial cancer.

Vulva

Thorough examination of the vulva – Women presenting with vulval symptoms must have a thorough examination of the vulva. It is easy to miss a smaller lesion within the labial and perineal skin folds.

Change in appearance or function – Diagnostic or therapeutic procedures involving the vulva can result in permanent changes in appearance, and may also have an impact on sexual, bladder or bowel function. In some circumstances it may even be necessary to remove the clitoris. No assumptions should be made regarding age and sexual function; however, discussions can be held sensitively and tailored to the individual patient. All potential consequences should be discussed with the patient, and their explicit consent obtained and documented prior to proceeding.

Biopsy for suspected vulval cancer – Stage IB vulval cancers under 4 cm in maximum diameter may be suitable for sentinel lymph node biopsy, rather than full staging lymphadenectomy [9]. Sentinel node biopsy is the management of choice for highly selected patients, as this approach has a markedly reduced incidence of immediate and significant long-term morbidity when compared to full lymphadenectomy. Excisional biopsy of vulval lesions must be avoided, as this usually results in the loss of opportunity for sentinel node biopsy. Although it is acceptable (and expected) that cancer unit clinicians take diagnostic biopsies for suspected cancer, when there are potential challenges with biopsy, the case should be referred directly to the cancer centre for planning of appropriate biopsy approaches.

Photographic documentation – It is often helpful and considered good practice to take photographs of vulval lesions as part of providing good quality care. Clinicians must remember that the vulva is a sensitive area for women. Written consent should be obtained and appropriate measures must be in place to make certain that the photographs are only seen by those directly involved in the woman's care. The GMC provides direct guidance on "Making and using visual and audio recordings of patients" [10].

Other Medicolegal Issues in Gynaecological Malignancy: Capacity and Best Interest Decisions at End of Life

Clinicians working in gynaecological oncology may need to seek advice from the courts regarding "best interest" treatment decisions, as women with mental health issues or cognitive impairment may present with symptoms suggestive of malignancy, or confirmed malignancy. They may lack capacity to give their consent to investigations or treatment. Although many decisions can be made in agreement after discussion with their GPs, carers, psychiatrists and independent mental health capacity advocate, occasionally the decision is more complex. Clinicians should seek advice or support from their local Clinical Ethics Committee if available. In a minority of cases it may be necessary to seek a Court ruling from the Family Courts. This may be required if the treatment is extensive, or when there is disagreement from the patient or members of the team making the decision. Individual clinicians caring for these women should seek advice from their organisation's legal team in any uncertain cases.

Avoidance of Litigation

- The provision of high-quality structure and processes by the healthcare organisation delivering cancer care is key to reducing the potential for litigation in gynae-oncology
- Individual clinicians have a responsibility to fulfil their roles within that service and to raise concerns if the organisational support is insufficient or dysfunctional
- Systems must be in place to ensure results of investigations are followed up, even in the absence of the requesting clinician
- Clinicians providing private services (non-NHS) to patients should be satisfied that their own infrastructure is sufficiently robust to deliver a quality service
- Good communication with the patient, supported by meticulous documentation, along all steps of the pathway is essential
- In cases of diagnostic uncertainty, women must be kept informed of the implications of potential management options, and given sufficient support to make their own choices about their treatment
- Persistent episodes of abnormal vaginal bleeding always warrant a pelvic examination to look for vulval, cervical or vaginal tumours, and should not be deferred because the patient is bleeding
- Cervical cancer can develop within the timeframe of a normal cervical screening interval
- Pelvic ultrasound will not usually pick up a cervical tumour and therefore must not be used as a substitute for physical examination
- Clinicians should be sensitive to the potential impact of treatment on sexual function, fertility, hormonal status, cosmetic appearance and emotional well-being
- Healthcare professionals working within gynaecological malignancy may occasionally require the support of Clinical Ethics Committees and legal services to support their care of women at the end-of-life, or when they need to make complex "best interest" decisions.

References

1. Department of Health. A policy framework for commissioning cancer services : a report by the Expert Advisory Group on Cancer to the Chief Medical Officers of England and Wales. 1995.

2. NHS Executive. A policy framework for commissioning cancer services. *Circular EL* 1995; (95)51.

3. Department of Health. The NHS cancer plan: a plan for investment, a plan for reform. 2000.

4. Independent Cancer Taskforce. Achieving World Class Cancer Outcomes: A Strategy for England 2015–2020. 2015.

5. NHS England. NHS Long Term Plan. 2019.

6. General Medical Council (GMC). Good Medical Practice. 2013.

7. World Health Organization (WHO). World Health Organization Surgical Safety Checklist. 2009.

8. Public Health England. Cervical screening: programme and colposcopy management. 2020.

9. British Gynaecological Cancer Society (BGCS). Vulval Cancer Guidelines: Recommendations for Practice. 2020.

10. General Medical Council (GMC). Making and using visual and audio recordings of patients. 2011.

Index